How to Design Studies and Write Research Proposals

How to Design Studies and Write Research Proposals

KADER PARAHOO

Emeritus Professor
School of Nursing and Institute of Nursing and Health Research
Ulster University
Northern Ireland

ELSEVIER

ISBN: 978-0-443-26163-3

Content Strategist: Robert Edward
Content Project Manager: Shivani Pal
Design: Amy Buxton

Printed in India

Last digit is the print number: 9 8 7 6 5 4 3 2 1

Working together
to grow libraries in
developing countries

www.elsevier.com • www.bookaid.org

ACKNOWLEDGEMENTS

■ ■

Research studies are journeys that we undertake to shed light on some of the many problems in our daily lives. Planning studies and writing proposals thoughtfully and meticulously can make our tasks a lot less challenging than they need to be. My own journey, in writing this book, was made easier by the many examples provided by those who shared their experience by publishing their research proposals. To them, I am very grateful.

There are others, closer to me, who have provided much needed 'sounding boards', motivation and encouragement. I am thankful to Hugh McKenna, Maurice Stringer, Roger Austin and Malcolm Murchison. I am particularly grateful to Roisín Parahoo for reading the manuscript many times over. Her sharp eye and insightful comments have enhanced the quality of the text enormously.

This book is dedicated to Ciarán, Yasmin and Roisín and to Eilís who, even in her absence, continues to support, sustain and inspire me.

CONTENTS

■ ■

LIST OF PROPOSAL EXAMPLES

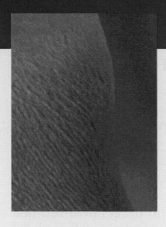

INTRODUCTION

We are all familiar with the term 'marriage proposal', a process that involves one person asking for another person's 'hand' in marriage. It is based on 'intention' and 'trust' (some would say love!). No more detail is usually required. A research proposal, on the other hand, requires more than intention and trust. Put simply, a research proposal is a written, detailed and succinct plan of a research project one is proposing to undertake. The proposal should provide answers to the following core questions:

- What is to be researched?
- Why is it important to do this research?
- Is it ethical?
- Who will undertake the study?
- Who will the participants be and how will they be recruited?
- How will the research be carried out?
- Where it will take place and when?
- How long it will take?
- What resources (time, equipment, expertise, etc.) will be required?
- How will the project be managed, and by whom?
- How will potential impact of the findings be achieved?

Research proposals may differ in length, structure, format and detail, depending on what each is required for. However, essentially each proposal should serve the same purpose: to describe what is to be done and how.

A written research proposal is an effective way of communicating your plan, about a research study you want to undertake, to others (research supervisors, funders, ethical committees, research governance, employers, etc.). Once agreed, approved and funded, it is a form of contract between those undertaking the study and those funding, sponsoring or commissioning the research. This is the document that will be referred to in case of disagreement, especially if timetables are not adhered to or outcomes not being met.

THE DIFFERENCE BETWEEN PROPOSALS AND PROTOCOLS

These two terms are sometimes used interchangeably and sometimes cause some confusion. In lay terms, a protocol can be defined as an established code of procedure or conduct in a group, organisation or situation (Oxforddictionaries.com). For example, there are protocols on how to greet and address dignitaries, for example a royal family or a Head of State. There are also protocols on what to do if a fire alarm is triggered in a hospital or theatre, or on how to deal with aggression against staff in hospitals. This type of protocol is different from a research proposal; the latter is specifically about a research project.

Researchers sometimes develop a protocol for the research team and others involved in a project to be clear about what is required of them. This type of protocol is especially helpful for researchers and clinicians in multisite projects, to know what is expected of them and provide guidelines on recruiting participants and collecting data to order to avoid variations in the way the study is conducted at different sites. In this case, a protocol is a set of procedures to be followed during the research process. These protocols aim to ensure ethical conduct and safety, and provide instructions on what to do if unexpected events occur.

More often, however, in research terms 'proposals' and 'protocols' are used interchangeably to refer to a detailed plan of a study, written before it is conducted. When proposals are published in journals they are invariably referred to as 'protocols'. Throughout this book, we will use the term 'proposal' to describe researchers' plan of how their studies will be conducted.

TYPES OF PROPOSAL

There are different types of research proposal depending on what purpose they are expected to serve. The most common ones are:

- research proposals as an assignment as part of an undergraduate or Master's programme
- research proposals as part of the application process for entry into a doctoral programme
- research proposals to apply for funding.

The Proposal as an Assignment in a Degree Programme

As part of the assessment scheme for the final year of a Bachelor's or Master's degree, students may be required to write a research proposal for a project they wish to undertake. This is sometimes called a 'dissertation'. The aim is normally to assess students' knowledge of the research process, their ability to formulate research questions or hypotheses, and to select appropriate designs and methodologies, as well as their knowledge of the topic through their critical use of the literature. Detailed guidelines are normally provided, including how marks are allocated for each section of the proposal.

The Proposal as Part of the Application Process for a Doctoral Programme

As part of the application process, potential students are often asked to write a proposal to outline the research project they would like to undertake for a PhD or other doctoral degree. This type of proposal helps universities to assess whether they have the capacity, expertise, facilities and resources when making decisions regarding admission. These decisions are based on the viability and originality of the project and its potential contribution to knowledge and society. At this stage of the application, the research proposal will help to match students with suitable supervisors. It will also give an indication of the extent to which the proposed study has been thought out, the amount of preparation (e.g. reading the literature) the applicants have carried out and their ability to think and write coherently.

While decisions regarding admission are usually made on number of factors, including qualifications, the proposal is a key part of the assessment of the suitability of students for a doctoral study and the suitability of the university to supervise the project. This type of proposal will also form the basis of further discussion on how the study will be conducted, in particular the choice of design, the selection of data collection and the analysis methods. Unlike a proposal written for the purpose of seeking funding, a proposal to gain entry to a PhD programme will still need to be further developed and refined. This is because a PhD study is primarily to train students to carry out research studies in order to make a significant contribution to knowledge. Most universities provide guidance on how to structure and write this type of proposal and how long the proposal should be. For example, the University of Edinburgh has produced an excellent guide on 'How to Write a Good Postgraduate Research Proposal' (http://www.ed.ac.uk/files/imports/fileManager/HowToWriteProposal090415.pdf). As it explains:

> *This guide highlights the "Golden Rules" and provides tips on how to write a good research application. Prospective research students may find it useful when asked to provide a research statement as part of their university application or an informal enquiry form.*

This type of guide can provide advice on the content, structure (headings, subheading etc.), style, format and length of the proposal. Some universities may require more detail than others. Other postgraduate students, such as those undertaking a Master's degree, may also be expected to produce outline proposals prior to undertaking a study. Applicants are strongly advised to consult their target universities' websites when seeking admission to a doctoral or Masters' programme.

Research Proposals to Seek Funding

There is increasing pressure on universities and similar organisations to attract funding for their activities. In such a competitive environment, the importance of writing excellent proposals cannot be overemphasised. Proposals seeking funding are expected to contain sufficient information for funders to decide whether or not they can fund the project. Such proposals are normally well thought out, comprehensive, detailed and refined before they are submitted. As with other academic activities (such as writing for publication), one has to learn, practise and develop the necessary skills and knowledge to do this.

Although proposals can differ in length, structure and format, the core purpose of these three types of proposals is the same. They describe:

- the proposed study and its importance;
- how it will be carried out;
- the resources, including time, expertise and funding required to do so.

This book is primarily aimed at nursing, allied health and social care students. It is a resource to guide them through the process of developing quality proposals as part of their assignments. Teachers, professionals and new researchers in nursing, health and social care will also find it useful in their work. On some undergraduate and postgraduate programmes students may be expected to undertake a small-scale study. This guide will help them to design their studies.

The type of research carried out in nursing, allied health and social care is normally not laboratory based and involves designs such as trials, surveys or case studies using quantitative, qualitative and mixed methods approaches. This book does not cover proposals for a systematic review or other type of review. It is for those using research methods to collect and analyse primary data or analyse secondary data to answer research questions. Primary data are information that researchers collect for their own studies. Secondary data are information that has already been collected by others (e.g. censuses, hospital records, etc.) that can be used to answer research question(s).

Poor proposals waste time and resources for everyone involved. Poorly developed proposals can cause frustration, stress and low self-esteem for those who spend considerable time and effort in producing them. On the other hand, successful proposals can be rewarding and lead to impactful findings and successful careers.

AIM AND SCOPE OF THE BOOK

Developing a research proposal starts with designing a study. One cannot design a research project without a basic understanding of the language and process of research, the main research designs, data collection and data analysis methods. Undergraduates developing research proposals as a dissertation would be expected to have completed an introduction to research module. Others (Master's and PhD students) may have acquired more advanced research skills during their course. While this book will refresh readers on some core research concepts, principles and methods, it will focus mainly on designing studies and writing research proposals. It will take them through the key steps of designing research studies and writing proposals, and offer advice and tips on what examiners, reviewers and funders look for in proposals.

No proposal can be developed without first designing the study. This is why this book covers both study design and research proposals. However, developing a proposal is more than designing a study. For example, a strong rationale for the study and plans for managing the project and its team have to be provided. Plans to involve patients and the public in the study and strategies to disseminate the findings and promote impact are also part of the proposal. Identifying, estimating and costing resources are as much an integral part of a proposal as is the methodology of the study. All these aspects of a proposal are discussed and explored in this book. The chapters follow closely the main sections of a generic proposal: formulating research questions; literature review and background to the study; selecting research designs, methods of data collection and analysis; samples and sampling; and ethical considerations. Additionally, there are separate chapters on impact, patient and public involvement and resources. The final chapter offers advice to those applying for funding. It is recognised that not everyone will develop proposals to seek funding. Students, in particular, or someone doing an in-house project may not need to do so. However, they may, at a later time in their career (e.g. as a postdoctoral researcher) apply for a grant.

Each chapter starts with issues related to the design of a study, followed by what should go into a proposal. One of the key features of this book is the provision of examples from actual proposals, published in (mostly open access) journals. There are also numerous references to key resources for designing studies and developing proposals that readers may also find useful. Although this book addresses the needs of students and new researchers, some sections may also appeal to seasoned researchers and teachers of research. Finally, checklists of what to include in the different sections of a proposal are provided throughout the book.

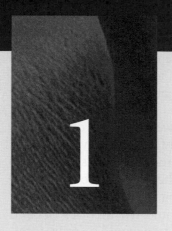

1

HOW TO DEVELOP RESEARCH QUESTIONS FOR PROPOSALS

INTRODUCTION

There is no research without questions, if not explicit, then at least implied (as in aims and objectives or hypotheses). A research question is the *raison d'être* (the reason) why a study is carried out. Every subsequent decision taken (e.g. choice of design, sampling, methods of data collection and analysis) is for the purpose of finding valid and reliable answers to research questions. This is why questions are at the heart of research.

Developing a research question does not happen in a vacuum. There are many factors and issues that researchers have to consider in the process of selecting and formulating research questions. One has to think about the practical, logistical, ethical and other issues that would make a project feasible or not. Failure to do this could, at best, hinder the study and, at worst, lead to non-completion of the research project.

In this chapter, we will explore sources of research questions, the importance of writing clear, researchable and comprehensive questions, as well as the different types of, and ways in which, research questions can be formulated. A framework to facilitate the development of specific questions from broad topics will be described.

SOURCES OF RESEARCH QUESTIONS

Researchers may already have research questions before they start designing studies and write research proposals. However, others may find it hard to think about a question, especially if it is for an assignment as part of a course. More often, they can think of a topic but cannot narrow it down to specific questions. There are many sources that provide or trigger ideas for research. These include our own curiosity and observations, the literature and talking (and brainstorming) with other people.

Curiosity and Observation

Humans have always been curious about the world they live in. The scientific and technological progress we have achieved is a testament to our desire to question, understand, change and control our environment in order to make our lives better. For most of us, our questions come mainly from what we experience and observe in our daily lives. For example, we may question the effects of 'being glued' to screens such as mobile phones, tablets or computers for long periods of time. We may also ask ourselves whether this behaviour affects our eyesight, our concentration or our social relationships.

Our conversations are full of lay theories, derived mainly from what we hear, read, observe and experience. During the COVID-19 pandemic, lay theories about the infection and vaccinations flourished. Even in 'normal' times, it is not unusual to hear that certain foods (such as coconut or turmeric) or remedies containing aloe vera or lemongrass are good for the heart or the skin. There are lay theories regarding the causes of diseases such as cancer, including the food we eat (in particular red meat or additives). Through our observation, we formulate our own 'theories' of child development and behaviour. For example, some people believe that children would be more intelligent if, as fetuses in their mothers' wombs, they listened to classical music (the 'Mozart effect'). Some children's behaviours are attributed (selectively) to hereditary factors and others to environmental ones. Some of these lay theories can, of course, be tested by research.

What we read in the media, in particular controversial issues, can trigger ideas for research. Issues such as the effects of legal highs (legal psychoactive drugs), the high prevalence of diabetes or the increase in the older people population raise questions that could be explored through research. The media is full of contradictory issues. On 1 August 2017, the British newspaper the *Daily Telegraph* ran a front page headline, 'Statins "needlessly doled out to millions" simply because of their age'. On the same day, another British newspaper, the *Express*, carried a front page headline 'STATINS: 6 million "miss out" on life-saving statins'. The latter newspaper added that doctors should be offering statins to almost every man aged over 60 years and all women over 75.

Media reports that butter is better than margarine (or the other way round) can confuse people. For researchers, it is an opportunity to ask questions about how people perceive such contradictory news and what factors influence their choice of butter or margarine. Of course, researchers can, and do, study the effects of these products on our health. Their findings can help to fuel the debate on what we should consume.

Professional practice is a fertile arena for questions. Professionals interact with people from a variety of backgrounds and conditions, and they engage in countless interventions with them. Thus they can become curious as to why some people behave differently from others or why some treatments and interventions for the same condition work and others do not. There is no doubt that many research studies started life as researchers' curiosity and/or interest.

The Literature as a Source of Research Questions

Reading the literature generally, and in one's own field of practice in particular, is useful for triggering ideas for research. Since the body of literature is vast and increasing at a very fast rate, it is best to start with one or two topics; the narrower the topic, the less time will be spent fishing for ideas. Do not be discouraged to find that some of your ideas have already been studied. There are always opportunities to build upon what others have done or to research it differently (e.g. using different designs and methods, with different populations or in different settings).

The place to look for such ideas in an article is usually in the 'limitations of this study' section. In a cross-sectional survey on 'Frequency and circumstances of falls for people with Charcot–Marie–Tooth disease', Ramdharry et al. (2017) pointed out that their sample was from one single specialist centre and that it might not be representative of people in different areas or countries. There is therefore scope for other researchers to build upon this study and use a different sample. Ramdharry et al. (2017) also pointed out that their study was retrospective and that there could have been recollection difficulties as participants were asked to recall their three last falling events. They suggested that a prospective study might overcome this limitation.

Another example is from Fenwick et al. (2018), whose study focused on the influence of personal and professional factors on rates of burnout among midwives. They recommended that future research 'explore workplace factors that have an impact on stress and strategies to enhance resilience'(p. 861).

Other Sources of Research Questions

Any source of information can be useful for researchers to think of research questions. Conferences, in particular, bring together large numbers of people to disseminate, discuss and share ideas. They provide ample opportunities to meet people who are equally, if not more, fascinated by the issues and concerns that you want to explore.

The internet is increasingly becoming the forum where discussion take place and ideas expressed and shared. For example, one blogger was interested in the Haka, the traditional Maori war dance performed by the New Zealand rugby team, the All Blacks, before their games. The blogger explained the reasons for undertaking a study on rugby:

> After being told by yet another 'Northern Hemisphere' poster that the Haka gives the All Blacks an unfair advantage, I decided to see if there was any substance to this belief. I honestly did not know what the results would be, but hoped they would be neutral.

No matter where ideas for research come from, it is important to read the literature on the topic and 'discuss' it with others, in particular mentors, practitioners, supervisors and other experienced researchers. There is much useful information on universities' websites giving advice on how to contact prospective supervisors, who may have ideas, based on their own research.

This is how one researcher (Gaetano, 2022) explained what her favourite part of being a scientist was:

> My favorite part about being a scientist is that I get to ask really interesting questions. I think there's a misconception that science is all about generating answers. However, I have found that projects and papers are most exciting when they create even more questions than we had before. It's very rewarding to find one of those new questions that frames your work in a slightly different perspective and allows it to evolve. I also love brainstorming about these big questions with my peers. Everyone has a different set of skills and expertise, so even an hour long conversation with a group of excited collaborators can advance a project by huge leaps!

Gaetano advised that researchers read as much as they can about the topics that interest them, 'whether it be in books, scientific journals, blog posts by other scientists etc.'.

The James Lind Alliance (JLA; https://www.jla.nihr.ac.uk/) is a very useful source of research questions. The JLA describes itself as 'a non-profit making initiative set up to identify and prioritise unanswered questions or evidence uncertainties' that patients, carers and clinicians agree 'are the most important, so that health research funders are aware of the issues that matter most to the people who need to use the research in their everyday lives'. The JLA has a list of the top 10 Priorities in almost all the health and social care professions and health conditions.

A Framework for Brainstorming Research Ideas and Questions

A brief overview of the literature in nursing, health and social care research shows that researchers tend to focus mainly on the following areas: professionals, practice, policy, patients, carers and their families, diseases and conditions, education and methodology. This list is by no means exhaustive and some of the topics/areas overlap. However, these areas can be thought of as potential thematic sources for questions (Table 1.1).

TABLE 1.1	
Potential Areas for Research in Nursing, Health and Social Care	
Core Themes	**Examples of Potential Areas for Research**
Professionals	Roles; personal attributes; attitudes; knowledge; beliefs; skills; competence; education and training; job satisfaction; bullying; burnout; communication; decision making; interdisciplinary working; professional development; professional identity
Practice	Assessing, planning, implementing and evaluating care; all types of interventions (e.g. treatment, rehabilitation, education); primary, secondary and tertiary care; managed care; palliative care; community care, mental health care, intensive care, care of people with learning disability; person-centred care; counselling; evidence-based practice; care of the dying and the bereaved family; midwifery care; care of the newborn
Policy	Organisation of health and social services; recruitment; retention; workload; regulations; guidelines; pay, health and safety; costs, technology; reforms; resources; policy interventions; advanced directives; governance, ethical issues; health service management; leadership
Patients, carers and families	Needs assessment of patients, carers, families; experience of care, treatment, rehabilitation and counselling; disease and illness perceptions; health beliefs, knowledge, attitudes; empowerment; privacy; dignity; relationship/interaction with health professionals; patients' wishes, hope, preferences, anxieties and concern; access to health services; adherence to treatment; lifestyles (including diet, nutrition, exercise and social activities)
Disease, illness and disability	All types of diseases, illnesses, disability and conditions (topical, rare, chronic or acute); physical, mental, psychological and social wellbeing; incidence and prevalence; disease patterns and pathways; death; bereavement, pregnancy; birth; substance abuse; gender and age differences; sexual identity and orientation; inclusion and exclusion; lifestyle; health promotion
Education	Teaching and learning methods and styles; mentoring; supervision; interprofessional education; student-focused learning; team-based learning; continuing education; curriculum development and evaluation; competencies; practice and placement education; e-learning

There are, of course, other themes such as methodology and theory-focused research. This framework can be a useful starting point for new researchers looking for a topic and ideas to research. As an exercise, I typed two keywords – 'role' and 'social worker' – in the 'title' section of Medline (at that point covering a date range from 1946 – 9 February 2022) and retrieved 271 articles when these two terms were combined. Not all of them were research studies but most were. A quick scan of their abstracts would show what specific aspects of the role of social workers researchers have focused on, what areas have not been researched, and the design and methods they have used. This can give an idea of gaps in research on this topic, as well as the potential to use different designs and methods for a future study.

FROM TOPIC TO SPECIFIC QUESTIONS

One of my earliest tasks as a lecturer was to facilitate final-year students on an undergraduate course to formulate questions for a research study. This exercise involved one-to-one consultations with students to explore topics and finalise research questions. For the most part, this exercise went rather well, as most of the students had well developed topics or even questions. One student, however, posed a particular challenge when she 'revealed' that her selected topic was 'death'. She could not think of any aspect of death to research. I do not recall what the outcome of our meeting was, but as all the students successfully completed their degree, and I can only think that, together with the student, we were able to formulate a research question on the topic of 'death'.

That was more than 30 years ago, when databases were not available on the internet. If we approached this topic today, we would use the framework in Table 1.1 to begin the process of brainstorming for potential areas for research questions. Table 1.2 gives an example of how this specific topic of death can lead to broad areas and specific research questions.

The table outlines a simplified account of how to narrow a topic and formulate specific questions. In real life, this exercise is a process involving researchers' own ideas and interests, a literature search and consultations/discussions with other people, in particular mentors and supervisors. For example, if you have an idea, you can go directly to the literature and then discuss it with your supervisor or an experienced colleague. This discussion may lead to more reflection on your part and to you going back to the literature again. This iterative process continues until the research question is formulated and refined. This is depicted in Figure 1.1.

Talking with experienced others and gatekeepers (i.e. those who have control over access to potential participants) is recommended, even if you have only a tentative research question. This will help you to understand some of the practical and ethical challenges that the proposed study may face. Taking into account the concerns and advice of practitioners will help you to develop a more realistic and relevant study matched to their needs, and they are also likely to assist in recruiting participants to the study. When undertaking a research project you should not feel that you are alone.

Using the literature efficiently requires the ability to search the internet and databases without being overwhelmed by the mass of information that is available. If the topic reveals an unmanageable amount of literature, it is a good idea to narrow your search by restricting it to

	TABLE 1.2		
	Developing Specific Research Questions on the Topic of 'Death'		
Broad Themes	**Potential Areas for Research**	**Broad Questions**	**Specific Questions**
Education	Attitudes, knowledge of health professionals regarding death	Effects of education on professionals' attitudes to death?	Does a 2-day educational intervention enhance newly trained occupational therapists' attitudes to death?
Disease, illnesses, conditions	Good death	Exploring the concept of a 'good death'	What is the meaning of 'good death' among general practitioners (doctors) and nurses?
Policy	Staffing and mortality in care settings	Effects of staffing on death rates	Is there a relationship between nursing staffing levels and mortality rates on intensive care units?
Health Professionals	EOLC	Health professionals' role in EOLC	How do social workers help patients in EOLC prepare for death?
Practice	Child death, bereavement, loss	How parents cope with a child death	What strategies do community nurses use to help clients who have experienced a recent child death?
Patients, carers and families	Death anxiety	Death anxiety among older people	Do older care home residents have anxieties about death and dying alone?

EOLC, end-of-life care.

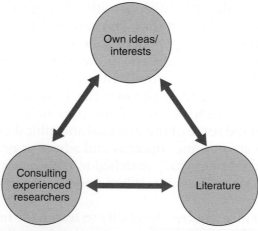

Fig. 1.1 ■ Depiction of the iterative process that continues until the research question is formulated and refined.

the last 3 or 4 years and/or combining relevant search terms. However, it takes less time and effort if you start with an idea or two.

Finally, there is sometimes a tendency to try to answer all imaginable questions on a particular topic. This is based on the belief that answering simple questions may be too little for a dissertation, but the slogan 'less is more' applies to research as well. New researchers in particular can sometimes underestimate what it takes to carry out a small study.

Researchable Questions

While there is no research without questions, not all questions can be answered by research. There are moral, political, ethical, practical and logistical reasons why it may not be feasible or possible to collect and analyse data in order to answer research questions. Consider this question: 'Should men have the same rights to make abortion decisions as their pregnant partners?' Research cannot provide the answer to this question but it can provide findings that will help society, in particular politicians, to decide whether men and women should have the same rights. Research can make a valuable contribution by, for example, exploring men's and women's perception on this issue. Ultimately, however, this is a moral, political and human rights issue that requires a collective decision.

Issues such as whether the government should spend more money on the 'care of older people' than on the 'care of people with mental health problems' are not resolvable by research. One can though ask the public and/or health and social care professionals about their views and preferences, and use this information to make informed political decisions on how to allocate funding. Research can also provide data on how much is currently spent on these two groups and the impact of expenditure on older people or those with mental illness. These findings can inform subsequent debates, but the allocation of funding is ultimately a political decision.

There are some topics such as using embryos or stem cells for research purposes that are ethically controversial to research. This is because people have different views on what stem cells represent to them. Some believe that an embryo is a person with the same moral status as an adult or a live-born child; others believe that an embryo becomes a person in a moral sense at a later stage of development than at fertilisation (Lo and Parham, 2009).

Research that involves concealing the real purpose of the study to participants is unethical. One of the most infamous studies in which researchers did not reveal the purpose of their research was the Tuskegee Syphilis Experiment between 1932 and 1972. No informed consent was obtained from the participants (approximately six hundred Afro-American sharecroppers, most of whom were illiterate) and they were not informed of their diagnosis (syphilis) but were instead told they were being treated for 'bad blood' (Newsome, 2021). There were other unethical practices as well, including the withholding of treatment known to be effective for syphilis, for the purpose of completing the study.

All research studies have ethical implications that need to be taken into account at all stages of the research process, from the development of the research questions to the dissemination of the findings. There are, however, research questions that would present significant ethical dilemmas requiring careful thought and approval from ethical committees before the study can be undertaken (see Chapter 13 for more discussion on the ethical implications of research studies).

Some studies may be difficult to carry out for practical reasons. The most common reason lies in accessing and recruiting participants (people) to the study or getting access to secondary data (data already collected for other purposes). People involved in illegal drugs or activities may not want to disclose this behaviour and information may be difficult to access. The incidence of some diseases or conditions may be so low that it can take a long time before an adequate sample is obtained. For example, if a sample size of 200 men newly diagnosed with prostate cancer is required for a 12-month study, it may be difficult to recruit this number if fewer than 200 are diagnosed each year in the setting where this study is to be carried out. The problem may be compounded by the possibility that not all newly diagnosed men will agree to take part or to stay in the study until it is completed.

Certain phenomena may be difficult to observe or to obtain access to in order to observe them. A study of the incidence of abuse in nursing homes may pose particular challenges in that 'abuse' may not take place at the time of observation as instances may occur infrequently. More likely, some nursing home owners may feel threatened by such a study and refuse access. Similarly, aggression or medication errors do not necessarily happen when observations are being undertaken. These difficulties can, however, be offset by the use of methods other than direct observation.

Questions such as 'What is the most effective treatment for radiography-induced skin burns?' are more appropriately answered by means of a systematic review. This is because it is not possible to test 'all' treatments in one study. However, if there is no study on the effectiveness of treatments for this condition, a primary research study (comparing the effectiveness of two or three treatments) is a good starting point.

The moral, political, ethical and practical considerations of a proposed study should be taken into account during the process of selecting topics and formulating questions. Failure to do so may affect the conduct of the study and its successful outcome.

Clear Questions

The research question has to make sense to readers without them having to read the rest of the proposal. The research question is a clear statement of the core issues, problems or concerns that the study will answer. Choosing clear and unambiguous words, phrases and language is crucial to avoid misunderstanding or confusion. Every word, verb or phrase should be chosen carefully. In this section, examples of poor questions (taken and adapted from the literature and from actual proposals) will be given.

Broad questions can sometimes be vague. For example: 'What can be done to prevent domestic abuse in Ireland?' Apart from being too broad, there is no indication of who will be expected to provide the answer. Is it the public, or health professionals such as social workers or community nurses? A clearer question is 'What is the public perception of how domestic abuse can be prevented in Ireland?' This is likely to be a large study, involving a representative sample of the 'public' (a term that will require to be defined prior to the study).

Vague phrases, in particular common expressions, should be avoided. Consider this: 'What is the current state of play regarding sexual health education in schools?' The phrase 'current state of play' is a common expression used in lay conversation. Whoever wrote this question no doubt understood what it means to them and how to go about getting the answer, but few readers would understand what exactly the researcher wants to know. A clearer question would be: 'How is sexual health education currently delivered by teachers in primary school curricula in country A?' This primary or main question may have to be supplemented by subquestions relating to the content of the curriculum that refers to sexual health education, the proportion of time allocated, who delivers this education, and the teaching and learning methods that are used. The clearer questions also let the reader know what, who, how and where. These pronouns will be returned to later.

Sometimes a word or a term in a research question can be ambiguous or vague. Consider, for example, the question 'What are the training needs of school staff with regards to sexual health education in schools?' The term 'school staff' could mean everyone from the cleaner to the headmaster. It is possible that the researcher means 'all' school staff, but it is also likely that not much thought has been given to the term 'school staff' in this context.

A word placed incorrectly in a sentence can also give a different meaning to a research question than that intended by the researchers. Consider this question: 'Do carers of stroke patients looking after them have problems?' The answer to this question is potentially 'yes' but they may have problems (e.g. financial worries or gambling) that have little or nothing to do with looking after people with stroke. A clearer question could be: 'What problems or challenges do carers experience when looking after people with stroke in Scottish care homes?'

When words or phrases are used inaccurately in research questions to describe participants, they can potentially create difficulties when recruiting them. This question, taken from a rehabilitation journal, shows how the use of an ambiguous phrase can be potentially problematic: 'Is therapeutic exercise of benefit in reducing impairment for people who would be expected to consult a physiotherapist?' Apart from other problems with this question, how would the researcher operationally define and recruit 'people who would be expected to consult a physiotherapist'? Also, would participants be from all different age groups?

It is helpful to think about how words, terms or phrases will be operationally defined while research questions are being developed. For example, in the above question on therapeutic exercises, the term 'of benefit' can be reworded in terms of the outcome of the exercises. In fact, if the words 'of benefit' is removed, the question can be worded with more precision, such as 'Do therapeutic exercises reduce physical and mental impairment in people over 65 years old?' However, this type of question is more appropriate for a systematic review as it involves more than one form of therapeutic exercise.

Words like 'useful' or 'helpful' are sometimes used in research questions. However, these words beg the question 'What is meant by 'useful' in this context?' It is better to think in terms of outcomes that can demonstrate 'usefulness'. For example, the question 'Are educational interventions useful for women newly diagnosed with breast cancer?' can be made more precise by asking: 'Do educational interventions reduce anxiety and uncertainty among women newly diagnosed with breast cancer?' Similarly, the words 'suffering from' can be superfluous and difficult to justify when used in the following question: 'What strategies do people suffering from diabetes use to control their blood sugar levels?' One could ask how we know if they are 'suffering'? 'People with diabetes' or 'newly diagnosed with diabetes' would suffice.

Finally, researchers should only state the questions or aims that the study will address. An objective such as 'to enhance practice' is superfluous or irrelevant if the study does not aim to change practice by, for example, implementing and evaluating an intervention in practice. All research aims to make a contribution to knowledge that may or may not be used to enhance policy, practice or other behaviour.

In a review of the rehabilitation literature, Mayo et al. (2013) found that 'a sizable' proportion of the research questions 'were poorly formulated: 65% did not indicate what the researchers wanted to know and 30% needed to be reworked' (p. 517).

Complete Research Questions

For research questions to be comprehensive, they have to be complete as well as clear. Complete research questions or hypotheses should have a number of basic, essential components for readers to understand without having to search the rest of the paper or report. To help researchers write complete questions, a number of frameworks have been developed (Davies, 2011).

One of the most popular framework is the PICO formula (Richardson et al., 1995). PICO is an acronym for Population (P), Intervention (I), Comparator I and Outcome (O). PICO has been extended to PICOT (T for Timeframe) and PICTOS (S for Setting). The following examples show how the PICO formula can ensure that the essential components are included in a research question and a hypothesis.

Research question: Do tutorials lead to higher exam marks than lectures among final year social work undergraduates?

P (Population):   Final year social work undergraduates
I (Intervention):   Tutorials
C (Comparator):   Lectures
O (Outcome):   Exam scores

Hypothesis: 'Twenty weeks of isometric handgrip home training will significantly reduce systolic blood pressure in hypertensive older men and women compared to usual care' (Jorgensen et al., 2018).

P (population): Older men and women. In the proposal, the age group was described as over 50 years of age. This information could have been included in the question to provide more precision. Instead of 'older men and women' it would have been more accurate to say 'men and women over 50 years of age'.

I (Intervention): Twenty weeks of isometric handgrip home training. The information regarding the duration and the setting of the intervention helps to make the hypothesis complete.

C (Comparator): Usual care

The PICO formula was originally designed to help researchers develop clinical questions for systematic reviews. It is particularly useful for studies evaluating the effectiveness of interventions (such as drugs, treatment, surgical procedures, and psychosocial, behavioural, educational and other therapies). It is best suited to studies using controlled trials (involving two or more groups). It has been adapted for use for other designs, such as qualitative ones, where P stands for Population, I for Interest and C for Context.

Qualitative studies tend to explore people's perception, experience or behaviour of some phenomenon or other. To ensure completeness when developing qualitative research questions, one can use the PEP acronym: P is for Population (patients, clients, families, carers, etc.), E is for Experience (this can include perception, views, attitudes, beliefs, etc.) and the second P is for Phenomenon (this can be a disease or condition such as diabetes or cancer, an event such as use of services, a behaviour or action such as decision making, etc.).

Survey designs, in particular correlational studies, are often used to test the relationship between variables. The research question can be expressed in the form of hypotheses (see the next section for more detail). Hypotheses should, at the very least, have four components: the dependent variable (D), the independent variable (I), the relationship between them (R), and the population (P).

A number of other frameworks or tools have similarly been developed to help (if not, confuse!) researchers develop their questions. They are more or less the same but new researchers should be aware of them, and choose the ones they feel comfortable with. Some of the other frameworks (see University of Leeds, 2023) are: CLIP (Client, Location, Improvement, Professional); CIMO (for realistic synthesis questions; Context, Intervention, Mechanism and Outcome); ECLIPSE (for health service management questions; Expectation, Client group, Location, Impact, Professionals and SErvice); SPICE (for social sciences questions; Setting, Perspective, Intervention, Comparison, Evaluation); and SPIDER (for qualitative evidence synthesis; Sample, Phenomenon of Interest, Design, Evaluation, Research type).

Although research questions should be complete, they should not, however, be cumbersome and long. Operational definitions and inclusion/exclusion criteria normally follow the section on research questions or aims and objectives, and these add more refinement to the research questions.

The importance of clear and complete questions should not be underestimated. While this may seem obvious to most researchers, there is some evidence that essential components of research questions are sometimes missing even in studies that have been published. Mayo et al. (2013), in their review of papers in rehabilitation journals, found that key information was missing in research questions and that 'the designs which most often had poorly formulated research questions were randomized trials, cross-sectional and measurement studies' (p. 513). Thabane et al. (2009) systematically reviewed 313 articles published in four key anaesthesia journals. They found that the percentage of papers that failed to adopt each PICOT element were as follows: Population (39%); Intervention (12%); Comparator (54%); Outcome (16%); and Timeframe (89%).

Question Format

There are different ways in which research questions can be formulated. It is preferable to phrase these in question form because that leaves no doubt as to what the research aims to achieve (i.e. find answers to the question). However, as explained earlier, 'aims', 'objectives' and 'hypotheses' are frequently used to express what researchers set out to do. Aims and objectives statements imply that there are questions to be answered. If the aim is to explore the effectiveness of a policy, then the question to answer is: 'Is the policy effective?' Too often, however, the aim of the study is confused with the potential benefit of the study. It is not unusual to see that the aim of a study is to improve practice but in reality the study is only seeking answers to one or more questions.

For an example of aims and objectives, see the proposal by Henery et al. (2021) for a study on 'Ethnic and social inequalities in COVID-19 outcomes in Scotland'. For hypotheses in a proposal, see the study by Cousins et al. (2021) on 'Preventing adverse drug reactions after hospital discharge'.

Types of Question

In everyday life, we constantly ask questions using words such as what, why, when, how, etc., and asking questions is not much different for researchers. Researchers also want to know what happens, why, under what conditions? Additionally, they want to describe, identify, compare, evaluate, examine, explore, interpret, assess, test or explore phenomena. To make sense of the many different types of question that researchers ask, we can group research questions into three categories: descriptive, correlational and causal.

Descriptive Questions

Descriptive questions usually start with the 'what' pronoun. Researchers may want to know *what* people's knowledge, attitudes, beliefs and practices are. They may also wonder *how* things happen, for example how a new policy or practice was introduced. Researchers are also interested in the prevalence or incidence of diseases and conditions (e.g. 'What is the prevalence of type 2 diabetes among athletes?'). They may also want to know the extent and level of patient/client satisfaction with their care and services. Descriptive questions can be used to compare people, phenomena or events (e.g. the prevalence of smoking between male and female adolescents or the frequency of the use of smart phones between teachers and students).

Descriptive questions can be quantitative or qualitative. Quantitative descriptive studies tend to use terms such as scores, percentage, proportion, prevalence, incidence, etc. to describe the phenomena they investigate. An example of a quantitative descriptive study is from Reis et al.'s (2015) study of 'Sports injury profile of a first division Brazilian soccer team'. The objective of study was 'To establish the injury profile of soccer players from a first division Brazilian soccer team' (p. 390). This is how Reis et al. describe what they found:

> *The incidence of injuries was 42.84/1000 hours in matches and 2.40/1000 hours in training. The injury severity was 19.5± 34.4 days off competition or training. Lower limb was the most common location of injury and most injuries were muscular/tendinous, overuse, non-recurrent, and non-contact injuries. Player's age correlated with the amount and severity of muscle and tendon injuries. Defenders had more minimal injuries (1–3 days lost), while forwards had more moderate (8–28 days lost) and severe injuries (>28 days lost). Furthermore, wingbacks had more muscle and tendon injuries, while midfielders had more joint and ligament injuries.*

> *Reis et al. (2015, p. 390)*

An example of a qualitative descriptive study comes from Timmins et al. (2018). The aim of the study was to 'describe the facilitators and barriers for nurses to perform quality wound care in three surgical wards of a hospital in Port-au-Prince, Haiti'. The researchers observed nursing staff on a number of wards while they performed 'routine dressing changes' and interviewed a number of nurses to enquire about their perceptions of facilitators and barriers for nurses to perform quality wound care. They used words to describe what they observed and heard. This excerpt from the abstract is a description of their findings:

A number of wound care practices appeared well integrated including using gloves to remove dressings, applying sterile dressings, properly disposing of soiled materials, inspecting wounds for signs of infection and employing comfort and privacy measures. Areas that may need improvement included aseptic technique, hand hygiene, pain assessments, patient education and documentation. We identified four themes related to barriers and facilitators to perform quality wound care: (i) materials and resources; (ii) nurse-to-patient ratios, workload and support; (iii) roles and responsibilities of nurses; and (iv) knowledge and training of nurses.

(p. 542)

Descriptive studies are sometimes undervalued. Manuscripts for publication may be rejected for being too descriptive. However, these type of studies can be very useful when there is a lack of data on which to base policy or practice. Descriptive data are needed to develop interventions, construct a profile of patients and health professionals, and increase our understanding of phenomena. For example, Kitt et al. (2016) carried out a qualitative descriptive study to 'assist the development of a group-based rehabilitation programme' to increase opportunities for activity in the inpatient stroke rehabilitation setting (p. 58).

Proposal Examples 1.1 and 1.2 show how questions and aims/objectives are formulated in proposals for quantitative descriptive and qualitative descriptive studies, respectively.

Correlational Questions

Nursing, health and social care professionals often wonder if demographic factors and/or socioeconomic status play a part in how patients or clients perceive the care they receive or in the way they access services. In research terms it means researchers may want to know if there is a correlation between, for example, age (younger or older) and health behaviour (e.g. accessing services). This type of question is termed correlational because it seeks to find out if there is a relationship between two variables (here, 'age' and 'accessing services'). This type of question is asked not just to satisfy curiosity, but to use this knowledge to identify, for example, people who are at risk or should be targeted in the future for health promotion interventions. Correlational questions can lead to the identification of 'predictors' of behaviour and other outcomes. For example, Oldfield et al. (2018) studied the 'Psychological and demographic predictors of undergraduate non-attendance at university lectures and seminars'. The aim of their study was to identify 'whether any demographic or psychological variables can predict their non-attendance levels'.

In its simplest form, a correlational research question seeks to establish whether there is a relationship between two variables (dependent and independent). Parahoo (2014) defined a variable as 'anything that varies or can be varied'. In the example 'Does obesity increase the risk of depression in patients with diabetes mellitus type 2?', the two variables are 'obesity' and 'risk of depression' (De la Cruz-Cano et al., 2015). In this correlational question, 'obesity' is the independent variable that is linked with 'risk of depression' (dependent variable). The independent variable (obesity) is more accurately called the 'predictor' variable because it does not

---

PROPOSAL EXAMPLE 1.1
QUANTITATIVE DESCRIPTIVE QUESTIONS

Zingela et al. (2020), 'Protocol for a prospective descriptive prevalence study of catatonia in an acute mental health unit in urban South Africa'.
The aims and objectives were stated as follows:

AIMS

This study aims to determine the prevalence of catatonia in an acute MHU [mental health unit] in urban SA and research its assessment and management in this setting.

OBJECTIVES

The two main research objectives are:
1. Screening of consenting participants admitted to the MHU in DNH [Dora Nzinga Hospital] using the BFCSI [Bush Francis Catatonia Screening Instrument] for catatonia, over a 12-month period from the 1 September 2020 to the end of August 2021, to describe the prevalence of catatonia in this setting.
2. Description of demographic and clinical information, including response to treatment, in participants diagnosed with catatonia based on their BFCSI scores and clinical assessments performed by the admitting doctor.

COMMENTS

The authors formulated aims and objectives rather than questions. They are in fact asking the following questions:
1. What is the prevalence of catatonia in an acute mental health unit in urban South Africa?
2. How is catatonia assessed and managed in this setting?
Both formats are acceptable and the choice depends mostly on personal preferences.

'cause' depression in people with type 2 diabetes; it may only increase the risk of depression (i.e. it can be a contributory factor).

There are at least three types of relationship between variables that correlational questions can reveal: positive, inverse or null (no) relationship. In the example 'Does anxiety affect undergraduate students' examination marks', a positive relationship would be one that reported 'the higher the anxiety, the higher the marks'. An inverse relationship would be the 'higher the anxiety, the lower the marks', and a null relationship would be a case where anxiety does not affect students' marks in the examination.

Researchers tend to investigate relationships between a number of variables. In the study by Oldfield et al. (2018) of undergraduate non-attendance at university lectures and seminars, they investigated the correlation between 'non-attendance' and a host of other variables (predictors) including 'sense of belongingness to university', 'working more hours in paid employment', 'having more social life commitments', 'facing coursework deadlines' and 'experiencing mental health issues'. From the knowledge gained from this study, Oldfield et al. (2018) recommended targeting interventions at the students most at risk of these predictors.

As explained above, correlational questions do not seek to establish cause and effect, mainly because researchers are not able to make things happen (such as asking students not to attend

---

PROPOSAL EXAMPLE 1.2
QUALITATIVE DESCRIPTIVE QUESTIONS

Stone et al. (2021), 'ASK a midwife: a qualitative study protocol'.
The aims and questions were formulated as follows:

The aim of this study is to reveal the knowledge and skills necessary for midwives' post-certification to provide safe care at low intervention births in free-standing birth centres in Germany. The phenomena under study are the skills and knowledge acquired by midwives post-qualification to care for women within a birth centre setting.

The main research questions are:
1. What are the experiences of midwives when they begin to work independently in a free-standing birth centre to support women to achieve a physiological birth?
2. What are the different formal and informal training procedures and methods that birth centres in Germany use to prepare new midwife colleagues to work independently to support and facilitate physiological birth?
3. What is the practical knowledge that is necessary to work at free-standing birth centres? Which skills are developed?

COMMENTS

Qualitative studies tend to state a broad aim. In this protocol, the authors were precise and clear what exactly they were focusing on. This is very helpful as the aims can lack the information for readers to know what aspects of the phenomenon the researchers were exploring.

---

classes) or to control other factors that may lead to non-attendance. Researchers undertaking correlational studies tend to collect data in the natural environment and not in a 'laboratory' setting.

Marker (2014) gave this real-life example to show the difference between correlation and causation. She used this excerpt from an article published by the TV news channel CNN:

Doctors have been less willing to prescribe medications, especially in states like Florida, formerly known for its pill mills, where tighter restrictions on prescribers led to a 23% drop in overdose death between 2010 and 2012.

The words 'led to' suggest a causative link between 'less prescriptions' and 'drop in overdose'. According to Marker (2014) this type of reporting 'creates an inaccurate and overly simplistic picture of the world for the reader'. She concluded that 'correlations are a great start in data generation, but getting to the bottom of why data correlate will allow us to build better practices for business, governments, and schools'.

Correlational questions are answered by means of quantitative methods and statistical analysis. The aim is to measure variables and establish links between them based on statistical tests. Qualitative research can indicate whether some phenomena are linked. For example, a qualitative study may give an indication that younger patients may use different strategies to cope with diabetes than older ones. However, this finding should be further tested by quantitative methods with a representative sample of patients before this link can be established. Proposal Example 1.3 shows how questions are formulated in proposals for correlational studies.

PROPOSAL EXAMPLE 1.3
CORRELATIONAL RESEARCH QUESTIONS

Limardi et al. (2016), 'Caregiver resilience in palliative care: a research protocol'.

RESEARCH QUESTIONS

- What are the prevailing socio-demographic aspects of principal informal caregivers in end of life (EoL) care and how do they relate to resilience?
- What are the relationships between resilience and psychological and behavioural characteristics of the main informal caregivers in EoL?
- How much and in what way do the clinical conditions of EoL patients impact the resilience of principal informal caregivers?
- What relationships exist between aspects of palliative care settings and the resilience of principal informal caregivers?

COMMENTS

1. It is clear from these questions that the authors are interested in the relationships between 'resilience' and a number of other factors including psychological and behavioural characteristics.
2. In this proposal, the authors also state these questions in the forms of aims and objectives. Only one format is required.

Causal Questions

While correlational questions seek to establish links between variables, causal questions aim to find out how one variable affects or causes another to change. In the above example of the 'drop in overdose deaths' (Marker, 2014), many other reasons than a change in prescription behaviour could have contributed to the 'drop'. There could have been a political and health promotion campaign to raise awareness of the issue and educate the population or individuals' socioeconomic circumstances could have changed. Professor Louise Richardson, at the time Vice-Chancellor of the University of Oxford), was asked in 2017 whether the rise in her salary from the post was linked to an increase in tuition fees, she replied 'that's correlation without a causation' (Grierson, 2017). She went on to say that 'Oxford University was operating in a "global marketplace" ' and competing with high remuneration packages offered at institutions overseas'.

Clinicians and practitioners may also want to know if their policies or interventions produce the effects they are designed for. They can ask causal questions and test their ideas in a controlled environment. For example, Wang et al. (2016) carried out a trial on the effects of a mindfulness-based intervention programme for people with schizophrenia. Their aim was to find out if the intervention had an effect on patients' 'functioning and rehospitalisation rate' and their 'insight into illness, symptom severity and progress of recovery' (Wang et al., 2016, p. 3098). This type of question is normally answered by means of randomised controlled trials.

Classifying research questions as 'descriptive', 'correlational' or 'causal' is only for the purpose of explanation. However, it can be seen as oversimplification of a rather more complex topic. For example, some researchers call their studies 'descriptive correlational'. Descriptive studies can have correlational elements. For example, if a researcher wants to create a profile of patients who do not adhere to medication prescriptions, they would collect demographic data for these patients to see whether, for example, 'educational level' is linked to non-adherence. What we normally call 'correlational' questions are those that focus intentionally on finding a link between variables, as in the study by Wang et al. (2022) that investigated correlations between the spiritual care competence, spiritual care perceptions and spiritual health of Chinese nurses.

A descriptive study can also explore correlations and cause and effect. For example, in a qualitative descriptive study by Kieft et al. (2014), the aim of this study was 'to understand from the perspective of nurses how the nursing work environment is related to positive patient experiences' (p. 3). They identified a number of 'essential elements', including 'clinically competent nurses', 'managerial support', 'patient-centred culture' and 'autonomous nursing practice', from the perspective of these nurses, that contribute to positive patient experiences. What this study does is to identify influential factors that can be further tested in quantitative correlational and causal studies.

Proposal Example 1.4 shows how causal questions are formulated in proposals for causal studies.

PROPOSAL EXAMPLE 1.4
CAUSAL QUESTIONS

Chan et al. (2020), 'The effects of a brief hope intervention on decision-making in chronic kidney disease patients: a study protocol for a randomized controlled trial'.

The aim of the study is:

To examine the effectiveness of a brief hope intervention in reducing the decisional conflict and improving the quality of life of chronic kidney disease patients who must plan for receiving dialysis therapy.

The hypothesis is:

Increasing hope will lead to a stronger decision for the selected treatment option, less decisional conflict, and reduced emergency room visits or hospitalization.

Cox et al. (2022), 'Evaluating the effectiveness of e-cigarettes compared with usual care for smoking cessation when offered to smokers at homeless centres: protocol for a multi-centre cluster-randomized controlled trial in Great Britain'.

Objectives

Primary:

To determine the 24-week sustained, biochemically validated abstinence rates in smokers offered e-cigarettes (EC) compared with usual care (UC).

Secondary:

1. Among those who have not achieved full abstinence, to compare the number reporting at least 50% smoking reduction at 24 weeks in the EC versus the UC arm.
2. To compare the number achieving 7-day point prevalence quit rates at 4-, 12- and 24-week follow-up in the EC versus the UC arm.
3. To document changes in risky smoking practices (e.g., sharing cigarettes, smoking discarded cigarettes) from baseline to 4, 12 and 24 weeks in both EC and UC arm.
4. To determine the cost-effectiveness of the intervention.

Continued

PROPOSAL EXAMPLE 1.4—cont'd

5. To document fidelity of intervention implementation; mechanisms of change; contextual influences and sustainability.

COMMENTS

From these two examples, one can see that research questions for trials can be formulated in different formats.

Checklist for research questions in research proposals:

Research is the systematic and rigorous collection and analysis of data for the purpose of answering research questions (Parahoo, 2014). Research questions, aims and objectives and hypotheses occupy a prime position in proposals (usually at the beginning or in a dedicated section of forms recommended by funders). It is normally a short section but it should be written in such a way that readers are in no doubt what the researchers intend to do. How the research questions are formulated will convey the first impression, and as such set the tone for the rest of the proposal.

The checklist for research questions in proposals is therefore:

1. Are the questions clear, unambiguous and complete?
2. Are the questions feasible and ethical?

SUMMARY AND CONCLUSIONS

In this chapter, we have shown how designing a study starts with one or more research questions. A framework to assist new researchers in the identification and formulation of research questions has been provided. The main aspects of clear, unambiguous, complete, feasible, ethical research questions have been highlighted. Examples from actual research proposals have been used to illustrate how this can be achieved.

REFERENCES

Chan, K., Wong, F. K., Tam, S. L., Kwok, C. P., Fung, Y. P., & Wong, P. (2020). The effects of a brief hope intervention on decision-making in chronic kidney disease patients: A study protocol for a randomized controlled trial. *Journal of Advanced Nursing, 76*(12), 3631–3640. https://doi.org/10.1111/jan.14520

Cousins, J., Parameswaran Nair, N., Curtain, C., Bereznicki, B., Wilson, K., Adamczewski, B., Barratt, A., Webber, L., Simpson, T., McKenzie, D., Connolly, M., & Bereznicki, L. (2022). Preventing Adverse Drug Reactions After Hospital Discharge (PADR-AD): Protocol for a randomised-controlled trial in older people. *Research in Social & Administrative Pharmacy: RSAP, 18*(8), 3284–3289.

Cox, S., Bauld, L., Brown, R., Carlisle, M., Ford, A., Hajek, P., Li, J., Notley, C., Parrott, S., Pesola, F., Robson, D., Soar, K., Tyler, A., Ward, E., & Dawkins, L. (2022). Evaluating the effectiveness of e-cigarettes compared with usual care for smoking cessation when offered to smokers at homeless centres: protocol for a multi-centre cluster-randomized controlled trial in Great Britain. *Addiction (Abingdon, England), 117*(7), 2096–2107. https://doi.org/10.1111/add.15851

Davies, K. S. (2011). Formulating the evidence based practice question: A review of the frameworks. *Evidence Based Library and Information Practice*, *6*(2), 75–80.

De la Cruz-Cano, E., Tovilla-Zarate, C. A., Reyes-Ramos, E., Gonzalez-Castro, T. B., Juarez-Castro, I., López-Narváez, M. L., & Fresan, A. (2015). Association between obesity and depression in patients with diabetes mellitus type 2; a study protocol. *F1000Research*, *4*, 7. https://doi.org/10.12688/f1000research.5995.1

Fenwick, J., Lubomski, A., Creedy, D. K., & Sidebotham, M. (2018). Personal, professional and workplace factors that contribute to burnout in Australian midwives. *Journal of Advanced Nursing*, *74*, 852–863.

Gaetano, M. (2022). Time scavengers. https://timescavengers.blog/2022/01/24/maddie-gaetano-phd-candidate/. Retrieved on 10/02/2022.

Grierson, J. (2017). Oxford vice-chancellor denies rising salary is linked to tuition fees. Published in the guardian (British Newspaper) on 06/09/2017. Retrieved on 25/01/2021.

Henery, P., Vasileiou, E., Hainey, K. J., Buchanan, D., Harrison, E., Leyland, A. H., Alexis, T., Robertson, C., Agrawal, U., Ritchie, L., Stock, S. J., McCowan, C., Docherty, A., Kerr, S., Marple, J., Wood, R., Moore, E., Simpson, C. R., Sheikh, A., & Katikireddi, S. V. (2021). Ethnic and social inequalities in COVID-19 outcomes in Scotland: Protocol for early pandemic evaluation and enhanced surveillance of COVID-19 (EAVE II). *BMJ Open*, *11*, e048852. https://doi.org/10.1136/bmjopen-2021-048852

Jørgensen, M. G., Ryg, J., Danielsen, M. B., Madeleine, P., & Andersen, S. (2018). Twenty weeks of isometric hand-grip home training to lower blood pressure in hypertensive older adults: A study protocol for a randomized controlled trial. *Trials*, *19*, 97.

Kieft, R. A. M. M., de Brouwer, B. B., Francke, A. L., & Delnoij D. M. J. (2014). How nurses and their work environment affect patient experiences of the quality of care: a qualitative study. *BMC Health Serv Res*, *14*, 249.

Kitt, C., Wang, V., Harvey-Fitzgerald, L., Kayes, N., & Saywell, N. (2016). Gaining perspectives of people with stroke, to inform development of a group exercise programme: A qualitative study. *New Zealand Journal of Physiotherapy*, *44*(1), 58–64.

Limardi, S., Stievano, A., Rocco, G., Vellone, E., & Alvaro, R. (2016) Caregiver resilience in palliative care: a research protocol. *Journal of Advanced Nursing*, *72*(2), 421–433.

Lo, B., & Parham, L. (2009). Ethical issues in stem cell research. *Endocrine Reviews*, *30*(3), 204–213. https://doi.org/10.1210/er.2008-0031

Marker, K. (2014). Correlation, causation, and qualitative research. https://www.keltonglobal.com/perspectives/correlation-causation-and-qualitative-research/

Mayo, N. E., Asano, M., & Barbic, S. P. (2013). When is a research question not a research question? *Journal of Rehabilitation Medicine*, *45*, 513–518.

Newsome, M. (2021). We learned the wrong lessons from the Tuskegee 'experiment'. https://www.scientificamerican.com/article/we-learned-the-wrong-lessons-from-the-tuskegee-experiment/

Oldfield, J., Rodwell, J., Curry, L., & Marks, G. (2018). Psychological and demographic predictors of undergraduate non-attendance at university lectures and seminars. *Journal of Further and Higher Education*, *42*(4), 509–523.

Parahoo, K. (2014). *Nursing research: Principles, process and issues*. Basingstoke: Palgrave.

Ramdharry, G. M., Reilly-O'Donnell, L., Grant, R., & Reilly, M. M. (2017). Frequency and circumstances of falls for people with charcot-marie-tooth disease: A cross sectional survey. *Physiotherapy Research International*, *23*, e1702. https://dx.doi.org/10.1002/pri.1702

Reis, G. F., Santos, T. R., Lasmar, R. C., Oliveira Júnior, O., Lopes, R. F., & Fonseca, S. T. (2015). Sports injuries profile of a first division Brazilian soccer team: A descriptive cohort study. *Brazilian Journal of Physical Therapy*, *19*(5), 390–397.

Richardson, W. S., Wilson, M. C., Nishikawa, J., & Hayward, R. S. (1995). The well-built clinical question: a key to evidence-based decisions. *ACP Journal Club*, *123*(3), A12–A13.

Stone, N. I., Thomson, G., & Tegethoff, D. (2021). ASK a midwife: A qualitative study protocol. *International Journal of Qualitative Methods*. https://doi.org/10.1177/16094069211048383

Thabane, L., Thomas, T., Ye, C., & Paul J. (2009). Posing the research question: Not so simple. *Canadian Journal of Anesthesia 56*, 71. https://doi.org/10.1007/s12630-008-9007-4

Timmins, B. A., Thomas Riché, C., Saint-Jean, M. W., Tuck, J., & Merry, L. (2018). Nursing wound care practices in Haiti: Facilitators and barriers to quality care. *International Nursing Review, 65*(4), 542–549.

University of Leeds. (2023). PICO and other tools for developing research questions and search concepts. http://information-specialists.leeds.ac.uk/information-specialists/search-concept-tools/.

Wang, L. Q., Chien, W. T., Yip, L. K., & Karatzias, T. (2016). A randomized controlled trial of a mindfulness-based intervention program for people with schizophrenia: 6-month follow-up. *Neuropsychiatric Disease and Treatment, 12*, 3097–3110.

Wang, Z., Zhao, H., Zhang, S., Wang, Y., Zhang, Y., Wang, Z., Li, X., Xiao, L., Zhu, Y., Han, G., Yan, Y., Wang, J., Zhang, Y., & Pang, X. (2022). Correlations among spiritual care competence, spiritual care perceptions and spiritual health of Chinese nurses: A cross-sectional correlational study. *Palliative & Supportive Care, 20*, 243–254.

Zingela, Z., Stroud, L., Cronje, J., Fink, M., & van Wyk, S. (2020). Protocol for a prospective descriptive prevalence study of catatonia in an acute mental health unit in urban South Africa. *BMJ Open*, 10, e040176. https://doi.org/10.1136/bmjopen-2020-040176

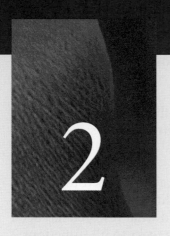

2

BACKGROUND AND LITERATURE REVIEW IN RESEARCH PROPOSALS

■ ■ ■ ■ ■ ■ ■ ■ ■ ■ ■ ■ ■ ■ ■ ■ ■ ■

INTRODUCTION

We have seen, in the previous chapter, how the literature can help to identify topics, issues or research questions for research studies. The design stage of a study can also benefit from the literature in terms of finding out the different ways in which the proposed study can be carried out and the implications of the selected design.

In this chapter, we will focus on the purpose and content of the introduction and background sections of a research proposal. Together they serve to highlight the need for the study and to inform others how much knowledge, if any, we already have on the topic and (more importantly) the gap in knowledge that the proposed study seeks to fill.

RELATIONSHIP BETWEEN LITERATURE AND PROPOSALS

The term 'literature' in nursing, health and social sciences refers to published work, in all different formats or genres (e.g. research studies, reports, guidelines, policy papers, blogs, X (formerly Twitter) posts, discussion papers, poems, etc.). Together, the literature represents the billions of contributions that individuals or groups have made to the body of knowledge in the world, on millions of topics. Some are original work (primary source) and others are reported, repeated or re-interpreted (secondary source). When used wisely, they all have important functions. To make a contribution to knowledge, however small, is a contribution to humankind, although we may not immediately appreciate it. *Clichés* such as 'standing on the shoulders of giants' or 'every little helps' may sound hollow when used too often, but they reflect the incremental nature of the growth of knowledge.

In the previous chapter, the importance of consulting the literature and discussing with others when formulating research questions was emphasised. In particular, the discussion and limitations sections of research articles and reports were identified as potential sources of ideas for future research. Students, in particular, are often unsure of how to carry out a literature review for their proposals or their dissertations. To avoid complicating things, they should ask themselves the following question: 'Why do I need a literature review, or what is the purpose of literature review in designing a study and writing a proposal?' Apart from searching the literature for research ideas, the literature review for a proposal has four functions (Parahoo, 2014). These are:

1. to provide a rationale for the current study;
2. to put the current study in the context of what is known about the topic;
3. to review relevant research studies carried out on the same or similar topics;
4. to discuss the conceptual/theoretical basis for the current study.

These four functions can be grouped into two sections in a proposal: 'introduction/rationale' and 'literature review'. In the introduction/rationale section, the literature is used to provide evidence for the significance of the study (function 1, above). In the literature review section, the literature is used to show what we already know about the topic and what research has been carried out, and to identify gaps in knowledge that the proposed study seeks to fill (functions 2 and 3, above). The fourth function is to identify and discuss the conceptual or theoretical basis upon which the study (or part of a study, e.g. data analysis) is constructed (see Chapter 3).

A number of terms or labels, such as 'introduction', 'context', 'rationale', 'background' and 'literature review', are used to describe the purpose of a literature review in the context of designing a study and writing a research proposal. Funding bodies or course guidelines will dictate exactly what headings or subheadings you should use. However, it is important to differentiate between the section that justifies the study and the section that puts the study in the context of what we know already and how this (proposed) study aims to build on previous knowledge. Therefore, the two sections will be discussed separately to emphasise the different ways in which the literature is used.

INTRODUCTION/RATIONALE FOR THE STUDY

The main purpose of this section is to provide a justification or rationale for the proposed study. This is a section that gives the reasons *why this study is needed, why it is needed now, what benefits the study will bring* and *for whom*. In nursing, health and social care the aim of research is mostly to provide evidence in order to prevent ill health, reduce suffering, promote wellbeing and increase the cost-effectiveness of services. Research can impact directly or indirectly on policy, practice and education (see Chapter 14). Research can also provide answers to theoretical and methodological questions.

The introduction will usually state the significance of the problem to be investigated. This can be shown by providing figures on the incidence, prevalence and frequency of the specific condition or illness to be investigated (e.g. liver cancer, diabetes, depression, self-harm or non-adherence to professional advice). Figures from reliable sources (e.g. statistical data collected by organisations such the World Health Organization [WHO] and American Cancer Society, charitable organisations, governments and research studies) are often used to show the magnitude or size of the problem. These figures are helpful to put the problem in a broad context.

However, just because the incidence of a condition or disease is increasing does not always mean that the study is justified. For example, studies on older people generally tend to cite figures on the increase in size of this population. This does not mean that all studies on older people are justified. There are many issues related to older people that could be investigated (e.g. depression, dementia, diabetes, heart disease, etc.). Therefore, it is important to provide appropriate, up-to-date and relevant data to justify the claim that your particular study is needed.

Apart from statistical and epidemiological data from official sources, evidence can come from research studies, reports (e.g. from government and non-government organisations) and policy documents. Discussion papers, expert opinions and even newspaper articles as well as one's own experience or observations form part of the 'collection' or array of evidence to justify the study. Newspaper articles often reflect topical issues with which people are concerned. However, relying on newspapers or expert opinion may not be sufficient to provide a robust and convincing rationale for why a study should be carried out. While it is acknowledged that not all proposals will include evidence from all of the above sources, efforts should be made to give as many reasons and valid arguments as possible, backed up by credible and up-to-date information.

It is also important, especially when applying for funding, to put the proposed study in context of the funder's research priorities and agendas. These priorities are often found in their policy documents. It is advisable to consult the relevant websites, which often provide this information. For example, AUTISTICA, an autism research charity, has published a list of research priorities relating to people with autism and their carers. Below are their top five priorities:

1. *Which interventions improve mental health or reduce mental health problems in autistic people? How should mental health interventions be adapted for the needs of autistic people?*
2. *Which interventions are effective in the development of communication/language skills in autism?*
3. *What are the most effective ways to support/provide social care for autistic adults?*
4. *Which interventions reduce anxiety in autistic people?*
5. *Which environments/supports are most appropriate in terms of achieving the best education/life/social skills outcomes in autistic people?*

AUTISTICA (2022)

The challenge of providing reliable and up-to-date figures is also recognised. This is why a thorough search should be carried out. If no figures or updated data are available, this should be stated to avoid reviewers or readers wondering whether or not figures are available.

To say that the proposed study has not been carried out in your hospital, community or country is sometimes not enough to justify the study, especially if funding is being sought. If it has been done elsewhere, reviewers may well ask why are the findings not applicable to your setting. For example, if there is an abundance of research to show that exercises lift the mood of people who are depressed, one may well ask why a similar study is needed. On the other hand, people from different countries may have different ways to cope with depression. Therefore, if your study is about policies and strategies to help people cope with depression, you should explain the differences in the setting (e.g. health and social care systems, cultural and socioeconomic factors etc.) that may produce findings more relevant to your setting.

There is also a case for replicating studies. For example, the effectiveness of an intervention cannot rely on one study only. There is a need to test them in different settings in order to produce robust evidence on their effectiveness. Therefore, replicating a study should, and can, be justified. There is a strong and growing movement asking that research studies should be reproduced using the same design and methods because the findings from some studies cannot be confirmed by other researchers.

The introduction is the first substantial section of a proposal that reviewers will read. It should be written in such a way (succinct, logical, jargon-free and clear) that readers will be interested in the proposed study and be convinced that it is needed. Whether the proposal is an assignment for a course or a response to a funding call, convince yourself and others why the study is relevant, worthwhile, value for money and likely to be of benefit to people, practitioners, policy makers or others.

Below is an example of an introduction/rationale for a proposal for a study on 'The decision-making process of young adult women in the UAE regarding food choice and the factors that influence their choice'. It was written as part of an assignment for a course and reproduced with the student's permission.

> **Title of proposal:** *The decision-making process of young adult women in the United Arab Emirates regarding food choice and the factors that influence their choice.*
>
> **Introduction and rationale**
> *The last four decades have seen a global increase in diet-related diseases and conditions. Worldwide, obesity has nearly tripled since 1975 (WHO, 2017). In 2016 more than 1.9 billion adults (18 years and older) were overweight, out of these 650 million were obese (WHO, 2017). Diet-related problems are largely preventable through individual will, government actions, and health promotion (Genius, 2005). The consequences are however very serious. Obesity increases the risk of all causes of death, high blood pressure, type 2 diabetes, coronary heart disease, stroke and osteoarthritis, among other illnesses and conditions. Overweight is associated with breathlessness, increased sweating, difficulty doing physical activities, joint and back pain, and may lead to low quality of life and depression.*
>
> *The Middle East has recently been experiencing a triple burden of disease, characterised by the simultaneous presence of undernutrition, micronutrient deficiencies, overweight and obesity (Hwalla et al, 2016). In a systematic review of published papers between 1990 and 2011, Musaiger (2011) reported that obesity had reached an alarming level in all age groups of the Eastern Mediterranean countries. The prevalence of overweight and obesity among preschool children (<5 years) ranged from 1.9% to 21.9%, while it ranged from 7% to 45% in school children, and 25% to 81.9% among adults (Musaiger, 2011). Al Nohair (2014) reviewed studies on the prevalence of obesity and its associated illnesses in the Gulf countries (Bahrain, Kuwait, Qatar, Oman, Saudi Arabia, Lebanon and the United Arab Emirates). The review showed that the prevalence of obesity in Gulf countries among children and adolescents ranged from 5% to 14% in males and 3% to 18% in females. The highest prevalence was among adult females (2% to 55%) compared with 1% to 30% in adult males (Al Nohair, 2014).*
>
> *A common pattern shown in these studies is the much higher (almost double) prevalence of obesity and overweight among women compared to men. According to Sarant (2013), obese women are more prone to miscarriages and can experience difficulties becoming pregnant. They also have a key role in the food consumption of the family. While a marked change in diet*

seems to be a common thread among Arab countries, the cause of the increase in obesity "varies between Arab countries depending on socio-economic, geographical and cultural differences" (Sarant, 2013).

Diet-related problems in the United Arab Emirates (UAE)

One of the gulf countries that has, in the last 30 years, experienced significant social, economic and cultural changes is the UAE. Predictably, overweight and obesity have also increased. On 18th February 2015, The National (a Middle East English language newspaper) carried the headline "Obesity rate in the UAE double world average" (The National, 2015). Figures from WHO (2016) show that 8% of the population were diagnosed with diabetes. The figures for overweight were 70.5% (males) and 70.9% (females). Obesity was higher for women (41.2%) than for men (31.6%).

A small number of studies have provided evidence to support the rise in obesity and diabetes in the UAE. Al Hourani et al (2003) who investigated the prevalence of overweight among 898 females aged 11–18 in the UAE reported that the proportion of the sample who were overweight or at risk of overweight were 19% and 15%, respectively. In another study of 628 randomly selected households in the UAE, Ng et al (2011), using a battery of measurements, found that 65% of adult females were overweight or obese. The study also reported that adult females and adolescents were more at risk of obesity and overweight than their male counterparts.

A few studies have investigated the prevalence of overweight and obesity as well as food consumption patterns. These have used quantitative measures and have focused almost exclusively on the 'captive' population of school children or adolescents. Their findings have been consistent in showing a higher prevalence of obesity and overweight among females. Only one study on young adult women in the UAE was found after a literature search. Trainer (2012) explored how young Emirati women negotiated weight and body image. She reported that there was concern among those who were underweight, about their body image. Overall, she reported that there was a marked trend towards nutritionally poor diets and sedentary living. Trainer's finding that more women in her sample were underweight than overweight, ran contrary to the prevalence figures reported earlier. Trainer's sample consisted of university students; these were educated women, most likely from families who were economically able to pay for their education. There is a lack of studies on young adult women in the UAE, other than those in education. In fact, despite being the most at risk group for obesity, overweight and other eating disorders, there is no study on their eating behaviour, other than Trainer's. As Musaiger (2011) noted, 'while we know that there are several dietary, social, lifestyle and cultural factors associated with overweight and obesity, there is a lack of comprehensive and in-depth studies on the role of these factors in the occurrence of these conditions'. There is a need to explore how young adult women in the UAE make decisions regarding food choice and the factors that influence their choice.

This study has the potential to generate knowledge that could have global significance. Food-related problems such as overweight, obesity and eating disorders and the increasing trend in the consumption of processed fast foods are not restricted to the UAE. More directly, findings of this study have the potential to inform health promotion interventions for this population of young women in the UAE who are at high risk of overweight, obesity and other eating *disorders. According to Musaiger (2011), despite obesity being at epidemic proportions in the Arab countries, there are no comprehensive, multi-sectoral programmes directed towards this problem. Inadequate understanding of the factors associated with eating behaviours has been behind the failure of interventions to modify eating patterns and behaviour (Story et al, 2002).*

Comments on the Introduction/rationale:

■ Obesity is put in the global context because it is a problem that affects other countries as well. It is also put in a Middle Eastern context because these countries seem to be facing similar health issues. Finally, figures for obesity in the United Arab Emirates (UAE) (the setting for the proposed study) are provided. Therefore one can see how the author (of this proposal) moves from the general (global) to the specific (i.e. the country where the study will take place).

■ A variety of literature sources are used: WHO reports, research studies and a newspaper (*The National*).

■ To make the case for focusing on adult women, figures on obesity and overweight from reliable sources (WHO), and research studies are cited to show the higher prevalence of these problems among women when compared with men in the UAE. The case is reinforced by suggesting that young adult women have a key role in influencing diet in the family.

■ Finally, a case is made for the use of a qualitative approach in the proposed study by explaining that there is a need for in-depth studies to inform interventions to address obesity and overweight.

Below is another example of an introduction/rationale section of a proposal (I wrote) for a study to develop 'a self-management psychosocial intervention for men with prostate cancer and their partners and to test the feasibility of a RCT for evaluating the effectiveness of the intervention'.

Introduction

Prostate cancer is the second most common cancer in men and the fifth most common cancer in the world among individuals of both sexes combined (Cancer Research UK, 2013). About one in six men will be diagnosed with prostate cancer during their lifetime (American Cancer Society, 2013), and incidence rates in the Western developed countries continue to rise. In the United Kingdom (UK), prostate cancer is the most common cancer in men, with around 41,000 new cases reported in 2010 (Cancer Research UK, 2013). In Northern Ireland, there were just over 1000 men diagnosed with prostate cancer in 2011 (Cancer Research UK, 2013). Over the past 25 years, the five-year relative survival rate (adjusted for normal life expectancy) for all stages of prostate cancer combined has also increased from 68% to 100% (American Cancer Society, 2013). The 18-year prostate cancer prevalence at the end of 2012 in Northern Ireland was 6,646 (Northern Ireland Cancer Registry, 2013). This had led to an increasing focus on survivorship issues, which researchers have started to address over the past two decades. A large body of evidence suggests that a diagnosis of cancer and the treatment that follows give rise to significant psychosocial problems, including distress, anxiety and depression.

The quality of life in men with localised prostate cancer, especially in the first six months post-diagnosis, may be reduced. Reeve et al (2012) reported significant decrements in physical, mental and social aspects of cancer patients' lives when compared with men without cancer. The cancer journey, however, does not end with treatment. Several studies have reported problems related to sexual function (Baniel et al., 2000; Mehrdad et al., 2011), urinary incontinence, relationships (between partners and within the family) and financial strain. Anxiety and uncertainty about disease recurrence and spread of the cancer are constant worries for some. Previous work conducted by the authors of this study demonstrated that the partners of men with prostate cancer were an integral component of the cancer journey (McCaughan et al., 2011). A recent review of the literature on psychosocial adjustment of female partners of men with prostate cancer shows that prostate cancer can have marked repercussions for the partner (Couper et al., 2006). Partners can often be more distressed than the men themselves (Couper et al., 2006), experiencing a lack of information and uncertainty about the future (Mason 2005; Ezer et al., 2011). In another study by Northouse et al (2007), spouses reported significantly less self-efficacy and social support than patients. Some couples report concerns about communication, sexuality, and intimacy (Sanders et al., 2006; Manne et al., 2010). They may not discuss erectile dysfunction and the loss of sexual intimacy with each other (Boehmer and Clarke, 2001) and can experience different perceptions related to these sexual symptoms (Ezer et al., 2011). Creating an environment that encourages discussion may reduce couple distress and uncertainty and improve their relationship (Manne et al., 2010).

Most men with prostate cancer adapt and cope with the disease and with its treatment, but a significant minority (almost a third) have moderate and severe unmet needs for psychosocial support (Ames et al., 2009; Ernstmann et al., 2009; McCaughan et al., 2011; White et al., 2012). Health professionals and researchers are rising to the challenges presented by prostate cancer by developing and testing psychosocial interventions designed for those men with cancer and their partners who need help and support.

Rationale for this study

Most psychosocial interventions for men with prostate cancer have been developed in the United States (Parahoo et al., 2013). To date there is no published account on the development and evaluation of psychosocial interventions for this population in the UK. While there is a lot to learn from the US experience, their findings are not readily generalisable to the Northern Irish context because of differences in health systems and because of socio-economic and cultural differences between these two countries. Caution should also be exercised when generalizing from these studies as they used a variety of interventions and strategies both in terms of content, delivery, duration, outcome measures, sample size, and composition (Parahoo et al., 2013).

In Northern Ireland, there is no evidence of any psychosocial intervention designed specifically for men with prostate cancer and their partners, post-treatment. However, they can access services offered by statutory and voluntary organisations in the form of support groups, counselling and information provision. To date there is no published data on the effectiveness of these services or support groups. There is the danger that interventions not based on evidence could, at best, be ineffective (and therefore a waste of precious resources) or, at worst, harmful. The stockpiling and prescribing of the drugs 'Tamiflu' and 'Relenza' for influenza in adults and children in the UK (Jefferson et al., 2014) is a recent example of how millions of pounds were wasted in the absence of evidence of their effectiveness (Gallagher, 2014).

There are few studies of psychosocial interventions designed for men with prostate cancer and their partners. A recent systematic review of psychosocial interventions for couples concluded that further investigation in the area was warranted (Chambers et al., 2011). This view has been reiterated by Galbraith et al (2011) who concluded that there is currently a paucity of literature determining how best to help couples improve their communication about intimacy, coping strategies, psychosexual functioning, and obtaining information on managing long-term treatment side effects. According to Aranda (2008), there is a lack of in-depth descriptions of psychosocial intervention development that is hindering the identification of which interventions (or which components of an intervention) work.

Psychosocial interventions

There are different types of psychosocial interventions including psycho-educational therapy, cognitive behavioural therapy or supportive group therapy (Newell et al., 2002). Cognitive behavioural change interventions commonly include goal setting, problem-solving, coping skills training, behavioural contracting in addition to the provision of information (Peyrot and Rubin, 2007). Most psychosocial interventions are based on theories that emphasise the importance of self-management and positive coping strategies in maintaining or enhancing the person's self-efficacy and competence to deal with the effects of the illness.

Compared with drug or surgical interventions, psychosocial interventions are relatively more difficult to implement in a randomised controlled trial. This is why psychosocial interventions have been described as complex interventions by the Medical Research Council (Craig et al., 2008). There are three main factors influencing the delivery of psychosocial interventions, each of which presents significant threats to the internal and external validity of randomised controlled trials of these types of interventions. Firstly, the personality, competence, motivation and the interpretation of the intervention by the facilitators (defined as the person/s delivering the intervention) can all affect the outcomes. When the same intervention is delivered by more than one facilitator on different sites, the potential for introducing bias can be high. Secondly, the intervention itself may look easy, on paper, to implement but may present difficulties when implemented in the real world of practice. Thirdly, the participants' personalities, motivation, interests, perceptions and ability to function in a group format can all have consequences on how the intervention is delivered.

A feasibility or pilot study, prior to the evaluation of complex interventions, is recommended (Craig et al., 2008). This provides a valuable opportunity to explore the process of implementing and testing the intervention, enabling a better insight into the practical and logistical issues of delivery, costs, recruitment and retention issues, as well as the views of facilitators and participants on how the intervention can be improved. Such 'process' evaluations can provide explanations for the findings and on how these interventions move from research to practice (Craig et al., 2008).

There is a lack of information on psychosocial interventions and the process of their implementation in reports of randomised controlled trials. Randomised controlled trials of these types of interventions have also been described as the 'black box' since little information is provided in the papers or reports in which the studies are reported (Grant et al., 2013). This study aims to provide knowledge in this area to address this gap.

As the incidence and the prevalence of prostate cancer continue to rise, the need for evidence-based interventions for men with prostate cancer and their partners, increases as well. "A cultural shift in the approach to care and support is needed for people affected by cancer to a greater focus on recovery, health and well-being after treatment" (DoH, 2010). The aim of the National Cancer Survivorship initiative "is to ensure that those living with and beyond cancer get the care and support they need to lead as healthy and active a life as possible, for as long as possible"(DoH, 2010). In Northern Ireland, initiatives such as 'Transforming Your Care: A review of health and social care in Northern Ireland' (HSC, 2011) is designed to address the challenges of cancer survivorship, as well as other health and social care issues.
The aims of this study were:

1. *To develop a psychosocial intervention for men with prostate cancer and their partners.*
2. *To test the feasibility of a randomised control trial for evaluating the effectiveness of the intervention.*

Comments on the above excerpt:

- The incidence of prostate cancer is put in a global, national (UK) and local (Northern Ireland) context. However, these figures on their own do not justify a study on the psychosocial aspects of prostate cancer. One can use the same figures to support a proposal on radiotherapy or chemotherapy related to prostate cancer. Therefore, a case is made specifically to show that survival rates have increased, leading to more men facing psychosocial problems, in the aftermath of diagnosis and treatment.
- This case is supported by figures from reliable and recognised sources (the American Cancer Society and Cancer Research UK).
- Higher prevalences of prostate cancer and higher survival rates are also not enough to justify a study on psychosocial interventions. Therefore evidence from a number of studies and literature reviews is used to show how men and their partners are psychosocially affected by prostate cancer.
- It was also important to explain why it was a feasibility study and why interventions should be developed for men and their partners. Therefore, a number of reviews, studies and papers are cited to support the need to study the feasibility of developing and implementing a psychosocial intervention for men with prostate cancer and their partners.

THE LITERATURE REVIEW SECTION OF A PROPOSAL

There are two parts to this section. The first briefly explains or defines some of the key terms or concepts in the research question and informs the reader about what is known about the topic. For example, in a study of 'stress, burnout and engagement among social workers in child welfare settings', Travis et al. (2016) provided clarity on each of these concepts in the research questions. After defining the concept of 'burnout', Travis et al. (2016) explained that they were focusing on two dimensions of burnout: emotional exhaustion and depersonalisation. The reason for clarifying and defining these terms or concepts is for readers to understand how these terms are interpreted in the context of the proposed study. For example, there are different types of stress, such as occupational stress, acute and chronic stress, episodic stress, emotional stress, etc. Being clear which type of stress the proposed study addresses and how it is defined will convey clearly to readers what your perspective of the concept is in your study.

The second part of this section is a brief literature review of previous research on your topic (i.e. how much or how little there is on this topic and what new questions need to be answered). For example, when reviewing the literature on 'psychosocial interventions for men with prostate cancer', Parahoo carried out a literature review that showed briefly how 'research on psychosocial aspects of prostate cancer has developed and progressed over the years'. In particular, he noted that earlier studies on this topic focused on exploring the psychosocial effects of prostate cancer and the needs of these men after diagnosis and as a result of treatment. This was followed by studies on the 'development and testing of interventions' to help men with prostate cancer to cope with the psychosocial effects. Later, researchers recognised that prostate cancer can affect the partners of men diagnosed with the disease and this led to studies on the development and evaluation of intervention for couples. With increased online access, researchers began to test online interventions. By reviewing the literature on the topic, it is therefore possible to track the 'journey' that researchers have travelled on this particular topic.

Not all this information needs to be reported in the proposal. What is required is a brief review of studies similar to the proposed one. Questions that reviewers of proposals often ask are: 'Has this study been done before' and 'why do we need another one?' It is possible to answer these questions by searching for the same or similar studies. The aim is to carry out a brief content analysis of these papers. For example, before developing a self-management psychosocial intervention for men with prostate cancer and their partners, McCaughan et al. (2013) reviewed similar studies. They found that the interventions in these studies used a variety of approaches. They identified the main outcomes measured and found that there were contradictory findings (some reported positive results and others showed no benefits). McCaughan et al. (2013) agreed with other researchers that while much can be learned from these studies, there was a lack of studies specifically on how to help couples improve their communication about intimacy and cope with other issues related to prostate cancer. This review was necessary in order to identify the lack of, or 'gap' in, research that the authors of the proposal wanted to fill.

Types of Literature Review for a Proposal

Students and new researchers often ask how they are expected to carry out a review of the literature when developing a proposal. They are sometimes confused by the number of different types of review and do not know which one to choose. Grant and Booth (2009) identified these 14 types of review:

critical review, literature review; mapping review/systematic map; meta-analysis; mixed studies review/mixed methods review; overview; qualitative systematic review/qualitative evidence synthesis; rapid review; scoping review; state-of-the-art review; systematic review; systematic search and review; systematized review and umbrella review.

It is clear from this list that some of these 'labels' are used interchangeably and that reviewers can be pedantic (excessively concerned with minor details) in their use of these labels. It would also be fair to state that the same review can be given different labels by different reviewers. To avoid getting lost in this 'jungle' of reviews, it is important to focus on what you want to achieve when reviewing studies similar to the one you are proposing. If the aim is to examine closely (and compare) key aspects of these studies, for example, their designs, methods, samples and findings, a scoping review would be appropriate. On the other hand, if the aim is to evaluate the effectiveness of interventions in terms of specified outcomes (e.g. quality of life, resilience, etc.), a systematic review is the most appropriate design. A scoping review that uses systematic search strategies would be appropriate and sufficient for a review of the literature for a research proposal. The term 'systematic' is not confined to systematic reviews. One can carry out a systematic search without doing a systematic review.

Scoping reviews aim to 'map the literature on a particular topic or research area and provide an opportunity to identify key concepts; gaps in the research; and types and sources of evidence to inform practice, policymaking, and research' (Daudt et al., 2013). While a scoping review can be systematic, it should not set narrow inclusion criteria (e.g. only RCTs) because it will not inform readers of other types of study design (such as qualitative or survey) that have been used to investigate this topic. The aim of a scoping review is intentionally broad, because it seeks to 'scope' or 'explore' what the body of literature offers. According to Grant and Booth (2009), 'scoping reviews are preliminary assessment of potential size and scope of available research literature' (p. 95). The aim of a scoping review for a proposal is to map the literature and identify gaps in research, to justify the proposed study. For examples of scoping reviews, see:

- Abbott (2022), 'Decision making by practitioners in the social professions involved in compulsory admission to mental health hospital'.
- Kelly et al. (2022), 'eHealth interventions to support self-management in people with musculoskeletal disorders'.
- Stimler et al. (2023), 'Current trends in occupational therapy for adolescent and young2adult cancer survivors'.

Differences Between Scoping and Systematic Reviews

Scoping reviews are different from systematic reviews in many ways. Scoping reviews tend to answer broader questions that can change during the review process, in comparison with systematic reviews in which questions tend to be narrow, focused and fixed. The questions/objectives of the systematic review are set in advance (as is the case in primary research). Outcomes (e.g. in studies of the effectiveness of interventions) in systematic reviews are also set in advance, while in scoping reviews the aim during the review process is to find out which outcomes these studies have focused upon. Since scoping reviews are a broad exploration of the literature, inclusion criteria tend to be broad and inclusive, in order to not exclude studies using a variety of designs (since the aim is precisely to find out the designs and methods researchers have used). Systematic reviews tend to focus on a specific design, such as RCTs, although more recently they have included studies with different designs. In scoping reviews, there is no need to appraise all selected studies individually and systematically (e.g. with the use of checklists). Finally, scoping reviews do not normally involve a meta-analysis or meta-synthesis of findings, although broad themes and trends can be identified.

Critiquing the Literature

Searching the literature is a first step. To review selected studies, one then has to make sense of them. This involves describing, analysing and critiquing/evaluating these studies. Although a certain amount of description is inevitable, it is important to critically review the literature. A descriptive literature review is often a summary of what was done and found in individual studies. Typically, the description will say what was done, what methodology was used and what was found (the findings) as in the example below from 'A scoping review of occupational therapy interventions in the treatment of people with substance use disorders', by Ryan and Boland (2021):

> *Wasmuth et al. (2016) used drama, where participants were involved in the production of a co-facilitated play. The occupational therapist used rehearsals to develop cognitive strategies with participants. Facilitated discussions linked character experiences to the participants' issues, which was an accessible medium for them to acknowledge the difficult impact of substance use in their lives. The community element provided a safe, supportive space, which facilitated participants who relapsed during rehearsals to return to gain support.*

(p. 110)

To review the literature, one has to analyse, synthesise and evaluate the literature. To 'analyse' means to break the literature into its constituent parts. Studies have many parts or components, such as 'research question', 'designs', 'methods', 'sample and sampling' and 'findings'. By analysing the types of question that researchers have used in their study, one can find the areas that have been researched the most, the least or not at all. By closely examining the designs in these studies, one is able to see the trends and patterns in the selection of designs for studies on this particular topic.

This is about more than separating these studies into quantitative or qualitative approaches. It involves, for example, examining the quantitative studies, comparing their methods and findings and looking at the rigour with which they have been conducted. By doing so, it is possible to uncover interesting trends. For example, in a review of 28 studies on a 'depression-specific online support group', Griffiths et al. (2009) found that studies of 'lower design quality' reported more positive outcomes (between depression and participation in these groups) than studies of higher quality.

This same exercise can be done for qualitative studies. However, for a research proposal, what you focus upon depends on the 'case' you want to make. As explained earlier, if you want to research an area in which there are few or no studies, you can examine the 'research questions' or 'aims' of the selected studies. If you want to test the effectiveness of a particular intervention that has been tested before, you will look at the findings of similar studies and, hopefully, be able to show that there is disagreement between them.

'Synthesis' means putting the parts back together to give an overall picture of the state of the research. This can show whether research is embryonic or advanced on this topic, and its strengths and limitations. Evaluation means making a subjective value judgement. It involves stating, for example, if the research is weak or strong, helpful or not helpful, and what needs to be done. The analysis is the 'objective' method that provides the evidence on which the 'subjective' judgement is made. Therefore, the analysis must be transparent for others to be able to replicate. For example, if you say that the samples in the quantitative studies you reviewed were small and not based on any sample size calculation, others should be able to arrive at the same conclusions if they analyse these studies. Below is an example of evaluation in 'A scoping review of online international student collaboration in occupational therapy education' by Hynes et al. (2022):

> *Sood et al. (2014) also sought to increase the cultural competence of their students and report that the programme was effective in increasing these perceived levels. Although they used a published measure to capture these data, the groups were too small to carry out the parametric analysis that was undertaken (e.g. n-4 [sic]; n = 9) and so the results reported are questionable.*
>
> **(p. 649)**

In this example, the authors of the review pointed out that the groups sizes were too small to draw reliable conclusions.

Finally, having reviewed individual studies, the review authors should come to a conclusion based on all the studies they included. For example, in a review of 'Family interventions in early psychosis service delivery', Day and Petrakis (2017) concluded:

> *This review highlights two main areas where there is a lack of research. The first is looking at ways to make early psychosis services more family inclusive, rather than looking at discreet one-off family interventions. This is touched upon in some of the studies reviewed here, but there is a general paucity of research in this area. The second is examining how family interventions can be effectively delivered to diverse populations, something that is almost entirely absent from the literature reviewed. Many early psychosis services operate in extremely diverse communities, and yet the research to date makes almost no acknowledgement of this. Additionally, the interventions themselves are not geared towards being inclusive. For example, group interventions tend to be delivered in one language (English in the Australian context).*
>
> **(p. 648)**

By stating that 'there is a lack of research' on different aspects of this topic, the authors made a judgement based on the analysis of the studies selected for review.

ADDITIONAL NOTES FOR THE INTRODUCTION/LITERATURE REVIEW IN PROPOSALS

The introduction and literature review and background to the study are the first sections that reviewers see when assessing a proposal. To convince and impress them, it is important that a good case is made for the study. This first impression is likely to influence reviewers as they read the rest of the proposal. If funding is being sought, it is advisable, when possible, to publish a literature review on the topic in the proposal.

Funding organisations normally set up panels to review proposals. They may also send proposals to experts on proposal topics for their views on the quality of the proposals and whether they would recommend funding. These experts are likely to be well aware of key literature on these topics. They may also have published in this area. Therefore it is imperative that the literature review is up to date and thorough. See Proposal Example 2.1 for an example of an 'introduction' and 'background' section in a research proposal. Watson (2018) also offers some good advice as to what goes in the 'introduction' and 'background' section'.

PROPOSAL EXAMPLE 2.1
INTRODUCTION AND BACKGROUND IN A RESEARCH PROPOSAL

Serrano-Ripoll et al. (2021), 'Effect of a mobile-based intervention on mental health in frontline healthcare workers against COVID-19'.

In this proposal, the authors provide an introduction and a background section (as per journal requirements).

COMMENTS

1. The 'introduction' consists of general statements (supported by up-to-date and relevant literature) about the challenges of COVID-19 to health systems and health care workers (HCWs). The authors make the link between the stress of caring for COVID-19 patients with the physical and mental health of staff. They cite a recent systematic review that reported high prevalence of acute stress, anxiety, burnout, depression and post-traumatic disorder among staff.
2. They also make the case that mobile health (mHealth) interventions are becoming popular and cite their benefits as being 'low cost, high scalability and sustainability'. They also cite recent trials on mHealth interventions and related topics and concluded that while systematic reviews have shown that 'they have potential for improving mental health symptoms, the available evidence is still scarce'(p. 2899), thereby justifying why this trial is needed.
3. The 'background' section is in two parts. The first is a brief summary of mHealth interventions. The authors cite literature that demonstrates how 'these interventions are well suited to help HCWs to combat the adverse effects of working in such high-pressure situations for a prolonged time period' (p. 2899). The second part makes the case of why this study is needed in Spain by citing up-to-date figures on mobile phone user rates in the country (98%), the cumulative number of COVID-19 infections among HCWs (20% of all HCW infections worldwide) and the impact of COVID-19 infections on the mental health of Spanish HCWs.
4. This is probably a shorter version than the one in the original proposal. This is because the journal in which it was published had word limits.

Checklist for the 'Introduction' and 'Background' sections in a proposal:
1. Has the gap in research and policy/practice been identified?
2. Has a strong case (rationale) for this study been made? Has the rationale included reference to any relevant policy/strategy?
3. How impactful is this study likely to be in terms of policy/practice etc.?
4. Has up-to-date literature been used to make a compelling case for the study?
5. Has a brief summary of a review of previous studies on this topic been provided? Does the review clearly lead to the research questions and to the chosen methodology?

SUMMARY AND CONCLUSIONS

The literature is a useful source for research ideas. A literature review can provide the arguments to justify the need for the proposed study and can inform readers of what we already know about the topic and what gap(s) the proposed study seeks to fill. This chapter has given examples of how to construct a rationale based on reliable sources and how to review similar studies on a topic. Both the 'rationale' and the 'literature review sections' should convince reviewers of the proposal that the authors have given much thought to the study, that they are well aware of the relevant and up-to-date literature on the topic and that they have something new to offer (in terms of filling a gap in knowledge or a new way to do research on their proposed topic). By providing a convincing rationale based on reliable, up-to-date evidence, the authors of a proposal can make a compelling case for why the study should be carried out and funded (if funding is being applied for).

REFERENCES

Abbott, S. (2022). Decision making by practitioners in the social professions involved in compulsory admission to mental health hospital: A scoping review. *The British Journal of Social Work, 52*(4), 1916–1933.

AUTISTICA. (2018). Your research priorities. https://www.autistica.org.uk/our-research/our-research/your-research-priorities. Accessed March 6, 2022.

Daudt, H. M., van Mossel, C., & Scott, S. J. (2013) Enhancing the scoping study methodology: A large, inter-professional team's experience with Arksey and O'Malley's framework. *BMC Medical Research Methodology, 13*, 48.

Day, K., & Petrakis, M. (2017). Family interventions in early psychosis service delivery: A systematized review. *Social Work in Mental Health, 15*(6), 632–650. https://doi.org/10.1080/15332985.2016.1271381

Grant, M. J., & Booth, A. (2009). A typology of reviews: An analysis of 14 review types and associated methodologies. *Health Information & Libraries Journal, 26*, 91–108.

Griffiths, K. M., Calear, A. L., & Banfield, M. (2009). Systematic review on Internet Support Groups (ISGs) and Depression (1): Do ISGs reduce depressive symptoms? *Journal of Medical Internet Research, 11*, e40. https://doi.org/10.2196/jmir.1270

Hynes, S. M., Hills, C., & Orban, K. (2022). A scoping review of online international student collaboration in occupational therapy education. *British Journal of Occupational Therapy, 85*(9), 642–652.

Kelly, M., Fullen, B., Martin, D., McMahon, S., & McVeigh, J. G. (2022). eHealth interventions to support self-management in people with musculoskeletal disorders, "eHealth: It's TIME"—A scoping review. *Physical Therapy, 102*(4), pzab307. https://doi.org/10.1093/ptj/pzab307

McCaughan, E., Prue, G., McSorley, O., Northouse, L., Schafenacker, A., & Parahoo, K. (2013). A randomized controlled trial of a self-management psychosocial intervention for men with prostate cancer and their partners: A study protocol. *Journal of Advanced Nursing, 69*(11), 2572–2583.

Parahoo, K. (2014). *Nursing research: Principles, process and issues* (3rd ed.). Basingstoke: Palgrave Macmillan.

Ryan, D. A., & Boland, P. (2021). A scoping review of occupational therapy interventions in the treatment of people with substance use disorders. *Irish Journal of Occupational Therapy, 49*(2), 104–114.

Serrano-Ripoll, M. J., Ricci-Cabello, I., Jiménez, R., Zamanillo-Campos, R., Yañez-Juan, A. M., Bennasar-Veny, M., Sitges, C., Gervilla, E., Leiva, A., García-Campayo, J., García-Buades, M. E., García-Toro, M., Pastor-Moreno, G., Ruiz-Perez, I., Alonso-Coello, P., Llobera, J., & Fiol-deRoque, M. A. (2021). Effect of a mobile-based intervention on mental health in frontline healthcare workers against COVID-19: Protocol for a randomized controlled trial. *Journal of Advanced Nursing, 77*(6), 2898–2907.

Sood, D., Cepa, D., Dsouza, S. A., Saha, S., Aikat, R., & Tuuk. (2014). Impact of international collaborative project on cultural competence among occupational therapy students. *The Open Journal of Occupational Therapy, 2*(3), 1–18.

Stimler, L., Campbell, C., Cover, L., & Pergolotti, M. (2023). Current trends in occupational therapy for adolescent and young adult cancer survivors: A scoping review. *Occupational Therapy in Health Care, 37*(4), 664–687.

Travis, D. J., Lizano, E. L., & Mor Barak, M. E. (2016). 'I'm So Stressed!' A longitudinal model of stress, burnout and engagement among social workers in child welfare settings. *British Journal of Social Work, 46*(4), 1076–1095.

Wasmuth, S., Pritchard, K., & Kaneshiro, K. (2016). Occupation-based intervention for addictive disorders: A systematic review. *Journal of Substance Abuse Treatment, 62*, 1–9.

Watson, R. (2018). I say "Introduction"; You say "Background". *Nurse Author and Editor, 28*(1), 4.

3 CONCEPTUAL FRAMEWORKS IN RESEARCH PROPOSALS

INTRODUCTION

Conceptual frameworks can help to guide researchers throughout the research process. They can also add theoretical credibility to the study. In this chapter, we will explore the meaning and importance of conceptual frameworks, and how researchers use conceptual frameworks in their studies. We will also stress the importance of showing clearly in the proposal which conceptual framework is chosen and why, as well as how it will underpin the proposed study.

In the first two chapters, we looked at how to develop research questions and review the literature when we design a study and write a proposal. One of the functions of a literature review is to identify and select an appropriate framework for one's study (Parahoo, 2014). However, one does not design a study first and then look for a conceptual framework. Developing research questions, reviewing the literature and selecting a conceptual framework are iterative, intertwined, overlapping and simultaneous activities to inform (or underpin) all aspects of the design of a study.

THE MEANING OF 'CONCEPTUAL FRAMEWORK'

The term 'conceptual framework' is made up of the two words: 'conceptual' and 'framework'. Conceptual is the adjective of the noun 'concept', which means a mental image of an idea (e.g. 'house') or phenomenon (e.g. 'grief'). We all have an idea, in our mind, of what 'health' is. We therefore have our own concept of 'health' or what it means to be healthy.

In 1948 the World Health Organization (WHO) defined health as 'a state of complete physical, mental and social well-being and not merely the absence of disease or infirmity' (WHO, n.d., para. 1). This has been described as an abstract and utopian concept that no human being can achieve or sustain. However, this example shows that a concept is not the real thing but an idea of it. It is in the realm of ideas; we imagine or mentally conceive or construct them in our minds. Some examples of lay concepts are 'happiness', 'strength', 'intelligence' and 'stupidity'. None of these is 'tangible' (perceptible by touch), but they help us to make sense of what goes on in our world and the people in it. Professionals, too, have invented or constructed a large number of concepts or constructs to help them in their practice. Examples of these concepts include empowerment, client satisfaction, disability, stress, wellbeing, caring, stigma, pain, anxiety, recovery and quality of life.

Although there are different ways in which each of these concepts can be imagined (e.g. there are different concepts of health), professionals aim to have consensus (or agreement) over their meaning to enable intra- and interprofessional communication. Therefore, these concepts are defined in ways that are more or less acceptable for nurses and health and social care professionals to use in their practice. Conceptual definitions are important as they convey the abstract ideas in words. Hence the WHO definition of health is actually a conceptual definition.

There are many definitions of 'frame' and 'framework'. A frame has been described as 'a rigid structure that surrounds something such a picture, door or window pane' (Dictionary.com). In this case, the frame defines or delineates a picture or painting. The frame 'holds' the painting and separates it from what else is on the wall. Another concept of a frame is that of a building such as house, which is made up of structures including the foundation, the floor, walls and a roof. These structures are the essential features of the concept of house. These features provide a frame to work from (a conceptual framework) for the builders when they set out to construct a house.

Similarly, health and social care professionals can use conceptual frameworks to guide and inform their practice. For example, in her paper: 'Practice frameworks: conceptual maps to guide interventions in child welfare', Connolly (2007) explained that her framework integrates three perspectives: child-centred; family-led and culturally responsive; and strengths and evidence based. She described her framework as a tool to provide a clear understanding of what underpins interventions with children and families. In this example we can see that the framework has three main components or pillars that provide a structure to the *framework*. For another example, see Hudon et al. (2015) 'The contribution of conceptual frameworks to knowledge translation interventions in physical therapy'.

An example of a policy framework comes from Northern Ireland, where the Department of Health, Social Services and Public Safety (DHSSPS) published a policy framework on 'Living with long term conditions' (DHSSPS, 2012). The framework listed six principles that practitioners can use to guide their practice when caring for people living with long-term conditions: working in partnership; supporting self-management; information to service users and carers; managing medicines, respect for carers; and improving care and services. These six principles form the main structures around which the framework is built. Unlike a framework for a picture, however, policy and practice frameworks are not rigid but are a guide, often based on sound theoretical and ethical principles. Professionals can interpret and modify them to suit their practice.

These policy and practice frameworks can also be used in research. For example, the six principles of living with long-term conditions (DHSSPS, 2012) can be used to develop a questionnaire/tool to find out if, and to what extent, these principles underpin practice in this area of care. Research questions can be developed from this framework, for example 'Are patients involved in decision-making about their care and treatment?' (Principle 1: working in partnerships) or 'What strategies do nurses use to teach patients how to manage their medications?' (Principle 4: managing medicines).

Most conceptual frameworks are developed to increase professionals' understanding of the concepts they deal with in their work. A search on MEDLINE (from 1946 to 6 October 2022), using 'conceptual framework' as a keyword, revealed 15,141 'hits'. These were conceptual frameworks developed mainly for policy and practice. For example, Biswas et al. (2019) developed a conceptual framework of 'barriers and solutions for increasing hand hygiene compliance in a low-resource neonatal intensive care unit'. Alshyyab et al. (2019) described how they carried out a literature review to 'explore the concept of patient safety culture as it may apply to emergency health care'. They developed a conceptual framework to 'assist managers and researchers to take a comprehensive approach to build an effective culture in emergency department setting' (p. 42).

Conceptual frameworks are also developed specifically for research studies. Sawatzky et al. (2015) developed the Conceptual Framework for Predicting Nurse Retention to 'explore and describe factors that predict the retention of nurses working in critical care areas' (p. 2316). This framework was based on previously published research evidence, as well as empirical models related to predictors of nurse retention and it represents the conceptual links between influencing factors, intermediary factors, and the primary outcome of interest: intention to leave (Sawatzky et al., 2015).

CONCEPTUAL FRAMEWORK, THEORETICAL FRAMEWORK AND CONCEPTUAL MODEL

The WHO definition of health describes their concept of 'health'. Similarly, the policy framework for long-term care (DHSSPS, 2012) represents the authors' concept of 'long-term care'. While both these conceptual frameworks are underpinned by research evidence and theories, they are not, in themselves, theories of health or long-term care. Therefore both the WHO definition of health and the DHSSPS (2012) principles of long-term care can be described as conceptual frameworks because these frameworks are based on 'concepts' rather than on 'theories'. A *conceptual framework* is a description or explanation of a mental image of idea or phenomenon (concept) that can be used as a frame of reference for policy, practice or research.

A *theoretical framework* can be developed from one or more theories. A theory is defined as 'a set of interrelated constructs (concepts), definitions, and propositions that present a systematic view of phenomena specifying relations among variables, with the purpose of explaining and predicting the phenomena' (Kerlinger, 1986, p. 9). The theory of 'diffusion of innovations' (Rogers, 2003) explained how a new idea is spread and adopted by people in different settings. Rogers' theory explains, among other things, how, when, why, in what circumstances and by whom innovations are, or are not, adopted. For example, 'innovators' are described as the first individuals to adopt an innovation as they are those most willing to take risks, are from the higher social classes, are economically successful, interact with other innovators, etc. Rogers (2003) went on to describe other types of adopter and the variables (such as personality, attitudes and ability) that influence adoption behaviours. This theory can be used as a framework for studies exploring or predicting change.

Zhang et al. (2015) identified a number of studies that used Rogers' (2003) theory to conceptualise 'technology adoption in the context of e-health' (p. 4). Zhang et al. (2015) used Rogers' theory as a theoretical framework to 'examine and explain the impact of factors, in particular, the characteristics of innovations and innovation decision-making processes, on patient acceptance and ongoing usage of an EAS (e-appointment scheduling) service' (p. 4). Therefore, one can see that the use of a theory as a framework can help to develop questions such as which factors impact on a patient's acceptance and use of a new service. In Zhang et al.'s (2015) study, Roger's theory was used as a framework to test propositions and hypotheses within the theory in the real-life setting of a health service. This is what Miles et al. (2014) meant when they stated that a conceptual framework explains the main things to be studied – the key factors, concepts, or variables – and the presumed relationships among them.

Ideas for 'factors', 'relationships' and 'outcomes' can come from existing theories, such as Rogers' (2003) theory of 'diffusion of innovations'. A *theoretical framework* is a description of a theory or theories that can be used as a frame of reference to inform or underpin policy, practice or research, whereas a *conceptual model* is a term used to describe graphically how a conceptual or theoretical framework is used in a particular study. Diagrams or graphical representations can convey more clearly what a large volume of words or text cannot. For an example of a conceptual model graphically depicting 'stages and typical learning activities in a reflective practice', see Heymann et al. (2022, p. 383).

In the literature, the three terms conceptual framework, theoretical framework and conceptual model are often used interchangeably. It is not very important to get the label right; it is more important to justify, describe and explain why and how a framework is used in your research study.

COMMON CONCEPTUAL AND THEORETICAL FRAMEWORKS USED IN NURSING, HEALTH AND SOCIAL CARE RESEARCH

Any theory or concept can be used (wholly or partly) as a framework for research studies; the choice depends on what the researchers want to study. Health and social care professionals are interested in patients' characteristics such as attitudes and personality as well as their beliefs and perceptions (of disease, treatment, services, etc.). They are involved in the organisation, delivery and evaluation of their services. They are often also engaged in changing the behaviour of their patients and clients. Other areas of professional interest include the education and training of personnel and issues such as staff's attitudes, knowledge, competence, job satisfaction and health and social wellbeing. There is an abundance of theories that explain all these areas.

Some of the common theories used by researchers in the nursing, social work and health professions include the Health Belief Model and Sick Role Behavior (Becker, 1974), Theory of Planned Behaviour (TPB; Ajzen, 1991), Social Learning Theory (Bandura 1977a), Stress, Appraisal and Coping Theory (Lazarus and Folkman, 1984), Self Efficacy Theory (Bandura, 1977b) and Diffusion of Innovations theory (Rogers, 2003). These theories come from the social sciences and other disciplines, but they have been widely applied to policy, practice and research in nursing, health and social care fields.

There are also theories specific to particular disciplines. For example, the Hub of Occupational Therapy Theory (HOTheory) is 'a database that contains theories, models, frames of reference, and frameworks that are developed specifically by occupational therapists or for use in occupational therapy'. The purpose of this database is to 'help occupational therapy practitioners and students to find theoretical knowledge to inform their practice and learning' (HOTheory, 2022). Nursing has many theories and conceptual frameworks including Interpersonal Relations Theory (Peplau, 1952), Transcultural Nursing (Leininger, 1988) and the Adaptation Model (Roy and Andrews, 1999). Some of the theories relevant to social work include the cognitive behavioural studies mentioned above as well as Family Systems Theory (Kerr and Bowen, 1988; Brown, 1999), the Crisis Intervention Model (Roberts, 1991) and the Recovery Model (Davidson 2005). Physiotherapists have used the Self-Determination Theory (Strempfl et al., 2022), the Dynamic Systems Theory (Darabi and Svensson,2021) and Motor Skills Acquisition Theory (Leech et al., 2022).

One of the best known frameworks that has been used to evaluate the quality of health care services and the effectiveness of interventions is the Donabedian Model, which involves structure, process and outcome (Donabedian, 1966). An example of the use of the Donabedian Model as a framework in a study will be given in the next section.

HOW CONCEPTUAL AND THEORETICAL FRAMEWORKS ARE USED IN RESEARCH STUDIES

In this section we will explore how researchers have used conceptual and theoretical frameworks to inform part or all aspects of their studies. A brief examination of the literature shows that conceptual or theoretical frameworks help researchers mainly to:

- develop research questions/hypotheses and inform the design of the study;
- analyse and interpret data;
- inform all aspects of the study (including the research questions, design, analysis, discussion and interpretation);
- develop and evaluate interventions;
- use (or adapt) existing frameworks in order to develop their own conceptual frameworks for their study.

Each of these will be explored below with examples from actual research studies.

Using Frameworks to Develop Research Questions or Hypotheses and Guide the Design of the Study

One of the main uses of a conceptual or theoretical framework in a study is to help develop research questions, aims or hypotheses. These frameworks have a number of components or concepts that provide structures to inform the development of research questions. For example, Gardner et al. (2014) used the Donabedian Model to examine the quality and safety of a nursing service innovation.

The Donabedian Model has three components (structure, process and outcomes) that together provide a holistic framework to evaluate the quality of health services. 'Structure' refers to the context in which the services are provided, including resources, equipment, facilities, personnel, etc. 'Process' refers to the actual delivery of services, including the interaction between staff and patients/clients, and 'Outcome' refers to the impact of the services on patients in terms of, for example, recovery, cure or rehabilitation. Gardner et al. (2014) explained how they used the Donabedian Model to develop the following questions for their study:

The nurse practitioner service is both a clinical care model and a service innovation; accordingly, evaluation included (1) the setting for nurse practitioner service (Structure); (2) the clinical service provided by the nurse practitioner (Process) and (3) the influence of nurse practitioner service on patients (Outcome). Data were collected, analysed and reported related to these three elements guided by the following audit questions:

1. *To what extent was the service/facility prepared to incorporate nurse practitioner service in terms of the multidisciplinary team (MDT) and the organisation of the service structure?*
2. *What impact does the nurse practitioner role have on service quality and processes, including the use of diagnostic resources, prescribing practices and perceived impact on service indicators?*
3. *Does nurse practitioner practice meet standards of safety and quality of patient care in terms of perceptions of clinical competence, patient satisfaction with care, conformity to scope of practice and best evidence?*

(p. 146)

The Donabedian Model has also been used to evaluate interventions. For example, McCaughan et al. (2013) used it to evaluate 'A randomized controlled trial of a self-management psychosocial intervention for men with prostate cancer and their partners'. The authors explained how the three components of the model were used to inform the aims of their study:

1. *To evaluate the cost of implementing the intervention. (Structure)*
2. *To explore the perceptions, experience, and satisfaction of men with prostate cancer and their partners of taking part in the intervention. (Process). This could also be an outcome.*
3. *To explore the reasons for refusal of men with prostate cancer and their partners who decline to take part in the intervention. (Process)*
4. *To explore the perceptions and experience of facilitators in delivering the intervention. (Process)*
5. *To test the effectiveness of the intervention in terms of achieving its proposed outcomes. (Outcome).*

McCaughan et al. (2013, p. 2574)

The Donabedian framework is a well-accepted and well-recognised tool to evaluate services, as it provides a 'holistic view' of what an evaluation of services should comprise (i.e. structure, process and outcome). Without a framework, researchers evaluating services would make up their own questions, which might be difficult to justify. A conceptual or theoretical framework can help to guide the formulation of questions and provide a justification for why these aspects of services are explored.

Frameworks can also help to guide the choice of research designs. Aldrich et al. (2018) used the TBP (Ajzen, 1985) to assess the 'effectiveness of a suicide prevention training'. As they explained:

The TPB also assumes background factors such as individual characteristics (e.g. personality, mood, intelligence, values, experience), social factors (e.g. education, age, gender, income, race), and informational considerations (e.g. knowledge, media, and intervention) can potentially affect beliefs, in this case about suicide intervention, which may indirectly influence behaviour.

The purpose of this study was to assess the effectiveness of the QPR (Question, Persuade, Refer) gatekeeper training in individuals' ability to recognise the warning signs of suicide, intention to question someone they think is suicidal, persuade the suicidal person to stay alive, and know how and where to get help for the person.

(p. 968)

Aldrich et al. (2018) developed the following hypotheses:

H1. Upon completion of QPR gatekeeper training, participants will recognise common suicidal warning signs.

H2. Completion of QPR gatekeeper training will increase intention to (a) address the presence of suicidal thoughts and feelings, (b) persuade a suicidal individual to stay alive and (c) get help for the suicidal person.

H3. Completion of QPR gatekeeper training will increase one's (a) positive attitudes towards suicide intervention, (b) belief that important others support intervention, (c) PBC [perceived behavioural control] to intervene and (d) intention to intervene with a suicidal individual.

H4. Together, attitudes, subjective norms, and PBC will predict one's intention to intervene with a suicidal individual after completion of QPR training.

(p. 968)

These hypotheses, in turn, guided Aldrich et al.'s choice of study design. In this case, they chose a 'pre-test–post-test survey', as this type of design is appropriate for testing hypotheses and study correlations between the variables identified in the hypotheses.

Using Frameworks to Analyse and Interpret Data

In a study of self-efficacy in the context of heart transplantation, Almgren et al. (2017) used Bandura's Self Efficacy Theory as a framework to analyse data collected by means of qualitative in-depth interviews. They described their design as a 'directed content analysis' and explained the steps they used in their analysis of data and how they used key concepts from Bandura's theory (efficacy expectation, outcome expectation, performance accomplishment, vicarious experience, verbal persuasion, emotional arousal and contextual factors). Bandura's theory was 'scrutinised in detail to identify the main concepts'(Almgren et al. (2017, p. 3009). They then 'chose the main concepts of self-efficacy and the contextual factors from the theory and applied them to the data' by 'searching for meaning units (MU) that corresponded with the content of each main concept in Bandura's theory' (Almgren et al., 2017, p. 3009).

As this was a qualitative study, it seems that the aim was not to test Bandura's theory but to retrospectively explore self-efficacy in the context of heart transplantations (Almgren et al., 2017). In this study, Almgren et al. justified the choice of theory by pointing out that 'Bandura is the one who developed the concept of self-efficacy, and it is the only available theory that comprehensively describes the concept' (p. 3008). While using an existing theory to inform and interpret the data, the authors were also able to make comments on the strengths and limitations of the theory when applied to practice and to make their own contributions towards adapting (or improving) the theory. This is an excellent example of the use of a theoretical framework in a study to provide practical as well as theoretical knowledge.

In a qualitative study of health eating behaviours in Ecuadorian adolescents, Verstraeten et al. (2014) used two conceptual frameworks, the Attitude, Social Influences and Self-efficacy Model (De Vries et al., 1988) and the Socio-Ecological Model (Green et al., 1996), to develop semistructured questions for focus groups with adolescents. They carried out a content analysis of the data based on 'both the literature and the theoretical framework' (p. 2) that they used in the study. Consistent with the aim of their study, they developed their own conceptual framework for Ecuadorian adolescents' eating behaviour that took into account 'culture-specific factors'. This is another example of how existing theories can be used to inform a study, and in particular to analyse and interpret data.

Using Frameworks to Inform All Aspects of a Study

Mock et al. (2007) used a conceptual model to develop an exercise intervention 'to mitigate cancer-related fatigue' (p. 1), formulate aims and objectives, identify data collection tools and select outcomes to be measured. The conceptual model they used was the Levine Conservation Model (Levine, 1996). Levine's model is based on four conservation principles: conservation of energy, conservation of structural integrity, conservation of personal integrity and conservation of social integrity (Levine, 1989).

> *Once the Levine Conservation Model was chosen to guide this study, the study variables were carefully selected to be congruent with the model, as were the tools used for data collection and the intervention being tested. This approach ensured that appropriate outcome variables were used in the evaluation, which includes measurement of the four components of this particular model. Also, it became clear that all four components should be addressed in implementing the intervention, as well as in interpreting the study data.*

> *Mock et al. (2007, p. 5)*

Using Frameworks to Develop Complex Interventions

Nurses, allied health professionals and social workers develop interventions such as those designed to encourage patients to adopt healthy lifestyles, prevent ill health, self-manage their conditions and change their behaviours. Some of these interventions are aimed at improving policy and practice, and enhancing practitioners' skills, knowledge and competence.

Interventions are an important part of what nurses, health and social care professionals do. Yet studies have shown that not all interventions are developed using theories or research evidence. Conn et al. (2016) carried out a systematic review of theory use in medication adherence intervention research. They concluded that only 18% of these studies reported using a theory or conceptual framework for developing interventions. Conn et al. (2016) concluded that 'clinicians may have minimal background in behavioral sciences to prepare them to apply behavioral theories to intervention design' (p. 12). Similarly, Alulis and Grabowski (2017) reviewed theoretical frameworks informing family-based and adolescent obesity interventions. They found that, out of 35 interventions, only 11 studies 'explicitly stated that theory guided the development' of their interventions (p. 627). Sinclair et al. (2016) also found, from their systematic review, that many e-learning interventions devised for clinicians were not developed based on theory.

Tebb et al. (2016) proposed a number of reasons for the non-use of theories in computer-based interventions to reduce alcohol use among adolescents and young adults, including 'some researchers/intervention developers may not fully appreciate how theory can be used to inform intervention approaches', 'more emphasis on outcomes than an intervention development' and lack of 'publication guidelines/standards for describing the use of theoretical frameworks in intervention studies' (Tebb et al., 2016, p. 30).

Although researchers may not always state the theories or parts of theories that underpin their interventions, they often make a number of implicit assumptions regarding how their interventions work and to what effect. For example, a counselling intervention involving six group sessions to stop people smoking and increase their resistance to stay off cigarettes makes a number of assumptions. These include: 'counselling may be effective in smoking cessation and in increasing resilience', 'group counselling is an effective way to achieve behaviour change' and 'six group sessions is sufficient to stop smoking'. A quick literature search would have informed the researcher that there are a number of theories they could use regarding group counselling, such as Adlerian group counselling, person-centred counselling, psychodynamic counselling and cognitive behavioural counselling (Chism, 2022).

Missler et al. (2018) make no mention of a conceptual or theoretical framework in their protocol on the 'Effectiveness of a psycho-educational intervention to prevent postpartum parental distress and enhance infant well-being'. They developed their own intervention and made the following assumptions or expectations:

We expect that the proposed intervention will reduce maternal parenting stress. Furthermore, we expect that the intervention will reduce paternal parenting stress and parental distress in general. Moreover, we expect that parental well-being will be enhanced. By psycho-educating parents during pregnancy, we expect parents to experience more self-efficacy and satisfaction in fulfilling their roles. In this way, parents should be better able to provide high-quality caregiving (including breastfeeding and co-sleeping), leading to enhanced infant well-being (less problems with sleeping, crying and feeding, and better well-being and health).

Missler et al. (2018, p. 3)

Some of these expectations are based on previous studies, but they are not linked to any existing theory or theories. One may well question the theoretical justification for these expectations and outcomes selected for this study. There is some evidence that interventions based on theories are more effective than those with no explicit use of theory. McCullough et al. (2016) carried out a systematic review of behaviour change theories used to develop adherence interventions in adults with chronic respiratory disease. They reported that 'behavior change theory was more commonly used to design effective interventions' (p. 78)

According to Pawson and Tilley (1997), all interventions are 'theories incarnate', although they may not use academic theories. Identifying relevant and appropriate theories to base our assumptions on can add theoretical credibility and guide research questions and design. By using a theoretical framework, researchers can link their study to, and add to, existing knowledge. More importantly a theoretical framework helps to explain how the different components of the intervention work together to produce the desired effects.

The types of intervention that nurses and health and social care professionals develop and use in their practice have been described as complex interventions. The Medical Research Council (MRC) has described complex interventions as those that 'contain several interacting components' (Craig et al, 2008). According to Skivington et al. (2021):

An intervention might be considered complex because of properties of the intervention itself, such as the number of components involved; the range of behaviours targeted; expertise and skills required by those delivering and receiving the intervention; the number of groups, settings, or levels targeted; or the permitted level of flexibility of the intervention or its components.

(p. 2)

Complex interventions can vary in the degree of complexity but most are likely to have a number of these dimensions. Nurses and health and social care professionals will recognise, from the description above, that these are the types of behaviour change intervention that they normally use with patients or clients. For example, Tickle-Degnen (2013) explained that interventions in occupational therapy do not have a 'single active factor inducing change' in clients but that a blend of active agents including 'person, environment and occupational factors' (p. 171) together contribute to the desired effects of the intervention. These dimensions add to the difficulty of developing, implementing and evaluating these interventions. Understanding why a complex intervention 'works' or not is not straightforward. This is why theories can be used to help to explain the process of behaviour change.

A good example of a theory-based intervention comes from Cherrington et al. (2015). The authors described in detail their choice of theory and how it was used to develop strategies to inform a peer-support intervention to achieve weight loss among Latina immigrants. Cherrington et al. also described how they used focus groups and semistructured interviews to explore the needs of participants and facilitators, their preferred strategies and the cultural context in which the intervention was to be implemented.

Using Frameworks to Evaluate Complex Interventions

Complex interventions require complex evaluation: apart from measuring outcomes, we need to know if the intervention works and if the theoretical assumptions underpinning it were valid. Other questions to ask include the following: Was the intervention implemented as proposed? Did all those who delivered the intervention (often to different participants/clients on different sites) implement it in the same way? Did participants find the intervention useful? These are some of the questions that need to be answered if we are to learn about the effectiveness of interventions. Therefore, the process of delivering the intervention is as important as its outcomes.

A number of theoretical frameworks have been used to evaluate complex interventions. The MRC has developed guidance on how complex interventions can be evaluated (see Craig et al., 2008; Moore et al., 2015). According to the MRC (Moore et al., 2015), a process evaluation should examine aspects such as these:

- **Implementation**: *The structures, resources and processes through which delivery is achieved, and the quantity and quality of what is delivered;*
- **Mechanisms of impact**: *how intervention activities, and participants' interactions with them, trigger change;*
- **Context**: *how external factors influence the delivery and functioning of interventions.*

(p. 2)

The MRC also recommends that process evaluations be conducted within a feasibility testing phase (Moore et al., 2015). Feasibility studies are essential to inform us whether the proposed methodology can be implemented and what potential difficulties, if any, there are. They can also tell us if, and how, the intervention works and how patients/clients respond to it. In the feasibility study of a 'psychosocial intervention for men with prostate cancer and their partners', McCaughan et al. (2013) explored the feasibility of recruiting participants and its associated issues (attrition, retention etc.), the participants' perceptions and experience of the intervention, the facilitators' perceptions of the delivery of the intervention, the cost of implementing the intervention and the potential effects of the intervention on selected outcomes.

A number of frameworks (apart from the MRC's) have been developed to help researchers to undertake feasibility or pilot studies (these two terms are sometimes used interchangeably in the literature). Thabane et al. (2010,) proposed the following four aspects that should be explored in a pilot study before a full-scale randomised controlled trial of a complex intervention is carried out. These are:

- Process: *This assesses the feasibility of the steps that need to take place as part of the main study. Examples include determining recruitment rates, retention rates, etc.*
- Resources: *This deals with assessing time and budget problems that can occur during the main study. The idea is to collect some pilot data on such things as the length of time to mail or fill out all the survey forms.*
- Management: *This covers potential human and data optimization problems such as personnel and data management issues at participating centres.*
- Scientific: *This deals with the assessment of treatment safety, determination of dose levels and response, and estimation of treatment effect and its variance.*

(pp. 2–3)

Bowen et al. (2009) have provided a number of key areas of focus for feasibility studies and possible outcomes: acceptability, demand, implementation, practicality, adaptation, integration, expansion and limited efficacy. In their article, they provide more detail on aspects of these that researchers can look at. For example, 'acceptability' includes 'satisfaction', 'intent to continue to use', 'perceived appropriateness', 'fit within organizational culture' and 'perceived positive or negative effect on organization' (Bowen et al., 2009). This framework is a useful guide for researchers to frame the questions or aim and objectives of their feasibility studies.

There are other frameworks (as well as Donabedian's mentioned earlier) that have been used to study the process or feasibility of complex interventions. One such framework is the RE-AIM framework (Glasgow et al., 2019). Each of the letters in RE-AIM refers to particular aspects to be explored when evaluating an intervention:

- *Reach* the target population
- *Effectiveness* or efficacy
- *Adoption* by target staff, settings or institutions
- *Implementation* consistency, costs and adaptations made during delivery
- *Maintenance* of intervention effects in individuals and settings over time.

More detail is available on the RE-AIM website (www.re-aim.org). For an example of the RE-AIM framework in a research proposal, see Schaller et al. (2016), a mixed methods study on 'Promoting physical activity and health literacy' (the AtRisk study).

Finally, Logic Models have been developed to provide:

a diagrammatic representation of an intervention, describing anticipated delivery mechanisms (e.g., how resources will be applied to ensure implementation), intervention components (what is to be implemented), mechanisms of impact (the mechanisms through which an intervention will work) and intended outcomes.

Moore et al. (2015, p. 8)

An example of the application of a Logic Model is from a 'Feasibility study of increasing social support to enhance a healthy lifestyle intervention for individuals with serious mental illness' (Aschbrenner et al., 2016). The UK government (https://www.gov.uk/government/publications/evaluation-in-health-and-well-being-overview/introduction-to-logic-models) has produced a useful guide on Logic Models for evaluating health and wellbeing. For examples of how to describe/report the use of Logic Models in proposals see Seismann-Petersen et al. (2022), 'Process evaluation of a multi-disciplinary complex intervention to improve care for older patients with chronic conditions in rural areas (the HandinHand Study)', and Lavertu et al. (2022), 'Fostering translational research in chronic disease management'.

CONCEPTUAL FRAMEWORKS IN QUALITATIVE STUDIES

Qualitative researchers may not want to be influenced by existing conceptual or theoretical frameworks. They may subscribe to the belief that the purpose of qualitative research is to develop new conceptual and theoretical understanding of phenomena. They may, however, use broad philosophical 'frameworks' to explain how they view reality and how phenomena should be studied. Thus, it is not unusual to read that 'phenomenology' or 'social constructivism' is being used to explain the researchers' worldview. They may also state their theoretical position on the topics they explore. For example, in their proposal for a qualitative study on loneliness and social isolation in emerging adulthood, Creaven et al. (2021,) explained that their study 'draws on macro-theories of development' and 'is also informed by several theories of loneliness' (p. 2). Another example is from a proposal for a study exploring the 'Good life', where the authors (Michel et al., 2021) explained that their study 'is based on a user-centred methodology characterised by 3 main approaches':

1. *An innovation approach: not for users but with or by users (regarded as actors in their own right).*
2. *A socio-anthropological approach to the analysis of needs in real-life, making it possible to observe and mobilise older persons in their living spaces, in relation to the people who support them in their daily life.*
3. *An approach to ageing as a social situation, as an evolution of ways of life structured by problems, concerns, as well as assets and motivations, which need to be defined with older persons, rather than exclusively viewing ageing as an accumulation of risks that need to be managed.*

(p. 2)

Michel et al. also provide the literature/evidence to support these approaches.

If a theoretical or philosophical perspective is used throughout a qualitative study, researchers should demonstrate how the philosophy or theory is used to collect, analyse and interpret the data. For example, if social constructivism is used as a framework, one would expect the researchers to show how knowledge was co-constructed, interpreted and reported.

Earlier in this chapter, examples were given regarding the use of theoretical frameworks to analyse qualitative data. Whether new knowledge is produced with or without the use of existing frameworks, it is important to discuss qualitative findings within the context of existing knowledge (concepts, theories, etc.) in order to make an original contribution to knowledge.

Below is an example of how a postgraduate student described her use of a conceptual framework in her proposal of a qualitative study of 'The decision-making process of young adult women in the United Arab Emirates regarding food choice and the factors that influence their choice':

Conceptual framework
Conceptual models or theories are useful in understanding and explaining the dynamics of health behaviours, the processes for changing behaviours and the effects of external influences on the behaviours (Story et al, 2002). Two of the common theories used to study behaviour are Social Cognitive Theory (Glanz et al., 1997) and the Ecological Theory (Bronfenbrenner, 1979). In the Social Cognitive Theory the whole behaviour is explained in terms of a 3-way dynamic and reciprocal interaction between personal factors, environmental influences and behaviour. The focus is on concepts such as self-efficacy, observational learning, reciprocal determinism, behavioural capability, expectations, functional meaning and

reinforcement (Story et al., 2002). In the Ecological theory, behaviour is viewed as affecting and being affected by multiple levels of influence. This model consists of four interacting levels: microsystems (e.g., the immediate environment such as family, peer, home etc.), the mesosystem (e.g., school, church, peer groups, clubs), the exosystems (e.g., media and community influences) and the macrosystems (e.g., culturally based belief systems, economic systems and political systems).

Story et al (2002) integrated these two theories to develop a framework "to understand the factors that influence adolescent eating behaviour". This model has four broad levels of influence: individual, social environmental, physical environment and macrosystem. Story et al's (2002) model will be used to underpin this study. The interviews will be based on questions on each of these levels. To explore individual influences, questions will focus on their attitudes, beliefs, knowledge and self-efficacy related to healthy eating and food choice. Social environmental influences will be examined by questions related to the influence of family, friends and peers in the choice of food. As part of the physical environmental influences issues of accessibility and availability of healthy food, access to food markets and outlets etc. will be examined. Macrosystem influences will be explored through questions related to social and cultural norms, availability and non-availability and cost of food, mass media and advertisements. This conceptual model will provide a structure to the interviews but the emphasis will be on how individuals negotiate these four levels and what factors facilitate and hinder their decisions to eat healthy food.

The student provided a diagram to simplify the explanation of conceptual framework.

LIMITATIONS OF FRAMEWORKS

The main argument against the use of conceptual frameworks in research studies is that they may stifle creativity. Using the same frameworks to answer the same research questions may not lead to new ways of exploring phenomena. Conceptual frameworks reflect the current knowledge of a phenomenon. To advance knowledge sometimes requires new thinking and this means challenging conventional wisdom. However, the decision not to use conceptual frameworks in research studies should be carefully considered and clearly justified.

Selecting conceptual frameworks may not be an easy task. Conceptual definitions of the same phenomenon may change over time. For example, Hawthorne et al. (2014) pointed out that there are conflicting definitions of the phenomenon of 'patient satisfaction' and that the 'major patient satisfaction theories were all published in the 1980's' (p. 527). This paper by Hawthorne et al. shows how the different definitions and theories of the same phenomenon (patient satisfaction) can pose a challenge to researchers selecting a framework for their studies. The relevance of a theory over time is also important. Should a researcher use Peplau's 1952 theory as a framework for explaining or predicting interpersonal interactions in the 21st century?

For an excellent example of conceptual framework in a proposal, see Wong (2022), 'Study protocol for a randomized controlled trial evaluating the effectiveness of a group-based self-determination enhancement intervention for adults with mild intellectual disability and their caregivers'.

Checklist for the use of frameworks in a proposal:
1. Is a conceptual framework used or does this study aim to develop one?
2. If a framework is selected, is a rationale/justification for the choice given in the proposal? Is this framework new or widely used in other studies?
3. Is a brief summary or overview of the framework given in the proposal? Is it based on one or more theories (or part of a theory)?
4. How does the framework underpin the study? (e.g. Does it guide the research questions, design or data analysis or is it used throughout the study?)
5. If an intervention is to be developed as part of the proposal, is the development of the intervention based on a conceptual framework?
6. If the proposal is on the evaluation of an intervention, will a specific framework (or a combination of frameworks) be used in the study? And how?
7. Is the framework introduced in the literature review section of the proposal but not referred to again?

SUMMARY AND CONCLUSIONS

In this chapter, the importance and benefits of using conceptual frameworks in research studies have been highlighted. Conceptual frameworks can help researchers to develop research questions, select an appropriate design and analyse and interpret the data. Conceptual frameworks also provide a link between the proposed study and the existing knowledge.

The challenge is to be judicious in the selection of frameworks. Justification should be provided for the selection of a particular framework, adapting an existing framework, using part of a framework, using more than one framework or developing one own's framework. There is scope to be flexible and creative in the use of frameworks. One does not choose a framework because one has to, but because it can make a meaningful contribution to one's study. Referring to his 'structure, process and outcome model', Donabedian once remarked that his model is 'a servant not a master'.

REFERENCES

Ajzen, I. (1985). From intentions to actions: A theory of planned behavior. In J. Kuhi & J. Beckmann (Eds.), *Action-control: From cognition to behavior* (pp. 11–39). Heidelberg: Springer.

Ajzen, I. (1991). The theory of planned behavior. *Organizational Behavior and Human Decision Processes, 50,* 179–211.

Aldrich, R. S., Wilde, J., & Miller, E. (2018). The effectiveness of QPR suicide prevention training. *Health Education Journal, 77*(8), 964–977.

Almgren, M., Lennerling, A., Lundmark, M., & Forsberg, A. (2017). Self-efficacy in the context of heart transplantation - a new perspective. *Journal of Clinical Nursing, 26*(19–20), 3007–3017.

Alshyyab, M. A., FitzGerald, G., Dingle, K., Ting, J., Bowman, P., Kinnear, F. B., & Borkoles, E. (2019). Developing a conceptual framework for patient safety culture in emergency department: A review of the literature. *The International Journal of Health Planning and Management, 34*(1), 42–55.

Alulis, S., Grabowski, D. (2017). Theoretical frameworks informing family-based child and adolescent obesity interventions: A qualitative meta-synthesis. *Obesity Research & Clinical Practice, 11*(6), 627–639.

Aschbrenner, K. A., Mueser, K. T., Naslund, J. A., Gorin, A. A., Kinney, A., Daniels, L., & Bartels, S. J. (2016). Feasibility study of increasing social support to enhance a healthy lifestyle intervention for individuals with serious mental illness. *Journal of the Society for Social Work and Research, 7*(2), 289–313.

Bandura, A. (1977b) Self-efficacy: Toward a unifying theory of behavioral change. *Psychological Review, 84*(2), 191–215.

Bandura, A. (1977a). *Social learning theory.* Englewood Cliffs, N.J: Prentice Hall.

Becker, M. H. (1974). The health belief model and sick role behavior. *Health Education Monographs, 2*(4), 409–419.

Biswas, A., Bhattacharya, S. D., Singh, A. K., & Saha, M. (2019). Addressing hand hygiene compliance in a low-resource neonatal intensive care unit: A quality improvement project. *Journal of the Pediatric Infectious Diseases Society, 8*(5), 408–413.

Bowen, D. J., Kreuter, M., Spring, B., Cofta-Woerpel, L., Linnan, L., Weiner, D., Bakken, S., Kaplan, C. P., Squiers, L., Fabrizio, C., & Fernandez, M. (2009). How we design feasibility studies. *American Journal of Preventive Medicine, 36*(5), 452–457.

Bronfenbrenner, U. (1979). *The ecology of human development: Experiments by nature and design.* Cambridge, MA: Harvard University Press.

Brown, J. (1999). Bowen family systems theory and practice: Illustration and critique [ebook]. *Australian and New Zealand: Journal of Family Therapy, 20*(2), 94–103.

Cherrington, A. L., Willig, A. L., Agne, A. A., Fowler, M. C., Dutton, G. R., & Scarinci, I. C. (2015). Development of a theory-based, peer support intervention to promote weight loss among Latina immigrants. *BMC Obesity, 2*, 17. https://doi.org/10.1186/s40608-015-0047-3

Chism, M. (2022). Group counseling theories. https://study.com/academy/lesson/group-counseling-theories.html.

Conn, V. S., Enriquez, M., Ruppar, T. M., & Chan, K. C. (2016). Meta-analyses of theory use in Medication Adherence Intervention Research. *American Journal of Health Behavior, 40*(2), 155–171.

Connolly, M. (2007). Practice frameworks: Conceptual maps to guide interventions in child welfare. *The British Journal of Social Work, 37*(5), 825–837.

Craig, P., Dieppe, P., Macintyre, S., Michie, S., Nazareth, I., & Petticrew, M. (2008). Developing and evaluating complex interventions: the new Medical Research Council guidance. *BMJ, 337*, a1655.

Creaven, A. M., Kirwan, E., Burns, A., & O'Súilleabháin, P. S. (2021). Protocol for a Qualitative Study: (ELSIE). *International Journal of Qualitative Methods, 20*. https://doi.org/10.1177/16094069211028682

Darabi, N., & Svensson, U. P. (2021). Dynamic systems approach in sensorimotor synchronization: Adaptation to tempo step-change. *Frontiers in Physiology, 12*, 667859. https://doi.org/10.3389/fphys.2021.667859.

Davidson, L. (2005). Recovery, self management and the expert patient: Changing the culture of mental health from a UK Perspective. *Journal of Mental Health, 14*, 25–35.

De Vries, H., Dijkstra, M., & Kuhlman, P. (1988). Self-efficacy: The third factor besides attitude and subjective norm as a predictor of behavioural intentions. *Health Education Research, 3*, 273–282.

DHSSPS. (2012). *Living with long term conditions: A policy framework.* Belfast: Department of Health, Social Services and Public Safety.

Donabedian, A. (1966). Evaluating the quality of medical care. *Milbank Memorial Fund Quarterly, 44*(suppl 3), 166–206. Reprinted in Milbank Q. 2005;83(4):691–729.

Gardner, G., Gardner, A., & O'Connell, J. (2014). Using the Donabedian framework to examine the quality and safety of nursing service innovation. *Journal of Clinical Nursing, 23*, 145–155.

Glanz, K., Lewis, F. M., & Rimer, B. K. (1997). *Health behaviour and health education* (2nd ed.). San Francisco, CA: Jossey Bass.

Glasgow, R. E., Harden, S. M., Gaglio, B., Rabin, B., Smith, M. L., Porter, G. C., Ory, M. G., Estabrooks, P. A. (2019). RE-AIM planning and evaluation framework: adapting to new science and practice with a 20-year review. *Frontiers in Public Health, 7*, 64. https://doi.org/10.3389/fpubh.2019.00064

Green, L. W., Richard, L., & Potvin, L. (1996). Ecological foundations of health promotion. *American Journal of Health Promotion, 10*, 270–281.

Hawthorne, G., Sansoni, J., Hayes, L., Marosszeky, N., & Sansoni, E. (2014). Measuring patient satisfaction with health care treatment using the Short Assessment of Patient Satisfaction measure delivered superior and robust satisfaction estimates. *Journal of Clinical Epidemiology, 67*(5), 527–537.

Heymann, P., Bastiaens, E., Jansen, A., van Rosmalen, P., & Beausaert, S. (2022). A conceptual model of students' reflective practice for the development of employability competences, supported by an online learning platform. *Education* + Training, *64*(3), 380–397.

HOTheory. (2022). Theories and models. https://ottheory.com/.

Hudon, A., Gervais, M. J., & Hunt, M. (2015). The contribution of conceptual frameworks to knowledge translation interventions in physical therapy. *Physical Therapy, 95*(4), 630–639.

Kerlinger, F. N. (1986). *Foundations of Behavioral Research* (3rd ed.). New York: Holt, Rinehart and Winston.

Kerr, M. E., & Bowen, M. (1988). *Family* evaluation: An approach based on Bowen theory. New York: W. W. Norton & Co.

Lavertu, G., Diendere, E., Légaré, F., Tchala, H., Zomahoun, V., Toi, A. K., Leblond, M., Rheault, N., Audet-Walsh, É., Beaulieu, M. C., Charif, A. B., Blanchette, V., Després, J. P., Gaudreau, A., Rhéaume, C., Tremblay, M. C., & Paquette J. S. (2022). Fostering translational research in chronic disease management: A logic model proposal. *Translational Medicine Communications, 7*, 13. https://doi.org/10.1186/s41231-022-00118-4

Lazarus, R., & Folkman, S. (1984). *Stress, appraisal, and coping.* New York: Springer.

Leech, K. A., & Roemmich, R. T., Gordon, J., Reisman, D. S., & Cherry-Allen, K. M. (2022). Updates in motor learning: Implications for physical therapist practice and education. *Physical Therapy, 102*(1), pzab250. https://doi.org/10.1093/ptj/pzab250.

Leininger, M. (1988). Leininger's theory of nursing: Cultural care diversity and universality. *Nursing Science Quarterly, 1*(4), 152–160.

Levine, M. E. (1996). The conservation principles in nursing: A retrospective. *Nursing Science Quarterly, 9*, 38–41.

Levine, M E. (1989). The conservation principles of nursing - twenty years later. In J. Riehl-Sisca (Ed.), *Conceptual models for nursing practice.* Norwalk, CT: Appleton-Lange.

McCaughan, E., Prue, G., McSorley, O., Northouse, L., Schafenacker, A., & Parahoo, K. (2013). A randomized controlled trial of a self-management psychosocial intervention for men with prostate cancer and their partners: A study protocol. *Journal of Advanced Nursing, 69*(11), 2572–2583.

McCullough, A. R., Ryan, C., Macindoe, C., Yii, N., Bradley, J. M., O'Neill, B., Elborn, J. S., & Hughes, C. M. (2016). Behavior change theory, content and delivery of interventions to enhance adherence in chronic respiratory disease: A systematic review. *Respiratory Medicine, 116*, 78–84.

McGowan, L. J., Powell, R., & French, D. P. (2020). How can use of the theoretical domains framework be optimized in qualitative research? A rapid systematic review. *British Journal of Health Psychology, 25*(3), 677–694.

Michel, H., Prévôt-Huille, H., Koster, R., Ecarnot, F., Grange, Z., & Sanchez, S. (2021). What is a "Good Life": Protocol for a qualitative study to explore the viewpoint of older persons. *PLoS One, 16*(12), e0261741. https://doi.org/10.1371/journal.pone.0261741

Miles, M. B., Huberman, A. M., & Saldana, J. (2014). *Qualitative data analysis: A methods sourcebook* (3rd ed.). Thousand Oaks, CA: Sage.

Missler, M., Beijers, R., Denissen, J., & van Straten, A. (2018). Effectiveness of a psycho-educational intervention to prevent postpartum parental distress and enhance infant well-being: Study protocol of a randomized controlled trial. *Trials, 19*(1), 4.

Mock, V., St Ours, C., Hall, S., Bositis, A., Tillery, M., Belcher, A., Krumm, S., & McCorkle, R. (2007). Using a conceptual model in nursing research—mitigating fatigue in cancer patients. *Journal of Advanced Nursing, 58*(5), 503–512.

Moore, G. F., Audrey, S., Barker, M., Bond, L., Bonell, C., Hardeman, W., Moore, L., O'Cathain, A., Tinati, T., Wight, D., & Baird, J. (2015). Process evaluation of complex interventions UK: Medical Research Council (MRC) guidance. *Medical Research Council.* https://mrc.ukri.org/documents/pdf/mrc-phsrn-process-evaluation-guidance-final/

Parahoo, K. (2014). Nursing research: Principles, process and issues (3rd ed.). Basingstoke: Palgrave Macmillan.

Pawson, R., & Tilley, N. (1997). *Realistic evaluation.* London: Sage.

Peplau, H. (1952). Interpersonal relations in nursing: A conceptual frame of reference for psychodynamic nursing. New York: G P Putnam's Sons.

Roberts, A. R. (1991). Conceptualizing crisis theory and the crisis intervention model. In A. R. Roberts (Ed.), Contemporary perspectives on crisis intervention and prevention (pp. 3–17). Englewood Cliffs, NJ: Prentice-Hall.

Rogers, E. M. (2003). Diffusion of innovations (5th ed.). New York: Free Press.

Roy, C, Andrews, H. A. (1999). The Roy adaptation model. Stamford, Conn: Appleton & Lange.

Sawatzky, J. V., Enns, C. L., & Legare, C. (2015). Identifying the key predictors for retention in critical care nurses. *Journal of Advanced Nursing, 71*(10), 2315–2325.

Schaller, A., Dejonghe, L., Alayli-Goebbels, A., Biallas, B., & Froboese, I. (2016). Promoting physical activity and health literacy: Study protocol for a longitudinal, mixed methods evaluation of a cross-provider workplace-related intervention in Germany (The AtRisk study). *BMC Public Health, 16,* 626.

Seismann-Petersen, S., Köpke, S., & Inkrot, S. (2022). Process evaluation of a multi-disciplinary complex intervention to improve care for older patients with chronic conditions in rural areas (the HandinHand Study): Study protocol. *BMC Nursing, 21,* 151. https://doi.org/10.1186/s12912-022-00858-6

Sinclair, P. M., Kable, A., Levett-Jones, T., Booth, D. (2016). The effectiveness of Internet-based e-learning on clinician behaviour and patient outcomes: A systematic review. *International Journal of Nursing Studies, 57,* 70–81.

Skivington, K., Matthews, L., Simpson, S. A., Craig, P., Baird, J., Blazeby, J. M., Boyd, K. A., Craig, N., French, D. P., McIntosh, E., Petticrew, M., Rycroft-Malone, J., White, M., & Moore, L. (2021). A new framework for developing and evaluating complex interventions: update of Medical Research Council guidance. *BMJ, 374,* n2061. https://doi.org/10.1136/bmj.n2061

Story, M., Neumark-Sztainer, D., & French, S. (2002). Individual and environmental influences on adolescent eating behaviors. *Journal of the American Dietetic Association, 102*(3), S40–S51.

Strempfl, J., Wutzl, T., Ün, D., Greber-Platzer, S., Keilani, M., Crevenna, R., & Thajer, A. (2022). Impact of self-determination theory in a physiotherapeutic training: A pilot-study on motivation for movement of obese adolescents. *Wiener Klinische Wochenschrift, 134*(5-6), 208–214.

Tebb, K. P., Erenrich, R. K., Jasik, C. B., Berna, M. S., Lester, J. C., & Ozer, E. M. (2016). Use of theory in computer-based interventions to reduce alcohol use among adolescents and young adults: a systematic review. *BMC Public Health, 16,* 517.

Thabane, L., Ma, J., Chu, R., Cheng, J., Ismaila, A., Rios, L. P., Robson, R., Thabane, M., Giangregorio, L., & Goldsmith, C. H. (2010). A tutorial on pilot studies: The what, why and how. *BMC Medical Research Methodology, 10,* 1. https://doi.org/10.1186/1471-2288-10-1

Tickle-Degnen, L. (2013). Nuts and bolts of conducting feasibility studies. *The American Journal of Occupational Therapy, 67*(2), 171–176.

Verstraeten, R., Van Royen, K., Ochoa-Avilés, A., Penafiel, D., Holdsworth, M., Donoso, S., Maes, L., & Kolsteren, P. (2014). A conceptual framework for healthy eating behavior in ecuadorian adolescents: A qualitative study. *PloS One, 9*(1), e87183. https://doi.org/10.1371/journal.pone.0087183

Wong, P. (2022). Study protocol for a randomized controlled trial evaluating the effectiveness of a group-based self-determination enhancement intervention for adults with mild intellectual disability and their caregivers. *International Journal of Environmental Research and Public Health, 19*(3), 1763. https://doi.org/10.3390/ijerph19031763

World Health Organization. (n.d.). Frequently asked questions. https://www.who.int/about/accountability/governance/constitution. Retrieved on 10/01/2024.

Zhang, X., Yu, P., Yan, J., Ton, A. M., & Spil, I. (2015). Using diffusion of innovation theory to understand the factors impacting patient acceptance and use of consumer e-health innovations: A case study in a primary care clinic. *BMC Health Services Research, 15,* 71. https://doi.org/10.1186/s12913-015-0726-2

4

SELECTING RESEARCH DESIGNS FOR DESCRIPTIVE AND CORRELATIONAL STUDIES

INTRODUCTION

The next step after developing research questions is to select an appropriate research design that can best answer the questions. Therefore research questions come before selecting designs. The literature review and the conceptual framework, as explained in the previous chapters, can help in the process of developing research questions and identifying appropriate designs.

In this chapter, we will define the term 'research design', provide a brief outline of the main research designs used in nursing, health and social care research and highlight the strengths and limitations of each. The purpose of this exercise is to provide enough information to enable new researchers to select a design that is fit to answer the research questions in their proposals and to understand the potential implications of their chosen design. Examples of how researchers have described the design section in proposals will also be provided.

METHODOLOGY AND DESIGN

As with many other research terms, 'methodology' and 'research design' are sometimes used interchangeably. For purists, one can describe the methodology as the overall philosophical, ethical and methodological assumptions that underpin the whole study, including the design. It includes the particular approach the study adopts to answer the research question. For example, if the aim is to find out how an intervention or service affects patients, researchers may select a qualitative approach to answer the question. The assumption here is that the answer to this question lies with patients and that a qualitative approach is more appropriate to get close to what patients think, feel or believe. Within this methodology, there are a number of research designs such as grounded theory (Glaser and Strauss, 1967), ethnography (Hammersley and Atkinson, 1989) or discourse analysis (Johnstone, 2008) from which researchers can select, depending on the particular research questions.

On the other hand, if the researcher's assumptions underpinning the same research question (how an intervention or service affects patients) is that such questions can best be answered by a quantitative methodology, the researcher may select a clinical trial. In this case the effects (or effectiveness) of the intervention will be measured in terms of specific outcomes (e.g. quality of life, length of hospital stay, etc.). Similarly, if the assumption is that this question can be answered by both qualitative and quantitative approaches, a mixed methods methodology will be selected.

The design of a study can be described as the plan or blueprint of what researchers will do in order to answer the research questions. This plan includes all the actions, decisions and resources required to successfully complete the study. The design includes selecting participants (sampling), the methods of data collection (interviews, questionnaires or observations, etc.), data analysis tools and the tests to be carried out, and how the results will be interpreted.

MATCHING DESIGNS TO QUESTIONS

A variety of research designs have been developed over the years to answer different types of questions. Therefore, the choice of design depends on the type of question. For simplicity we can use the three types of questions described in Chapter 2 – descriptive, correlational and causal – to explain how to select a study design. There are different types of design for different types of question. In this chapter we will explore the type of design that best suits descriptive (quantitative) and correlational questions. Designs for causal, qualitative and mixed methods questions will be dealt with in later chapters.

Quantitative descriptive questions typically investigate phenomena in terms of numbers, level, frequency, prevalence, incidence, trends or patterns (Parahoo, 2014). The data are presented in numerical forms and involve descriptive and inferential statistics in terms of mean, mode, median, ratio, standard deviations, probability, etc. Roggenkamp et al. (2018) carried out a study to describe the demographic and clinical characteristics of mental-health related Emergency Medical Services (EMS) presentations in Victoria, Australia, by analysing patients' records. Below is an excerpt from their findings:

> *Of the total 504,676 EMS attendances, 48,041 (9.5%) were mental health presentations. In addition, 4,708 (6.6%) cases managed by a paramedic or nurse via the EMS secondary telephone triage service also involved mental health complaints. EMS-attended mental health patients were younger and more often female compared to other patients attended by EMS. Most mental health patients were transported to hospital (74.4%); however, paramedics provided treatment to significantly fewer mental health patients compared to other EMS-attended patients (12.4% vs. 50.3%, $p < 0.001\%$).*

> *Roggenkamp et al. (2018, p. 399)*

Correlational studies aim mainly to explore relationships between variables. For example, Yarbrough et al. (2017) explored relationships of professional values orientation, career development, job satisfaction and intent to stay in recently hired mid-career and early-career nurses in a large hospital system. They reported, among other things, that there was 'a strong correlation between professional values and career development and that both job satisfaction and career development correlated positively with retention' (Yarbrough et al., 2017, p. 675).

Descriptive studies may have some elements of correlation. For example, in the study by Roggenkamp et al. (2018), the authors sought to explore the relationship between age and the most common presentation. They reported that patients aged 15 years or less presented more with social or emotional issues, while those aged 65 years or above presented more with anxiety. However, the main aim of the study was to describe, not correlate. On the other hand, the aim of Yarbrough et al. (2017) was to explore the relationships between 'retention' and 'professional values', 'job satisfaction', etc. To do this they described the mean age of participants or mean career development or job satisfaction before carrying out statistical tests to explore the relationships between these variables. Therefore, while correlational studies have some descriptive elements, their main aim is to explore the relationships between variables.

RESEARCH DESIGNS IN DESCRIPTIVE AND CORRELATIONAL STUDIES

The main designs in descriptive and correlational studies in nursing, health and social care research are surveys, cohort studies and case-control studies.

Survey Designs

A survey design typically involves using questionnaires or scales (such as quality of life scales or self-esteem scales) to sample whole or part of a population on issues such as attitudes, behaviour, knowledge, satisfaction with care services, prevalence, incidence, etc. The term 'survey' is sometimes used interchangeably with 'questionnaire' (Parahoo, 2014). Strictly speaking a survey is a research design, while a questionnaire is a data collection tool. A survey design includes plans regarding the development or selection of questionnaires or scales, how they are to be administered (face to face, online, by post or by telephone), the selection of participants (including inclusion and exclusion criteria), ethical considerations and how the data will be analysed and reported.

Data collection in surveys (see also Chapter 8) can be face to face, by post, by telephone or online. Each of these has their strengths and limitations. However, in general the advantages of surveys include their low cost and wide coverage, and the fact that the collection and analysis of data is relatively quick and easy. The limitations are the low response rates, difficulties for respondents in interpreting questions, uncertainty over who actually answered the questions and lack of opportunity for the researchers to probe. Good questionnaire design and pilot studies can overcome some of these limitations.

Online surveys have increased in popularity. One can develop one's own online system to collect survey data, and there are an increasing number of free or paid online software tools available to choose from. Some of the online survey tools include SoGoSurvey, SurveyMonkey, Typeform, Google Forms, Client Heartbeat, Zoho Survey and Qualtrics. It is advisable to read the reviews of these online software packages and/or ask the advice of those with experience using them before selecting one for your study.

When developing a research proposal involving surveys it is important to justify which delivery format is selected (e.g. a face-to-face questionnaire). This choice is often based on a number of factors including the need to obtain high response rates or the type of respondent (e.g. people who do not have access to the internet to complete an online questionnaire). If a particular online software package is to be used, this choice should also be justified. For an example of an online survey, see Proposal Example 4.1.

PROPOSAL EXAMPLE 4.1
AN ONLINE SURVEY STUDY

Gaikwad et al. (2016), 'Understanding patient perspectives on management of their chronic pain — online survey protocol'.

COMMENTS

1. The aim of this study, in this proposal, was to investigate the views, perceptions, beliefs and expectations of individuals who experience chronic pain on a daily basis, and the strategies used by them in managing chronic pain.
2. The design was described as an 'online survey'. This design was selected because it is appropriate for exploring patients' perspectives and experiences. In this case a quantitative approach was chosen. The same types of question can also be explored by means of qualitative interviews (see Chapter 9).
3. The rationale given for choosing the survey design was because it is cost-effective and easy to administer. As Gaikwad et al. (2016) explained:

   unlike face-to-face interviewing, a survey provides a standardized approach allowing uniformity of questions asked to all participants. It also provides access to individuals without geographical dependency thus allowing the collection of rich data. Although online surveys may limit participation from individuals without access to the internet the advantages of this method have been shown to outweigh the disadvantages in terms of external validity.

   (p. 32)

4. Descriptive studies, such as this one, are useful because they can provide a wealth of data on beliefs, attitudes and behaviours. In this case the authors expected this study to 'provide information on intake of complementary and alternative medicines, dietary supplements, nonpharmacological therapies, and educational sources most frequently used by the chronic pain patients for managing their pain' (p. 34).

Surveys can be cross-sectional, longitudinal, prospective or retrospective. With cross-sectional data collection, a cross-section of the population is selected to take part in the study. For example, if a researcher wants to know how patients cope after heart surgery, a cross-section of patients reflecting different ages, genders, social classes and types of heart disease can be interviewed or administered a questionnaire at one point in time (e.g. 1 month after discharge). The researcher will thus be able to compare, for example, younger patients' coping strategies with those of older people. Cross-sectional data collection is common practice in descriptive and correlational qualitative studies. It is particularly appropriate for looking at trends and prevalences at one point in time.

For example, in their study of 'Health-related quality of life in patients with lymphoedema', Klernäs et al. (2018) collected data from two lymphoedema units in Sweden and described their design as 'cross-sectional multicentre'. 'Three subgroups were recruited by strategic selection: secondary lymphoedema in the upper limbs/head and neck (n = 80), secondary lymphoedema in the lower limbs/genitalia (n = 60) and primary lymphoedema (n = 60)' (p. 635). In this study, data were collected at one point in time (although a test–retest procedure was followed) from a cross-section of the people with lymphoedema. The study provided a snapshot of the health-related quality of life (HRQoL) of the three different groups of patients at the time of data collection. This type of design does not, however, show if and how their quality of life changes over time in the disease trajectory. As this study shows, the cross-sectional design is useful for comparison purposes. In this study, the authors were able to compare HRQoL in the different subgroups and the 'general Swedish population'.

Cross-sectional designs can be used to generate large amounts of data in a relatively short time from large populations (e.g. in the case of national surveys) over wide geographical areas at a relatively lower cost than for other designs (e.g. longitudinal studies or randomised controlled trials). Cross-sectional designs provide an opportunity to explore relationships between two or more variables (e.g. differences in beliefs and attitudes to mental illness among different groups of the population in terms of education or occupation).

Cross-sectional designs are limited in that they can only explore relationships between variables (e.g. coffee consumption and lack of sleep) but cannot establish causation (e.g. that coffee consumption causes lack of sleep). They are also not appropriate for studies investigating changes in the same participants over time (e.g. long-term changes in quality of life). Cross-sectional designs are prone to low response rates, as is the case with most surveys. For example, Bonsaksen et al. (2017) used a cross-sectional design to study the associations between self-esteem, general self-efficacy and approaches to studying in occupational therapy students. The aim of their study was to 'explore associations between self-esteem, general self-efficacy, and the deep, strategic, and surface approaches to studying' (p. 326). Norwegian occupational therapy students ($n = 125$) completed questionnaires measuring study approaches, self-esteem and general self-efficacy. The authors commented on the limitations of the 'cross-sectional, correlational design', pointing out that it is 'difficult to infer causal relationships between the study variables' (p. 336). As they explained:

> For instance, we assume that general self-efficacy is related to approaches to studying. In turn, approaches to studying are believed to have an impact on academic performance. However, it may well be that high academic performance produces high self-efficacy, and ultimately shapes students' learning preferences.

> (p. 336)

They also pointed out that the cross-sectional design was unable to report on students' development over time.

Longitudinal Designs

When researchers are interested in how things change or evolve over a period of time, they can use a longitudinal approach that involves collecting data at several time points. For example, if the question is how patients cope with a disease or condition over time, it makes sense to collect data at different time points. The time points at which data are collected should be justified. For example, an intervention on healthy eating may have an immediate effect on knowledge, attitudes and behaviour soon after the intervention. This is because what participants have learnt is still fresh in their minds. However, one can question how long the effects will last. For example, according to de Ridder et al. (2017) 'many people are aware of the negative consequences of eating too much or eating an unhealthy diet but rarely manage to implement advice in their dietary routines over prolonged periods of time' (p. 931). While this may justify the need for collecting data well after the intervention is completed, the question is how we know whether we should collect data at 3, 6, 12 or 24 months after the intervention. The number of times and the intervals at which data should be collected depend on a number of factors, including whether the participants will continue to take part in the study if it lasts months or years, and the resources needed to complete the study.

As explained earlier, the main strength of the longitudinal design is the opportunity it provides to follow up participants and explore change over time. It is therefore possible to observe how the same individuals change or cope. The limitations or implications relate to the commitment of participants to continue with the study and difficulties in collecting data over a long period. The personnel involved in the study may change and participants may die or move to other addresses if the study lasts a long time. The financial cost can be high and the respondents' commitment to the project may diminish. Therefore, researchers should consider all the implications of this when designing a study.

Longitudinal studies can be quantitative and qualitative. Byun et al. (2017) measured the effects of uncertainty on perceived and physiological stress in caregivers of stroke survivors over a 6-week period. They explain the rationale for the choice of time-points for data collection as follows:

> *Caregivers were enrolled at the hospital within the first 2 weeks following their relatives' stroke (baseline: T1) and revisited 1 month later (4 to 6 weeks post-stroke: T2). Measuring uncertainty, perceived stress, salivary cortisol, and selected covariates in a natural clinical environment allowed examination of changes over time that occurred in the early weeks of the post-stroke period. Further, by 4 to 6 weeks following the event, stroke survivors are more likely to have been discharged (to home, rehabilitation hospitals, or nursing facilities) and family caregivers to be more directly involved in their care.*

> *(p. 31)*

The attrition rate (loss of participants to the study) was 38%. This was 'due to the high death rate of stroke patients' (Byun et al., 2017, p. 39). Attrition is a real problem in longitudinal studies. If this study's duration had been longer, it is likely that the attrition would have been higher. Therefore, when choosing a longitudinal design, researchers should be aware of the potential risk of high attrition when recruiting participants with conditions (such as stroke or heart disease) associated with mortality or morbidity.

Nash and Mitchell (2017) used a phenomenological approach to explore occupational therapy students' views of the value of frames of reference (FoR) as they progressed through the didactic portion of an occupational therapy programme. The research question was: 'How do occupational therapy students' perspectives of the value of FoR change over the course of the didactic portion of an occupational therapy program?' Data were collected over a 15-month period: 'during orientation and at the end of each of three courses that introduced FoR with a focus on pediatrics (after 5 mo in the program), adults (after 8 mo in the program), and geriatrics (after 15 mo in the program)' (p. 3). According to the authors, the rationale for choosing the longitudinal design was to provide an understanding of how 'students view the use of FoR and how these views change over time' (p. 2). They believe that this would 'inform educators as they seek to prepare students who make sound practice decisions grounded in a firm foundation of FoR and theory' (p. 2).

Only 2 out of 36 students withdrew from Nash and Mitchell's (2017) study. The loss of participants to the study was far less than in the study by Byun et al. (2017). This shows that the attrition rate can differ depending on the characteristics of the population (a captive population of students in Nash and Mitchell's study and stroke patients in Byun et al.'s) and the topic being studied. In addition Nash and Mitchell (2017) pointed out that 'changes in students' perspectives over time could have resulted from a variety of factors other than classroom and fieldwork experiences' (p. 6). One of the potential limitations of the longitudinal design is the possibility that changes may be affected by factors outside the control of the researchers.

Prospective and Retrospective Studies

In lay terms, prospective means something likely to happen in the future. For example, prospective students are those likely to apply for courses aimed at them. In research terms, prospective means collecting data starting in the present and continuing at one or more time- points in the future. Prospective studies share the same strengths and limitations of longitudinal designs, outlined above. An example of a research proposal for a study using a prospective design is 'The burden of gastroenteritis in Switzerland' by Schmutz and Mäusezahl (2018). These authors proposed a weekly follow-up of a cohort of 3000 participants to estimate the incidence of gastroenteritis and to explore 'the socio-economic impact of the disease including absence from work and inability to perform daily activities' (p. 1).

Retrospective studies, on the other hand, involve analysing and interpreting data already collected (i.e. in the past). Retrospective designs are useful when researchers can use available and accessible data to answer their research questions. An example of a proposal for a retrospective study relates to the analysis of data from former professional footballers in order to assess the incidence of neurodegenerative disease in this population (Russell et al., 2019). They proposed to analyse databases of all 'Scottish professional footballers held as the Record of Pre-War Scottish League Players (v2) and the Record of Post-war Scottish League Players (v6)' (p. 2). This proposal provides an excellent example of how data can be extracted from existing records.

Retrospective studies are particularly appropriate for looking at the incidence and prevalence of diseases and conditions as well as risk factors. They can also be useful for studying the use and outcomes of services. Most of the data analysed in retrospective studies were most likely for reasons other than for research. They are collected routinely as part of clinical practice or for administrative purposes. Therefore hospital and patient records as well as censuses are prime sources of data for retrospective studies. The strengths of these types of study lie in the availability of large amounts of data that researchers can start analysing as soon as ethical approval and access are obtained. Collecting data can be expensive; therefore if data are readily available, researchers can save time and money. However, extracting the required data and interpreting them are not without their own challenges. Records are often not complete and there can be missing data.

van Weel et al. (2019) analysed routinely collected data as part of the delivery of community home nursing and healthcare services in Victoria, Australia. This was for their retrospective study of home care service utilisation by people with dementia. The authors commented that their 'study shows that using routinely collected data is cost effective and can improve population reach, enable long-term follow-up and avoid both attrition and reporting bias' (p. 673). However, a number of limitations were also pointed out by the authors. They found that 'due to the parsimonious nature of the administrative data sets, the number of variables available for analysis were limited and measures of cognitive status, functional status and medical needs were not collected' (p. 673). The data set contained a small amount of missing data for a number of variables. They believe that 'diagnostic misclassification' may have occurred 'due to the diagnostic difficulties related to the insidious nature of dementia' (p. 673). These limitations point to the challenges that researchers may face when undertaking the analysis of data that were collected for reasons other than research.

The gap between the time the data were collected and the time they are analysed may affect the validity of the data. Difficulty in recalling events that happened and changes in disease classification and/or diagnostic procedures and technology over time can inflate or deflate the incidence and prevalence figures. For example, King and Bearman (2009) found that changes in practice for diagnosing autism led to substantial increases in the number of cases of autism.

When designing a retrospective study and developing a research proposal, it is advisable to explore, beforehand, if access will be granted to carry out the study (since much of the information collected is confidential) and what the quality of the available data is before undertaking the study. In addition, extracting and analysing secondary data requires training. It is worth pointing out that there is now greater emphasis in some countries, such as the UK and Australia, on using routinely collected data for research (van Weel et al., 2019). Data sharing is also increasingly being encouraged.

Cohort Designs

In lay terms 'cohort' refers to a group of people sharing common characteristics. For example, all the students on year 1 of a degree course are referred to as 'year 1 cohort' since they all started at the same time and undertake the same training. In research terms, a cohort refers to a group of people who share some characteristics and take part in a study. A cohort can be a sample or the whole population (e.g. all patients who had heart surgery in a particular hospital in a particular year). When the term 'cohort' is used, it normally means that the focus is on participants as a group and that they may be followed up in time to see, for example, how they 'journey' through their disease and treatment experience.

Cohort designs are particularly appropriate to study the incidence of diseases, risk factors and predictors. Cohort studies are mostly correlational as they seek to explore the links between outcomes (e.g. diabetes or smoking) and personal, behavioural and other factors (gender, social class, lifestyles, etc.). These types of study tend to study participants in their own environment. This is why they have been described as 'observational' studies.

For example, Feng et al. (2018) used a prospective cohort design to study the effects of black tea on cognitive decline among older US men. The objective of this study was to determine whether black tea consumption is associated with cognitive decline among older men. This was not an experimental study as the researchers did not introduce 'black tea drinking' – they studied the normal behavior of these men in their natural environment. While a non-significant relationship between black tea drinking and cognitive decline was reported, the authors recognised the limitations of their study. They relied on self-reports of tea-drinking behaviour and did not record the amount and frequency of tea drinking. Feng et al. (2018) suggested that a randomised controlled trial might be an appropriate design to report a cause and effect relationship between tea drinking and cognitive function.

Cohort studies can be prospective or retrospective. For example, Wu et al. (2020) used a prospective cohort design to evaluate the association between dietary cholesterol and gestational diabetes mellitus during pregnancy in a cohort of 2124 women in a province of China. Several measurements were used to collect data on a range of demographic, behavioural and clinical factors throughout the pregnancy period. On the other hand, Mbachi et al. (2019) used a retrospective cohort design to explore the 'Association between cannabis use and complications related to Crohn's disease' by extracting data from the National Inpatient Sample dataset (a yearly survey of 20% of total admissions from more than 4000 hospitals across over 30 US States and the District of Columbia). In Mbachi et al.'s (2019) study, they compared cannabis users with a matched cohort without recognised cannabis use. These two cohorts were similar in all identifiable aspects except with regards to cannabis use.

Matching cohorts is a strategy used by researchers for them to have some degree of control over bias in these types of study (although not all cohort studies have matched cohorts). Another example of 'matched controls' is from a study by Bourgeois et al. (2018) that aimed 'to determine if children with substantiated reports of sexual abuse were at higher risk than children from the general population of at least one psychotic disorder diagnosis between the substantiated report of abuse and the beginning of adulthood' (p. 124). They matched a cohort of 882 young people with a substantiated report of sexual abuse with another cohort of 882 youth from the general population over a 13-year period, in terms of 'birth year and month', gender and geographical area. Although 'matched controls' is not sufficient to establish 'cause and effect', they are particularly useful for developing hypotheses that can then be tested in experiments. For example, in the above study, matching participants from the same geographical area is an attempt to control socioeconomic factors that may influence child sex abuse.

Cohort designs share some of the same strengths and weaknesses of prospective and retrospective studies. A particular strength of cohort studies is that they can involve a large number of participants and can explore the relationships between health outcomes and a range of variables. They are particularly useful for developing hypotheses that can thereafter be tested in experiments. The limitations include the length of time and the amount of resources it takes to complete these studies. Changes over time and high rates of attrition may also bias the findings.

See Proposal Examples 4.2 and 4.3, respectively, for how prospective and retrospective cohort designs are reported in research proposals.

PROPOSAL EXAMPLE 4.2
A PROSPECTIVE COHORT STUDY

Bennett et al. (2020), 'Study protocol for a prospective, longitudinal cohort study investigating the medical and psychosocial outcomes of UK combat casualties from the Afghanistan war: the ADVANCE Study'.

COMMENTS

1. The objective of this '20-year cohort' study is to 'determine the long-term effects on both medical and psychosocial health of servicemen surviving this severe combat related trauma' (p. 1). 'A prospective cohort of 1200 Afghanistan-deployed male UK military personnel and veterans will be recruited and will be studied at 0, 3, 6, 10, 15 and 20 years' (p. 1). Half of the sample will be those who 'sustained combat trauma'. A comparison group consisting of non-injured personnel will also be recruited.
2. Participants will be 'followed' for a period of 20 years for researchers to find out what effects combat trauma could have on these soldiers in terms of cardiovascular disease, musculoskeletal disease, mental health and other conditions.
3. The longitudinal nature of this study is to provide data on how these conditions progress during the 20-year period. These types of data will be useful for anticipating the needs of this population and, in the future, plan for the care of similar populations.

PROPOSAL EXAMPLE 4.3
A RETROSPECTIVE COHORT STUDY

Wan et al. (2021), 'Retrospective cohort study to investigate the 10-year trajectories of disease patterns in patients with hypertension and/or diabetes mellitus on subsequent cardiovascular outcomes and health service utilisation: a study protocol'.

COMMENTS

1. While Bennett et al. (2020), in Proposal Example 4.2, seek to explore how conditions or diseases will develop in the future, this study (Wan et al., 2021) aims to look at 'the 10-year trajectory patterns of the clinical and treatment profiles' of patients, in primary care, with hypertension (HT) and/or diabetes mellitus (DM) in primary care, in the period 2016–19.
2. Wan et al. (2021) will extract data from existing databases during this period in order, among other things, 'to detect a difference in the 10-year relative risk of HT/DM-related complications between patients with and without continuity of care as a primary outcome' (p. 2).
3. According to the authors, 'the results can inform policy and practice on strategies to deliver primary care services more effectively and efficiently to achieve the best performance and outcomes for patients with HT and DM' (p. 2).
4. Wan et al. (2021) recognise that the 'misclassification' of diseases and 'missing data' will present challenges to researchers. These are common problems of collecting and analysing data retrospectively.
5. Finally, the authors point out that retrospective nature of the study design 'does not allow for any inferences be drawn regarding causality'.

Case-Control Designs

With case-control designs, researchers are interested in finding out which factors (genetic, personal, social, environmental, etc.) are likely to contribute to a condition, health outcome or behaviour (e.g. smoking). Therefore they start with an outcome (e.g. chronic obstructive pulmonary disease) and compare the cases with a group who did not develop the disease. In this way it is possible to identify the type of people and the environment that are more likely to be associated with the outcome. Therefore in case-control studies, researchers start with the outcome and work backwards to analyse the available data (retrospective analysis). Case-control studies are mostly retrospective but can be prospective as well. However, they should always involve a comparison group (often called a control group), preferably a matched cohort. Case-control designs are best suited to the study of rare conditions, as, prospectively, it may take years before there would be enough cases to establish statistically significant correlations. The strength of case-control designs lies in the availability of data to analyse. Therefore, case-control studies can be cheaper and require less time to complete than prospective cohort studies.

Case-control designs share some of the limitations of retrospective studies in relation to recall, misdiagnosis, misclassification, underdiagnosis and unreported conditions. They cannot establish cause and effect, but can point to associations between outcomes and risk factors. Matched controls can help to control some of the confounding variables but may be difficult to set up. See Proposal Examples 4.4 and 4.5, respectively, for how prospective and retrospective case study designs are reported in research proposals.

PROPOSAL EXAMPLE 4.4
A PROSPECTIVE CASE-CONTROL STUDY

Pastor et al. (2020), 'Remote monitoring telemedicine (REMOTE) platform for patients with anxiety symptoms and alcohol use disorder: Protocol for a case-control study'.

COMMENTS

1. As the authors stated, 'the primary objective of this study is to analyze the digital physiological patterns of two groups of participants—one group with symptoms of anxiety disorder and alcohol use disorder and one healthy control group without these disorders—using data collected from a mobile device (i.e., smartphone) and a wearable sensor (i.e., Fitbit) (p. 2).

2. Participants will be monitored, over a period of four months, on a range of factors, including sleep cycle, heart rate, movement patterns and sociability. As this is a prospective study, the researchers have more control over the choice of outcomes and how they will be measured than with a retrospective study.

3. Sixty participants will be recruited (30 with 'symptoms of anxiety disorder and alcohol use disorder' and 30 healthy volunteers). They will be matched for 'age' and 'gender'. Although the terms 'experimental' and 'control' were used to label these groups, this is not a trial as there is no intervention.

PROPOSAL EXAMPLE 4.5
A RETROSPECTIVE CASE-CONTROL STUDY

Balaji et al. (2020), 'The Young Lives Matter study protocol: A case-control study of the determinants of suicide attempts in young people in India'.

COMMENTS

1. In this proposal, the authors aim to find out about some of the factors (e.g. demographic characteristics, adverse life events, etc.) that could be associated with self-inflicted non-lethal injuries and poisoning, among a group of 15–29 year-olds. To do so, they intend to explore/ measure these factors with a number of questionnaires. The data required to answer the research questions will come from the responses of participants about events that led to the outcome (suicide attempts). Therefore, the study is retrospective. It is also a case-control design because the researchers start with the outcome and want to explore the circumstances that led to it. It also has a control group (those attending the general medicine outpatient department of the hospital with health complaints other than suicide attempts), matched for age and gender.

2. According to the authors, a case-control design was used because it 'is suitable for studying predictors of rare outcomes and for exploring multiple exposures simultaneously' (p. 3). They want to explore the link (correlation) between these factors and suicide attempts; hence it is also a correlational study.

3. One of the limitations of the study, pointed out by Balagi et al. (2020), is the possibility of recall bias as participants must answer questions about their past. The authors are aware of this and have listed the ways in which they will try to prevent or reduce this bias.

4. As part of the publication process of this paper (Balaji et al. (2020), two open reviews were published (see the end of their paper). One of reviewers asked for 'clearer justification for their choice of the suicide model underpinning their assessment battery' and suggested that 'other models, notably the Integrated Motivational-Volitional Model, may have greater empirical support and would be relevant to this study' (p. 14). This shows the importance that reviewers put on the use of conceptual frameworks/models to underpin research studies (see Chapter 3).

BLURRING TERMINOLOGIES

There are many examples in the literature of the different ways in which researchers interpret terms such as prospective, retrospective, cohort, case-control, etc. For example, some randomised control trials have been described as 'retrospective'. Kim et al. (2009) described their study of 'Treatment of early breast cancer in women over 65', as a 'retrospective trial'. They retrospectively analysed the data from 4990 early cancer patients. This type of study would normally be described as a 'retrospective cohort study'. The term 'retrospective' when used to describe a trial is a misnomer (wrongly named) since one cannot carry out a trial retrospectively. In a trial one has to introduce an intervention in order to test it; this cannot be done retrospectively.

Cohort studies should ideally collect data from large populations at different time points. Some researchers test their interventions in studies they describe as cohort studies when in fact they are 'quasi-experiments' (see Chapter 5). For example, Osborne et al. (2018) carried out 'an evaluation of an innovative specialist social worker-led model of care designed to identify and coordinate timely discharge of long-stay patients and those at risk of a long stay in a large teaching hospital' (p. 2). Patients were allocated into two groups: experimental and control. The researchers in this case introduced a change (a new model of care) and collected data before and after the intervention from the experimental and control groups. They described their study as a 'prospective cohort study with historical controls', whereas normally this design would be described as a 'before and after trial'.

Wrongly labelling the design of one's study does not invalidate the results. However, in a proposal (especially one competing for funding) naming the design of the study wrongly may not inspire confidence in experts on the panel who have to review the proposal.

Checklist for surveys, cohort and case-control studies:
1. Has a particular design been identified?
2. Why is this design appropriate for answering the research questions for this study? For example, is there a consensus in the literature that this type of research question is best answered by the chosen design?
3. If the selected design is to be modified or adapted, is a rationale or explanation given?
This section (naming and justifying the selected design) is normally no more than one or two paragraphs in the proposal. The rest of the design section, including methods of data collection, sampling and samples, and data analysis, will be dealt with in later chapters.

The Strobe Statement (von Elm et al., 2008) was developed to improve the quality of reporting of observational studies. The Strobe Statement consists of a number of checklists for research designs, including cross-sectional, cohort and case studies. While the Strobe Statement was developed to report these types of study, it can also be useful for researchers writing proposals.

SUMMARY AND CONCLUSIONS

This chapter has emphasised the importance of matching research questions to appropriate research designs. In particular, the common designs for answering descriptive and correlational research questions have been outlined, as well as their strengths and limitations. Research proposals should provide sufficient information on why particular designs are being selected and how the study will be conducted. In the next chapter, we will explore the common designs used in experimental studies that aim to answer causal questions (i.e. those examining cause and effect relationships).

REFERENCES

Balaji, M., Vijayakumar, L., Phillips, M., Panse, S., Santre, M., Pathare, S., & Patel, V. (2020). The Young Lives Matter study protocol: A case-control study of the determinants of suicide attempts in young people in India. *Wellcome Open Research, 5,* 262. https://doi.org/10.12688/wellcomeopenres.16364.1

Bennett, A. N., Dyball, D. M., Boos, C. J., Fear, N. T., Schofield, S., Bull, A., Cullinan, P., & ADVANCE Study. (2020). Study protocol for a prospective, longitudinal cohort study investigating the medical and psychosocial outcomes of UK combat casualties from the Afghanistan war: The ADVANCE Study. *BMJ Open, 10*(10), e037850. https://doi.org/10.1136/bmjopen-2020-037850

Bonsaksen, T., Sadeghi, T., & Thørrisen, M. M. (2017). Associations between self-esteem, general self-efficacy, and approaches to studying in occupational therapy students: A cross-sectional study. *Occupational Therapy in Mental Health, 33*(4), 326–341.

Bourgeois, C. A., Lecomte, T., & Daigneault, I. (2018). Psychotic disorders in sexually abused youth: A prospective matched-cohort study. *Schizophrenia Research, 199*, 123–127.

Byun, E., Riegel, B., Sommers, M., Tkacs, N., & Evans, L. (2017). Effects of uncertainty on perceived and physiological stress in caregivers of stroke survivors: A 6-week longitudinal study. *Journal of Gerontological Nursing, 43*(10), 30–40.

de Ridder, D., Kroese, F., Evers, C., Adriaanse, M., & Gillebaart, M. (2017). Healthy diet: Health impact, prevalence, correlates, and interventions. *Psychology & Health, 32*(8), 907–941.

Feng, L., Langsetmo, L., Yaffe, K., Sun, Y., Fink, H. A., Shikany, J. M., & Osteoporotic Fractures in Men (MrOS) Study Group. (2018). No effects of black tea on cognitive decline among older US men: A Prospective Cohort Study. *Journal of Alzheimer's Disease, 65*(1), 99–105.

Gaikwad, M., Vanlint, S., Moseley, G. L., Mittinty, M. N., & Stocks, N. (2016). Understanding patient perspectives on management of their chronic pain - online survey protocol. *Journal of Pain Research, 10*, 31–35.

Glaser, B. G., & Strauss, A. L. (1967). *The discovery of grounded theory. Strategies for qualitative research.* Chicago: Aldine.

Hammersley, M., & Atkinson, P. (1989). *Ethnography, principles in practice.* London: Routledge.

Johnstone, B. (2008). *Discourse analysis.* Oxford: Blackwell.

Kim, K., Jung, Y., Hur, L., & Kim, S. (2009). Treatment of early breast cancer in women over 65: What is important? Retrospective trial. *Cancer Research, 69*(Suppl. 2), 1125. https://doi.org/10.1158/0008-5472.SABCS-1125

King, M., & Bearman, P. (2009). Diagnostic change and the increased prevalence of autism, *International Journal of Epidemiology, 38*(5), 1224–1234.

Klernäs, P., Johnsson, A., Horstmann, V., & Johansson, K. (2018). Health-related quality of life in patients with lymphoedema - a cross-sectional study. *Scandinavian Journal of Caring Sciences, 32*, 634–644.

Mbachi, C., Attar, B., Wang, Y., Paintsil, I., Mba, B., Fugar, S., Agrawal, R., Simons-Linares, R. C., Jaiswal, P., Trick, W., & Kotwal, V. (2019). Association Between Cannabis Use and Complications Related to Crohn's Disease: A Retrospective Cohort Study. *Digestive Diseases and Sciences, 64*(10), 2939–2944.

Nash, B. H., & Mitchell, A. W. (2017). Longitudinal study of changes in occupational therapy students' perspectives on frames of reference. *The American Journal of Occupational Therapy, 71*(5), 7105230010p1–7105230010p7.

Osborne, S., Harrison, G., O'Malia, A., Barnett, A. G., Carter, H. E., & Graves, N. (2018). Cohort study of a specialist social worker intervention on hospital use for patients at risk of long stay. *BMJ Open, 8*(12), e023127. https://doi.org/10.1136/bmjopen-2018-023127.

Parahoo, K. (2014). *Nursing research: Principles, process and issues* (3rd ed.). Basingstoke: Palgrave Macmillan.

Pastor, N., Khalilian, E., Caballeria, E., Morrison, D., Sanchez Luque, U., Matrai, S., Gual, A., & López-Pelayo, H. (2020). Remote Monitoring Telemedicine (REMOTE) Platform for Patients With Anxiety Symptoms and Alcohol Use Disorder: Protocol for a Case-Control Study. *JMIR Research Protocols, 9*(6), e16964. https://doi.org/10.2196/16964

Roggenkamp, R., Andrew, E., Nehme, Z., Cox, S., & Smith, K. (2018). Descriptive analysis of mental health-related presentations to emergency medical services. *Prehospital Emergency Care, 22*(4), 399–405.

Russell, E. R., Stewart, K., Mackay, D. F., MacLean, J., Pell, J. P., & Stewart, W. (2019). Football's InfluencE on Lifelong health and Dementia risk (FIELD): Protocol for a retrospective cohort study of former professional footballers. *BMJ Open, 9*(5), e028654. https://doi.org/10.1136/bmjopen-2018-028654

Schmutz, C., & Mäusezahl, D. (2018). The burden of gastroenteritis in Switzerland (BUGS) study: A research proposal for a 1-year, prospective cohort study. *BMC Research Notes, 11*(1), 816. https://doi.org/10.1186/s13104-018-3916-2

van Weel, J. M., Renehan, E., Ervin, K. E., & Endicott, J. (2019). Home care service utilisation by people with dementia—A retrospective cohort study of community nursing data in Australia. *Health and Social Care in the Community, 27*(3), 665–675.

von Elm, E., Altman, D. G., Egger, M., Pocock, S. J., Gøtzsche, P. C., Vandenbroucke, J. P., & STROBE Initiative. (2008). The Strengthening the Reporting of Observational Studies in Epidemiology (STROBE) statement: Guidelines for reporting observational studies. *Journal of Clinical Epidemiology, 61*(4), 344-349.

Wan, E., Chin, W. Y., Yu, E., Chen, J., Tse, E., Wong, C., Ha, T., Chao, D., Tsui, W., & Lam, C. (2021). Retrospective cohort study to investigate the 10-year trajectories of disease patterns in patients with hypertension and/or diabetes mellitus on subsequent cardiovascular outcomes and health service utilisation: A study protocol. *BMJ Open, 11*(2), e038775. https://doi.org/10.1136/bmjopen-2020-038775

Wu, Y., Sun, G., Zhou, X., Zhong, C., Chen, R., Xiong, T., Li, Q., Yi, N., Xiong, G., Hao, L., Yang, N., & Yang, X. (2020). Pregnancy dietary cholesterol intake, major dietary cholesterol sources, and the risk of gestational diabetes mellitus: A prospective cohort study. *Clinical Nutrition (Edinburgh, Scotland), 39*, 1525–1534.

Yarbrough, S., Martin, P., Alfred, D., & McNeill, C. (2017). Professional values, job satisfaction, career development, and intent to stay. *Nursing Ethics, 24*(6), 675–685.

5 SELECTING EXPERIMENTAL DESIGNS

INTRODUCTION

In the last chapter, we saw how survey, cohort and case control designs can answer descriptive and correlational questions. While these types of study produce vital findings to inform policy and practice, they do not answer 'causal' questions. They explore relationships between variables (e.g. heart disease and exercise) but not the cause and effect between these variables. This is because researchers do not have control over the variables. When they want to find out if their interventions (treatment, therapies, behavioural programmes, etc.) work, they are in fact asking questions such as 'Does therapy X reduce depression?' (i.e. they want to find out if therapy X is the cause of the reduction in depression).

In correlational studies using cohort or case control designs, researchers do not introduce interventions; they study them after they have happened (e.g. as in retrospective cohort studies) or as they may happen in the future (e.g. as in prospective cohort studies). In either case, these changes happen in the natural environment, without being influenced by researchers. In such studies, researchers can establish a correlational relationship between exercise and heart disease, for example, but they cannot say for certain that exercise reduces the chance of heart disease, because there are many other factors or variables, such as diets, medication, pollution, lifestyle, etc., that can confound (confuse) the results. To control these variables, they can use what is known as an experimental design.

In this chapter, we will explore the different types of experimental design and find out about their strengths and limitations that we need to consider when designing a study. Examples of experimental designs in research proposals will be provided.

EXPERIMENTAL DESIGNS

'Experimental design' is an umbrella term for the different types of trial that researchers undertake. The terms 'experiment' and 'trial' are used because researchers 'experiment' on their patients by introducing an intervention whose effectiveness is not known. The new intervention is being 'tried' on patients. While this seems to be rather crude, in reality there are moral, ethical, legal and other principles that researchers have to comply with before they are allowed to carry out such research. The term 'trial' is used to describe the type of experiments conducted in nursing, health and social care. The main types of experimental design are the randomised controlled trial and quasi-experiments.

Randomised Controlled Trial

According to Bhide et al. (2018), 'a randomised controlled trial is a prospective, comparative, quantitative study/experiment performed under controlled conditions with random allocation of interventions to comparison groups' (p. 380). Qualitative data can also be collected alongside a trial. A randomised controlled trial has three main components (criteria): intervention, control and randomisation. Intervention, as explained earlier, can be a drug (or a combination of drugs), a procedure (e.g. surgery or a wound dressing), a therapy (rehabilitation, clinical, social or behavioural), a policy (a discharge service or a model of care), counselling sessions or an educational programme. Without the introduction of an intervention, there is no trial. Researchers can 'manipulate' or vary the intervention in terms of dosage, timing, frequency or duration.

'Control' is a procedure designed to prevent other variables from interfering with the 'experiment'. Researchers control these other variables by having at least two groups of participant: one group (the experimental group) receives the intervention and the other (the control group) does not. The groups are selected in such a way that they are similar in every way possible, with the exception that only one group receives the intervention. For example, both groups may be similar in age, sex distribution, stage of disease or socioeconomic status. The variables that researchers control are those that they believe (based on reliable information) may confound the results. By having a control group, the researcher may say, with some confidence, that the results/outcome were caused by the intervention and not by any of these other factors or variables. Therefore, 'control' is the process by which researchers ensure that known or potential factors (confounders) are accounted for when designing a randomised controlled trial. There can also be more than one experimental and control groups.

Randomisation is the process of allocating participants to either the experimental or the control group, by using a strategy or method that ensures researchers are not biased in the selection of participants. This can be done, for example, by using computer-generated random numbers or by using opaque envelopes for group allocation (e.g. 'A' for the intervention group and 'B' for the control group). The researcher/allocator is unaware which envelope is A or B when giving it to the participant. The aim of randomisation through concealed allocation is to prevent the potential for selection bias. There are different types of randomisation (see Chapter 11 for more detail).

The randomised controlled trial is 'the most rigorous and robust research method of determining whether a cause-effect relation exists between an intervention and an outcome' (Bhide et al., 2018, p. 380). This does not mean that the randomised controlled trial is better than other research designs. It is the 'gold standard' only for answering cause and effect questions. It is not appropriate to compare it with surveys or qualitative approaches, since their aim and purpose are different from those of a randomised controlled trial. For each type of question (descriptive, correlational and cause and effect), there are 'best' or 'appropriate' designs, and each design has its strengths and limitations. For a useful discussion on the hierarchy of evidence from different research designs, see Booth (2010).

In its basic form, the research process in conducting randomised controlled trials consists of formulating one or more hypotheses, identifying outcomes to be measured, setting inclusion and exclusion criteria, recruiting and randomising participants to the groups (intervention and control), collecting data before and after the intervention is implemented, analysing the data and reporting the findings. Researchers have to ensure that the trial has internal validity by controlling sources of bias through blinding (researchers, clinicians and participants, as far as possible are unaware of the group allocation). External validity is enhanced by ensuring that participants in the trial are similar to those in real-life situations, so that the findings have generalisability.

There are different types of randomised controlled trial design. The common ones are parallel, crossover and factorial. The parallel design is perhaps the most used trial design in health and social care research. The National Institute for Health Research (now the National Institute for Health and Care Research; NIHR, 2019) described the parallel group trial as:

> groups or individuals randomised to one of two interventions (A or B) with outcomes compared at the final endpoint (either by comparing differences in a pre-specified primary outcome at a pre-specified time point, or by comparing the disease severity between baseline and follow-up).

In a parallel design, one group of individuals is given the intervention while another similar group receives a placebo or usual treatment. A placebo is a substance that resembles the intervention but does not contain any active ingredient that could affect the outcome of a trial. The two groups (intervention and control/comparison) are compared with regards to the outcomes that the intervention is expected to achieve.

An example of a proposal for a study using a parallel design is given by Lubman et al. (2019), who proposed a parallel group randomised controlled trial to 'examine the efficacy of a stand-alone, structured telephone-delivered intervention to reduce alcohol consumption, problem severity and related psychological distress among individuals with problem alcohol use' (p. 1). The authors proposed recruiting 344 participants across Australia with problem alcohol use. The intervention group ($n = 172$) would receive the 'Ready 2 Change intervention' (delivered by telephone), a self-help resource, guidelines for alcohol consumption and stress management pamphlets; the control group ($n = 172$) would receive four brief check-in phone calls and would be provided with alcohol consumption and stress management pamphlets. The two groups were to be studied at the same time (in parallel). In a parallel group design, the aim is to ensure that the groups are similar in as many characteristics as possible.

In this study, the researchers reported that they stratified the groups by gender, to ensure that both groups had the same number of men and women. In this proposal, Lubman et al. (2019) explained that 'randomisation lists' for each gender stratum 'will be generated at the start of the study' by a statistician and linked to a unique identification code. To prevent selection bias, 'allocations will be concealed in individual envelopes labelled with the unique identification code and opened (in consecutive order) by a designated researcher (researcher 1) after baseline assessment' (p. 5). This researcher played no further part in the study. Data collection was carried out by another researcher who was unaware of individual allocations to the groups.

A parallel design can also involve more than two groups. For example, a new treatment (group 1) can be compared with the current treatment (group 2) and with a group receiving no treatment (group 3). For a checklist on what to include when reporting multi-arm trials, see Juszczak et al. (2019); their checklist is also useful when writing a proposal for a parallel design in a trial.

Proposal Example 5.1 shows how a parallel, randomised controlled trial is described in a proposal.

A crossover design is described by NIHR (2019) as a trial where groups or individuals are randomised to one of two treatments (A or B) followed by a wash-out period (not always needed) and then a switching of treatments (to B or A, respectively). With this design, the same participants in the trial receive both treatments, one after the other, with a short period of no treatment to allow for the effects of the first treatment to be over. Therefore, in crossover trials, participants act as their own experimental and control group. An example of a crossover trial is when, for example, half of the participants receive aloe vera cream for their skin burn caused by radiation treatment and the other half receive another ointment (such as a standardly used emulsion treatment). At the end of 6 weeks, there is a short period of 3 weeks when no treatment is administered (to allow for the effects of the cream to 'wash out'). Then the two groups switch treatment for another 6 weeks. It must be noted

---

PROPOSAL EXAMPLE 5.1
A PARALLEL RANDOMISED CONTROLLED TRIAL

Kato et al. (2020), 'Study protocol for a pilot randomized controlled trial on a smartphone application-based intervention for subthreshold depression: study protocol clinical trial (SPIRIT Compliant)'.

COMMENTS

1. As the authors explain, this is a 5-week, single-blind, two-arm, parallel-group, pilot randomised controlled trial to determine the effectiveness of the video playback application in reducing depression, anxiety and psychological stress. A total of 32 individuals with 'subthreshold depression' will be randomly assigned to the experimental or control group in a 1:1 ratio. The experimental group will receive a 10-minute intervention consisting of the video playback application per day, whereas the control group will receive no such intervention.

2. Participants will be randomised to the two groups using a list that will be 'generated using an Excel spreadsheet by a third party not involved in this study' (p. 4). 'The randomized list will be created using a reasonably sized permuted block method, the block size of which will not be disclosed until the end of this trial to ensure concealment' (p. 4).

3. In this study, it is not possible to blind the participants and the therapists to the intervention. Therefore, some therapist and participant biases may be present. However, the data collector will not be aware of which groups participants belong to.

4. Finally, in this study, the researchers will not control demographic variables such as age and sex (because it is a pilot study). They recognise that this is a limitation and recommend that future studies take this into account.

PROPOSAL EXAMPLE 5.2
A CROSSOVER DESIGN TRIAL

van Dam et al. (2018), 'Quality of life and paracetamol in advanced dementia (Q-PID): protocol of a randomised double-blind placebo-controlled crossover trial'.

COMMENTS

1. In this study, it is proposed that 95 patients with advanced dementia will be recruited to the study. All of them will receive the paracetamol and a placebo, but not at the same time. Some will receive the paracetamol first, followed by the placebo. Others will receive the placebo first, followed by the paracetamol. There will be a 'wash-out' period of 7 days between the two treatments to minimise the 'carryover of effects from one treatment period to another'. In this proposal, the authors explain in detail how randomisation to the two groups will take place. This includes putting randomisation numbers, 'generated by a computer random number generator', in sealed envelopes.

2. In this study, the participants will receive both interventions (paracetamol and placebo); they thus act as their own control. Therefore, as van Dam et al. (2018) explain, 'the characteristics of the participants of the two randomised treatment groups are the same at baseline' (p. 6). In this way 'confounding is minimised when comparing the two treatments' (p. 6).

3. van Dam et al. (2018) also point out that one of the advantages of using the crossover design is that '(on average) 73% fewer participants are needed to achieve the same satisfactory power as studies that have parallel groups without crossover of treatment' (p. 6). Another advantage is that since participants receive both treatments, the results can be compared within one individual.

4. Crossover designs can have more than two interventions. For example, Siegler et al. (2019) compared 'performance' and 'pleasure' among men using three types of condom: 'fitted', 'thin' and 'standard'.

here that withholding or stopping treatment during a trial may have ethical and safety implications.

Proposal Example 5.2 describes a randomised, double-blind placebo-controlled crossover trial study. For another example of a proposal using a crossover trial design, see Pudkasam et al.'s (2020) study of 'physical activity adherence, psychological health and immunological outcomes in breast cancer survivors'.

Factorial trials involve a number of groups or individuals, randomised to single or combined treatments, for the purpose of answering two or three questions at once (e.g. is treatment A more effective than treatment B, or is the combination of A and B more effective than A or B on its own?) (NIHR, 2019). Therefore, a factorial design is appropriate when testing combinations of treatments (as, in real life, people often receive a number of treatments at the same time).

An example of a study using a factorial design is that of Hopewell et al. (2021). They assessed the clinical effectiveness and cost-effectiveness of progressive exercise compared with best-practice physiotherapy advice, with or without corticosteroid injection, in adults with a rotator cuff disorder. This study involved four groups: (1) progressive exercise (six or fewer physiotherapy

---

PROPOSAL EXAMPLE 5.3
A FACTORIAL TRIAL DESIGN

Bradley et al. (2019), 'A 2 × 2 factorial, randomised, open-label trial to determine the clinical and cost-effectiveness of hypertonic saline (HTS 6%) and carbocisteine for airway clearance versus usual care over 52 weeks in adults with bronchiectasis: a protocol for the CLEAR clinical trial'.

COMMENTS

1. In this factorial trial, the authors explain that patients will be randomised to one of four groups: (1) standard care and twice-daily nebulised HTS (6%); (2) standard care and car-bocisteine (750 mg three times per day until visit 3, then reducing to 750 mg twice per day); (3) standard care and a combination of twice-daily nebulised HTS and carbocisteine; or (4) standard care. Standard care will be given in all the groups because the authors want to know which new treatment (or combination of treatments) together with standard care is the most effective. The primary outcome is the mean number of exacerbations over 52 weeks after randomisation.

2. Whatever type of trial is selected, it is important to provide a credible justification for this choice. In this proposal, Bradley et al. (2019) provided a strong rationale for the choice of the interventions and the comparator. They explained that the physiological rationale for the use of HTS in bronchiectasis is 'based on its osmotic effects on the airway surface layer that improves airway hydration and accelerates mucus transportability, especially when combined with airway clearance techniques' (p. 2).

3. The authors also point out that 'this trial's pragmatic research design avoids the significant costs associated with double-blind trials whilst optimising rigour in other areas of trial delivery'.

---

sessions); (2) best practice advice (one physiotherapy session); (3) a corticosteroid injection and then progressive exercise (six or fewer physiotherapy sessions); or (4) a corticosteroid followed by best practice advice (one physiotherapy session).

Proposal Example 5.3 gives an example of a proposal for a study using a factorial design.

Strengths and Limitations of Randomised Controlled Trials

Randomised controlled trials are generally considered to offer the best evidence for the effectiveness of interventions. This design has high internal validity (the extent to which the research has been able to exert control in the experiment – to conclude that the outcomes were caused by the intervention and not by other factors) because bias and flaws are kept to a minimum by having a control group, randomisation and blinding. However, randomised controlled trials can be low on external validity (the extent to which the findings are generalisable to other similar settings and populations).

It is believed that with randomised controlled trials, researchers create a 'laboratory type' of research because their samples are 'sanitised'. For example, when testing the effects of a psycho-social intervention on people with prostate cancer, researchers may set criteria to exclude those who have prostate cancer and dementia. In real life, people with cancer may also have other conditions. By controlling as many variables as possible (to enhance internal validity) there is increasing risk that external validity may be reduced. In the previous example, the population under study may, in the end, not resemble the general population of people with prostate cancer. For the strengths and limitations of randomised controlled trials, see Booth and Tannock (2014). For a discussion on the 'limitations of using randomised controlled trials as a basis for developing treatment guidelines', see Mulder et al. (2018).

The rationale for selecting one of these trial designs (parallel, crossover or factorial) depends on a number of factors including the research questions, the topic being researched, the outcomes to be measured, the potential participants, the ethical, legal and pragmatic issues, the scope of the trial (e.g. multicentre, longitudinal etc.) and the resources (time, funding etc.) needed to successfully complete the study. Each design has strengths, weaknesses and challenges. A crossover design has the advantage of the comparing treatment/intervention within the same population, as the participants act as their own 'control'. Therefore, fewer participants are needed than if a parallel design was used.

The challenges in crossover designs relate to the carryover effect and wash-out period (i.e. how long the wash-out should last) as well as what to do if the first treatment works (i.e. produces the cure). For example, if two creams are tested for a skin condition and the first cream is effective, should the participant be administered the second cream? Crossover designs may be more appropriate in cases where the condition is chronic rather than when there is potential for a cure. With the latter, a parallel design may be more appropriate. If the researchers have doubts about the carryover effect of the first intervention, it may be wise to use a parallel design. However, with parallel designs more participants need to be recruited to have an adequate sample size in the intervention and control groups. According to Evans (2010), 'a crossover study may reduce the sample size of a parallel group study by 60–70% in some cases' (p. 10). For a discussion of the advantages and disadvantages of parallel and crossover trials, see Dwan et al. (2019) and Krogh et al. (2019).

Factorial designs reflect real-life situations where more than one intervention or treatment is used to address a health problem. Therefore, factorial designs are high on external validity. However, a factorial design may not be able to differentiate which treatment has the most effect when a combination of two treatments is tested. Factorial designs would require even more participants (than parallel designs) as factorial designs tend to involve a number of groups. For a discussion on the choice of designs, see Evans (2010).

Randomised controlled trials are not always the most suitable, appropriate, ethical, practical or cost-effective design for testing interventions; therefore, researchers have turned to quasi-experimental designs for their trials.

Quasi-experimental Designs

It is not always possible to carry out a randomised controlled trial. For example, Verjans-Janssen et al. (2018) tested a 'physical activity and nutrition' intervention in 11 schools (8 intervention and 3 control). In this case it was not possible to randomise pupils or students to the intervention or control groups since this would cause major disruptions for the school and the students. Even the schools could not be randomised because the schools where the intervention was tested had actively participated in the development and implementation of the intervention (Verjans-Janssen et al., 2018). While efforts were made to choose similar schools and students in another city, the lack of randomisation makes this study a quasi-experiment rather than a randomised controlled trial. However, the rigour in which the quasi-experiment is carried out determines how valid and reliable the findings are.

Sometimes an intervention is tested with only one group of participants. For example, Letourneau et al. (2015) carried out a quasi-experiment to evaluate a telephone-based peer support intervention for maternal depression with only one group of participants. They explained why it was not possible or ethically appropriate to allocate participants to intervention and control groups. According to Letourneau et al., there is strong evidence that peer support, as a treatment, was effective and therefore could not be withheld from these mothers. They also explained that the 'ethical requirement to refer depressed mothers to professional care, makes it difficult to assess whether treatment effect is due to the intervention or to the referred treatment' (Letourneau et al. 2015, p. 1590). In this study they measured maternal depression before and after the intervention. When choosing a quasi-experimental design for a study, it is important to explain in the proposal why a true experiment was not feasible or appropriate.

From the above examples one can see that experiments without randomisation and/or a control group do not meet one or two characteristics of a randomised controlled trial (intervention, control and randomisation). They are referred to as quasi-experiments because they resemble experiments (e.g. they test interventions) but lack randomisation and, in some cases, a control or comparison group. To be called an experiment, it is essential for the study to meet the first criterion: the introduction of an intervention, whose effect is measured before and after it is implemented. Quasi-experiments may not have a control group, or if there is a control group, there is no randomisation involved in allocating participants to groups.

Quasi-experimental studies should not be considered as failed randomised controlled trials. A quasi-experiment is a viable and valuable design, on its own, to provide answers to questions that researchers need and/or randomised controlled trials are not suitable for. van Dellen et al. (2019), in their quasi-experimental study of the effect of a breastfeeding support programme on breastfeeding duration and exclusivity, reported that the reason why they chose the quasi-experimental design was because randomisation was impractical. They explained that a 'Dutch health insurance company offered the BSP to their clients at the time of the research' and that the researchers were 'able to carefully monitor the effects' but 'had no possibility to intervene' (p. 3). Crucially, van Dellen et al. (2019) believed that in this case, 'randomisation was considered to limit the ecological validity (women usually make a personal choice to participate in a breastfeeding programme or not; limiting personal choice could create unwanted bias in testing the effectiveness of such a programme' (p. 3).

There are three main types of quasi-experimental design: pre- and post-test involving two non-randomised groups (experimental and comparison), pre- and post-test involving one group, and time series.

Pre- and Post-Test Involving Two Non-Randomised Groups

This quasi-experimental design closely resembles the randomised controlled trial without randomisation. For example, in a quasi-experimental study of structured nurse-led follow-up for patients after discharge from an intensive care unit (ICU) (Jónasdóttir et al., (2017), the intervention was structured nurse-led follow-up that included a booklet, ward visits, contact after discharge and an appointment 3 weeks after discharge. There were two groups: the experimental group consisting of patients discharged from an ICU in one building, and the control group of patients discharged from ICU wards in another building. It was not practical or ethical to randomise patients to either the experimental or the control group as this would interfere with the services provided to these patients. Therefore, in this case, a quasi-experimental design with non-equivalent groups was chosen. However, the lack of randomisation meant there was no guarantee that the two groups were similar.

Proposal Example 5.4 comments on a proposal for pre and post-test trial involving two non-randomised groups.

Pre- and post-Test Design Involving One Group

The pre- and post-test one group design (also described as a one-arm trial) is sometimes used when it is not possible to set up a control group; researchers may collect data prior to and after

---

PROPOSAL EXAMPLE 5.4

A PRE- AND POST-TEST TRIAL INVOLVING TWO NON-RANDOMISED GROUPS

Burgos-Díez et al. (2020), 'Study protocol of a quasi-experimental trial to compare two models of home care for older people in the primary setting'.

COMMENTS

1. This proposal is about a quasi-experimental study that aims to compare two home care (HC) models in two primary centres in Barcelona, Spain. One centre was already using an 'integrated HC model' and the patients in this centre would constitute the control group. The other centre's patients (the experimental group) would receive the new HC model.

2. All patients aged over 65 years, 'irrespective of their cognitive status' would be selected for inclusion in the study. In this case, it is not practical or ethical to randomise participants to the groups or blind them (and the staff) to the group allocation. As the authors pointed out, the sample 'is naturally defined by patients attending one of the primary care units based on their location' (p. 8).

3. This study's design is quasi-experimental because it meets two of the three criteria for a randomised control trial: it has an intervention and a control group. However, it lacks 'randomisation'.

4. The authors recognise that 'active selection' was not possible. However, the data they have collected suggested that the characteristics of the participants in the two groups were 'very similar in terms of age and complexity'(p. 8).

5. This proposal shows that there are circumstances when it is not possible to randomise participants to groups. However, the quasi-experiment in this study, according to the authors, 'will permit assessment of health outcomes, feasibility, and resource utilization of new functional HC model and identify its strengths and weaknesses compared to the integrated model' (p. 8). Therefore, as they explain, the 'results obtained from this study may have important policy implications' (p. 8).

the intervention to evaluate its effects. However, it can be used as a preliminary or pilot study to explore whether there is some indication that an intervention is effective. Thereafter, the intervention can be tested in a randomised controlled trial. If it is part of a feasibility study, the pre-test, post-test one group design can be used to find out if it is possible to implement it and how it will be received by the participants (i.e. it can be a 'dress rehearsal' for a future randomised controlled trial). The main limitation of this design is the lack of a control group to compare outcomes. Therefore, it is not possible to attribute any outcome to the intervention alone. For a discussion of the use of the pre-test, post-test one group design in nursing education, see Spurlock (2018).

Many of these studies do not explain why a control group (even a non-identical, non-randomised one) was not used. This may be due to a lack of resources or other ethical or practical reasons. Most likely the studies may be being carried out as a preliminary study prior to conducting a randomised controlled trial. Many authors of the studies using the single-group, pre- and post-test design recommend testing their findings in controlled trials. For example, Brantingham et al. (2010), in their study of full kinetic chain manipulative therapy with rehabilitation in the treatment of patients with hip osteoarthritis, reported positive findings. However, they pointed out that 'fully powered clinical trials are necessary to report generalizable findings' (p. 445). Thereafter, Brantingham et al. (2012) conducted a randomised controlled trial on the same topic and concluded that 'there were no statistically significant differences in the primary or secondary outcome scores when comparing full kinematic chain MMT plus exercise with targeted hip MMT plus exercise for mild to moderate symptomatic hip OA [osteoarthritis]' (p. 259).

Kozlowski et al. (2017) used a 'single-group longitudinal' design to 'examine the feasibility, safety, and secondary benefit potential of exoskeleton-assisted walking with one device for persons with multiple sclerosis' (p. 1300). The authors used a single group pre- and post-test design because this was a preliminary study, the purpose of which was to test the feasibility of using this intervention, in particular in terms of accessibility, tolerability, learnability, acceptability and safety. This design is justified in this case as, to the authors' knowledge, this was the first trial to test the use of this intervention. According to Kozlowski et al. (2017), the results of this study provide a foundation for larger feasibility trials with this device. They recognise that their results are 'not generalizable to the larger population of persons with multiple sclerosis, given the small sample and unblinded single-group design' (p. 1305). They explained further that 'the convenience sample with no blinding or randomization to the intervention increases the likelihood for bias towards positive results' (p. 1305) in patient-reported outcomes and clinician-rated outcomes. The study showed that the device may not be suitable for many persons with multiple sclerosis, but it could provide opportunities for some individuals to benefit from its use. The findings of this study have provided useful information and insight that would be useful for testing in larger, controlled trials.

See Proposal Example 5.5 for an example of a proposal for a study using a single group pre- and post-test design.

Interrupted Time Series

Another design in quasi-experimental studies is the interrupted time series (ITS). As the name suggests, the experiment takes place over a period of time during which an intervention is

PROPOSAL EXAMPLE 5.5
A SINGLE GROUP PRE- AND POST-TEST DESIGN

Bickton et al. (2022), 'Protocol for a single-centre mixed-method pre–post single-arm feasibility trial of a culturally appropriate 6-week pulmonary rehabilitation programme among adults with functionally limiting chronic respiratory diseases in Malawi'.

COMMENTS

1. This a three-phase feasibility study comprising a 'pre-trial qualitative work to inform the modifications required to make pulmonary rehabilitation (PR) specific to the Malawi context (phase 1), a single group trial of the 6-week programme (phase 2) and a 'post-trial quantitative and qualitative evaluation to determine the feasibility and acceptability of PR among participants' (phase 3) (p. 2). Therefore, one can see that the trial is part of a larger investigation.
2. Ten patients will be 'consecutively sampled and recruited from the chest clinic and medical wards' and will receive the intervention. The size of the sample 'was chosen pragmatically based on previous PR studies of similar sample sizes' (p. 3). There will be no control group. The authors are aware that the lack of a control group means they will be unable to attribute any pre–post PR difference or change in clinical outcomes to PR. They plan to discuss the findings 'in relation to published minimal clinically important differences' (p. 5).
3. One can see why this type of design was selected in this proposal when the authors knew in advance that the results might not be conclusive in the absence of a control group. This is because the overall aim of the study is to investigate the 'feasibility and effectiveness of PR' (p. 2), in the context of health care in Malawi. According to the authors, 'the findings of this trial will inform the design of a multicentre randomised controlled trial of PR in Malawi' (p. 2).

repeated several times and 'before and after' measurements are taken. Ramsay et al. (2003) explain that ITS is used 'to detect whether the intervention has an effect significantly greater than the underlying secular trend' (p. 613). The ITS design can include one or two groups (control and experimental). It can be prospective or retrospective. There are variations in the design of ITS as well as in the analysis of the data. The difference between an ITS and experimental longitudinal studies is that, in the latter, the intervention is administered once, and its effects are measured at pre-specified intervals. In an ITS trial, the intervention is repeated and, after each one is completed, the outcomes are measured. The intervention can be implemented and then withdrawn many times (hence the term 'interrupted'), the outcomes are measured after each cycle (of implementation and withdrawal) and this process is repeated until the number of cycles, decided in advance, is completed.

The ITS is 'one of the strongest quasi-experimental designs' (Hategeka et al., 2020, p. 1) when it is not possible to undertake a randomised controlled trial. It has been used for different types of intervention including behavioural, educational, clinical, environmental and health policy. For a systematic review of ITS studies in healthcare settings, see Hudson et al. (2019). Despite the popularity of the ITS design, there are some limitations in that it is difficult to maintain control over the trial as other changes, in the setting and population, could account for the outcome. The more complicated the design, the more difficult it is to maintain rigour throughout the duration of the study.

The strength of the ITS design is that the participants can act as their own control (hence reducing the need for a control group). This design is suitable for data that are routinely collected as well as for prospective data collection. The ITS has stronger internal validity than 'before and after' quasi-experimental designs because the repeated measures can have more control over confounding factors. ITS designs rely strongly on the statistical analysis of multiple measurements over time and comparison with normal or secular trends. However, the choice of statistical methods and the interpretation of findings can be influenced by subjective preferences. From their systematic review of studies using the ITS design in healthcare, Hudson et al. (2019) found that, in addition to a poor reporting of ITS studies, there were numerous ways of analysing data from these studies. They pointed out that 'this can make interpretation of results difficult, for example presenting effect sizes as either relative or absolute' (p. 7).

For a detailed discussion of the value and limitations of ITS experiments, see Biglan et al. (2015), Kontopantelis et al. (2015) and Bernal et al. (2016). For a description of an ITS study in a proposal, see Proposal Example 5.6.

PROPOSAL EXAMPLE 5.6
INTERRUPTED TIME SERIES TRIAL

Kastner et al. (2011), 'Evaluation of a clinical decision support tool for osteoporosis disease management: protocol for an interrupted time series design'.

COMMENTS

1. This is a three-phase study evaluating the implementation of a clinical decision support tool for osteoporosis disease management. Phase 1 is the implementation of the tool to ensure that clinicians can use it. Phase 3 is a qualitative phase exploring 'participants' experiences and perceived utility of the tool and readiness to adopt the tool at the point of care'. In phase 2, an ITS design was to be used 'to determine if it can improve osteoporosis disease management at the point of care'(p. 1). This multicomponent tool (targeted at family physicians and patients at risk of osteoporosis) was developed to support clinical decision making in osteoporosis disease management at the point of care.

2. The design consists of a baseline phase, involving a 12-month chart review to determine standard practice, before implementing the tool (12 months). There would be 52 data collection points (26 before and 26 after the introduction of the tool).

3. The rationale, given by the authors, for the choice of this ITS design is that it is a particularly strong alternative to randomised controlled trials and is 'considered a useful and pragmatic tool, particularly for pilot studies where initial evaluations of interventions and their refinement need to be done before the testing of the tool on a wider scale is justified' (p. 3).

4. This is a pilot evaluation of the osteoporosis disease management tool. The authors pointed out that the ITS design 'is susceptible to several potential threats to internal validity'(p. 5) and has limited generalisability.

TRIALS IN RESEARCH PROPOSALS

A lot of effort has been put into developing guidelines on how to report trials (after completion) in order to enable the assessment of their quality. Perhaps the best known is the Consort Statement (Schulz et al., 2010), a 25-item checklist developed by a 'group comprising experts in clinical trial methodology, guideline development, biomedical journal editors, and research funders'. The Consort Statement has been extended to adapt to various clinical areas as well as different types of trial. While the checklist focuses on the reporting of trials, the items in the Consort statement and extensions can serve as a useful reminder to research proposal developers as well. In 2007, the Standard Protocol Items: Recommendations for Interventional Trials (SPIRIT) initiative was set up with the primary aim of improving the content of trial protocols (Chan et al., 2013). The SPIRIT 2013 Statement is a 33-item checklist accompanied by a flow chart and instructions. For more information, see https://www.spirit-statement.org/publications-downloads/.

It is important to describe complex intervention trials in proposals in sufficient detail to allow others to fully understand what the experimental and control groups will receive, and the implications of this for participants, clinicians/therapists and researchers. Dorling et al. (2014) reported that 'one of the most common reasons for rejecting research proposals in the National Institute for Health Research (NIHR) Health Services and Delivery Research (HS&DR) Programme is the failure to adequately specify the intervention or context in research proposals'(p. 1). To address this lack of information on this aspect of a trial, Dorling et al. (2014) carried out a mixed methods study to develop a six-construct checklist (relating to 'organisation', 'location', 'patient group', 'workforce and staffing', 'intervention' and 'other important contextual information').

These and other checklists, in particular those on universities and funding organisation websites, provide a framework that research proposal developers can use when checking whether all the crucial information regarding trials is included in proposals. The checklist of items discussed in this chapter relates to the design section of a proposal.

Checklist for the design section in proposals involving trials:
1. Has a trial design been identified?
2. Has a rationale been provided for the choice of design?
3. Has a particular guideline (e.g. the SPIRIT checklist) been used to inform the reporting of items?
4. Have the experimental and control groups been described? What will each receive? What implications will this have for the participants, health professionals involved in their care and others in the setting?
5. What are the outcomes and how will they be measured?
6. If the design is quasi-experimental, why is a controlled trial not feasible?
7. What type of quasi-experiment is it? Have the strengths, limitations and challenges been identified?
8. How will rigour be ensured for the study?

This section should include information about outcome measuring tools, inclusion/exclusion criteria, the sample, the sampling process (including randomisation) and ethical issues. These will be discussed in later chapters.

SUMMARY AND CONCLUSIONS

There are many types of trial design, and the choice of design depends on the type and nature of the intervention, the outcomes to be measured, the availability of and access to participants, the risk of attrition, and practical and ethical issues. The choice of design should be carefully thought out, fully justified and, as much as possible, well articulated in the proposal. As Evans (2010) pointed out

> 'most errors in clinical trials are a result of poor planning. Fancy statistical methods cannot rescue design flaws. Thus, careful planning with clear foresight is crucial. The selection of a clinical trial design structure requires logic and creativity' (p. 8).

REFERENCES

Bernal, J. L., Cummins, S., & Gasparrini, A. (2017). Interrupted time series regression for the evaluation of public health interventions: A tutorial. *International Journal of Epidemiology, 46*(1), 348–355.

Bhide, A., Shah, P. S., & Acharya, G. (2018). A simplified guide to randomized controlled trials. *Acta Obstetricia et Gynecologica Scandinavica, 97*(4), 380–387.

Bickton, F. M., Mankhokwe, T., Nightingale, R., Fombe, C., Mitengo, M., Mwahimba, L., Lipita, W., Wilde, L., Pina, I., Yusuf, Z. K., Ahmed, Z., Kamponda, M., Limbani, F., Shannon, H., Chisati, E., Barton, A., Free, R. C., Steiner, M., Matheson, J. A., Manise, A., ... Orme, M. (2022). Protocol for a single-centre mixed-method pre–post single-arm feasibility trial of a culturally appropriate 6-week pulmonary rehabilitation programme among adults with functionally limiting chronic respiratory diseases in Malawi. *BMJ Open, 12*(1), e057538. https://doi.org/10.1136/bmjopen-2021-057538

Biglan, A., Ary, D., & Wagenaar, A. C. (2000). The value of interrupted time-series experiments for community intervention research. *Prevention Science: The Official journal of the Society for Prevention Research, 1*(1), 31–49.

Booth, A. (2010), On hierarchies, malarkeys and anarchies of evidence. *Health Information & Libraries Journal, 27*, 84–88.

Booth, C. M., & Tannock, I. F. (2014). Randomised controlled trials and population-based observational research: Partners in the evolution of medical evidence. *British Journal of Cancer, 110*(3), 551–555.

Bradley, J. M., Anand, R., O'Neill, B., Ferguson, K., Clarke, M., Carroll, M., Chalmers, J., De Soyza, A., Duckers, J., Hill, A. T., Loebinger, M. R., Copeland, F., Gardner, E., Campbell, C., Agus, A., McGuire, A., Boyle, R., McKinney, F., Dickson, N., McAuley, D. F., ... CLEAR Study Group. (2019). A 2 × 2 factorial, randomised, open-label trial to determine the clinical and cost-effectiveness of hypertonic saline (HTS 6%) and carbocisteine for airway clearance versus usual care over 52 weeks in adults with bronchiectasis: A protocol for the CLEAR clinical trial. *Trials, 20*(1), 747. https://doi.org/10.1186/s13063-019-3766-9

Brantingham, J. W., Globe, G. A., Cassa, T. K., Globe, D., de Luca, K., Pollard, H., Lee, F., Bates, C., Jensen, M., Mayer, S., & Korporaal, C. (2010). A single-group pretest posttest design using full kinetic chain manipulative therapy with rehabilitation in the treatment of 18 patients with hip osteoarthritis. *Journal of Manipulative and Physiological Therapeutics, 33*(6), 445–457.

Brantingham, J. W., Parkin-Smith, G., Cassa, T. K., Globe, G. A., Globe, D., Pollard, H., deLuca, K., Jensen, M., Mayer, S., & Korporaal, C. (2012). Full kinetic chain manual and manipulative therapy plus exercise compared with targeted manual and manipulative therapy plus exercise for symptomatic osteoarthritis of the hip: A randomized controlled trial. *Archives of Physical Medicine and Rehabilitation, 93*(2), 259–267.

Burgos-Díez, C., Sequera-Requero, R. M., Tarazona-Santabalbina, F. J., Contel-Segura, J. C., Monzó-Planella, M., & Santaeugènia-González, S. J. (2020). Study protocol of a quasi-experimental trial to compare two models of home care for older people in the primary setting. *BMC Geriatrics, 20*(1), 101. https://doi.org/10.1186/s12877-020-1497-0

Chan, A. W., Tetzlaff, J. M., Gøtzsche, P. C., Altman, D. G., Mann, H., Berlin, J. A., Dickersin, K., Hróbjartsson, A., Schulz, K. F., Parulekar, W. R., Krleza-Jeric, K., Laupacis, A., & Moher, D. (2013). SPIRIT 2013 explanation and elaboration: Guidance for protocols of clinical trials. *BMJ (Clinical Research ed.), 346*, e7586. https://doi.org/10.1136/bmj.e7586

Dorling, H., White, D., Turner, S., Campbell, K., & Lamont, T. (2014). Developing a checklist for research proposals to help describe health service interventions in UK research programmes: A mixed methods study. *Health Research Policy and Systems, 12*, 12. https://doi:10.1186/1478-4505-12-12.

Dwan, K., Li, T., Altman, D. G., & Elbourne, D. (2019). CONSORT 2010 statement: Extension to randomised crossover trials. *BMJ (Clinical Research ed.), 366*, l4378. https://doi.org/10.1136/bmj.l4378

Evans, S. R. (2010). Clinical trial structures. *Journal of Experimental Stroke & Translational Medicine, 3*(1), 8–18.

Hategeka, C., Ruton, H., Karamouzian, M., Lynd, L. D., & Law, M. R. (2020). Use of interrupted time series methods in the evaluation of health system quality improvement interventions: A methodological systematic review. *BMJ Global Health, 5*(10), e003567. https://doi.org/10.1136/bmjgh-2020-003567

Hopewell, S., Keene, D. J., Heine, P., Marian, I. R., Dritsaki, M., Cureton, L., Dutton, S. J., Dakin, H., Carr, A., Hamilton, W., Hansen, Z., Jaggi, A., Littlewood, C., Barker, K., Gray, A., & Lamb, S. E. (2021). Progressive exercise compared with best-practice advice, with or without corticosteroid injection, for rotator cuff disorders: The GRASP factorial RCT. *Health Technology Assessment (Winchester, England), 25*(48), 1–158.

Hudson, J., Fielding, S., & Ramsay, C. R. (2019). Methodology and reporting characteristics of studies using interrupted time series design in healthcare. *BMC Medical Research Methodology, 19*(1), 137. https://doi.org/10.1186/s12874-019-0777-x

Juszczak, E., Altman, D. G., Hopewell, S., & Schulz, K. (2019). Reporting of Multi-Arm Parallel-Group Randomized Trials: Extension of the CONSORT 2010 Statement. *JAMA, 321*(16), 1610–1620. https://doi:10.1001/jama.2019.3087

Kastner, M., Sawka, A., Thorpe, K., Chignel, M., Marquez, C., Newton, D., & Straus, S. E. (2011). Evaluation of a clinical decision support tool for osteoporosis disease management: Protocol for an interrupted time series design. *Implementation Science, 6*, 77. https://doi.org/10.1186/1748-5908-6-77

Kato, Y., Kageyama, K., Mesaki, T., Uchida, H., Sejima, Y., Marume, R., Takahashi, K., & Hirao, K. (2020). Study protocol for a pilot randomized controlled trial on a smartphone application-based intervention for subthreshold depression: Study protocol clinical trial (SPIRIT Compliant). *Medicine, 99*(4), e18934. https://doi.org/10.1097/MD.0000000000018934

Kontopantelis, E., Doran, T., Springate, D. A., Buchan, I., & Reeves, D. (2015). Regression based quasi-experimental approach when randomisation is not an option: Interrupted time series analysis. *BMJ (Clinical Research ed.), 350*, h2750. https://doi.org/10.1136/bmj.h2750

Kozlowski, A. J., Fabian, M., Lad, D., & Delgado, A. D. (2017). Feasibility and Safety of a Powered Exoskeleton for Assisted Walking for Persons With Multiple Sclerosis: A Single-Group Preliminary Study. *Archives of Physical Medicine and Rehabilitation, 98*(7), 1300–1307.

Krogh, H. B., Storebø, O. J., Faltinsen, E., Todorovac, A., Ydedahl-Jensen, E., Magnusson, F. L., Holmskov, M., Gerner, T., Gluud, C., & Simonsen, E. (2019). Methodological advantages and disadvantages of parallel and crossover randomised clinical trials on methylphenidate for attention deficit hyperactivity disorder: A systematic review and meta-analyses. *BMJ Open, 9*(3), e026478. https://doi.org/10.1136/bmjopen-2018-026478

Letourneau, N., Secco, L., Colpitts, J., Aldous, S., Stewart, M., & Dennis, C. L. (2015). Quasi-experimental evaluation of a telephone-based peer support intervention for maternal depression. *Journal of Advanced Nursing, 71*(7), 1587–1599.

Lubman, D. I., Grigg, J., Manning, V., Hall, K., Volpe, I., Dias, S., Baker, A., K Staiger, P., Reynolds, J., Harris, A., Tyler, J., & Best, D. (2019). A structured telephone-delivered intervention to reduce problem alcohol use (Ready2Change): Study protocol for a parallel group randomised controlled trial. *Trials*, *20*(1), 515. https://doi.org/10.1186/s13063-019-3462-9

Mulder, R., Singh, A. B., Hamilton, A., Das, P., Outhred, T., Morris, G., Bassett, D., Baune, B. T., Berk, M., Boyce, P., Lyndon, B., Parker, G., & Malhi, G. S. (2018). The limitations of using randomised controlled trials as a basis for developing treatment guidelines. *Evidence-Based Mental Health*, *21*(1), 4–6.

NIHR. (2019). Clinical trials guide (Version 1). https://www.nihr.ac.uk/documents/clinical-trials-guide/20595. Retrieved on 18/08/2022.

Pudkasam, S., Pitcher, M., Fisher, M., O'Connor, A., Chinlumprasert, N., Stojanovska, L., Polman, R., & Apostolopoulos, V. (2020). The PAPHIO study protocol: A randomised controlled trial with a 2 x 2 crossover design of physical activity adherence, psychological health and immunological outcomes in breast cancer survivors. *BMC Public Health*, *20*(1), 696. https://doi.org/10.1186/s12889-020-08827-x

Ramsay, C. R., Matowe, L., Grilli, R., Grimshaw, J. M., & Thomas, R. E. (2003). Interrupted time series designs in health technology assessment: Lessons from two systematic reviews of behavior change strategies. *International Journal of Technology Assessment in Health Care*, *19*(4), 613–623.

Schulz, K. F., Altman, D. G., Moher, D., & CONSORT Group (2010). CONSORT 2010 statement: Updated guidelines for reporting parallel group randomized trials. *Annals of Internal Medicine*, *152*(11), 726–732.

Siegler, A. J., Rosenthal, E. M., Sullivan, P. S., Ahlschlager, L., Kelley, C. F., Mehta, C. C., Moore, R. H., Rosenberg, E. S., & Cecil, M. P. (2019). Double-Blind, Single-Center, Randomized Three-Way Crossover Trial of Fitted, Thin, and Standard Condoms for Vaginal and Anal Sex: C-PLEASURE Study Protocol and Baseline Data. *JMIR Research Protocols*, *8*(4), e12205.

Spurlock D. R., Jr. (2018). The Single-Group, Pre- and Posttest Design in Nursing Education Research: It's Time to Move on. *Journal of Nursing Education*, *57*(2), 69–71.

van Dam, P. H., Achterberg, W. P., Gussekloo, J., Husebo, B. S., & Caljouw, M. (2018). Quality of life and paracetamol in advanced dementia (Q-PID): Protocol of a randomised double-blind placebo-controlled crossover trial. *BMC Geriatrics*, *18*(1), 279. https://doi.org/10.1186/s12877-018-0974-1

van Dellen, S. A., Wisse, B., Mobach, M. P., & Dijkstra, A. (2019). The effect of a breastfeeding support programme on breastfeeding duration and exclusivity: A quasi-experiment. *BMC Public Health*, *19*(1), 993. https://doi.org/10.1186/s12889-019-7331-y

Verjans-Janssen, S., Van Kann, D., Gerards, S., Vos, S. B., Jansen, M., & Kremers, S. (2018). Study protocol of the quasi-experimental evaluation of 'KEIGAAF': A context-based physical activity and nutrition intervention for primary school children. *BMC Public Health*, *18*(1), 842. https://doi.org/10.1186/s12889-018-5764-3

6

SELECTING QUALITATIVE DESIGNS

INTRODUCTION

Selecting qualitative designs for descriptive studies requires careful consideration as there are a number of approaches from which to choose. The rationale for the choice of design, as well as a clear description of how the design underpins the selected approach, should be provided in the research proposal. In this chapter, we will examine the types of question that qualitative researchers seek to answer, the use of theories and conceptual frameworks to underpin qualitative studies, the use of the term 'design' in qualitative studies and the common qualitative approaches that designers of qualitative studies can choose. Examples of how researchers select and describe the design of their qualitative studies, in research proposals, are also provided.

QUESTIONS IN DESCRIPTIVE QUALITATIVE STUDIES

To select qualitative designs, we need to understand the types of question that qualitative research can or cannot answer. Qualitative research is appropriate for descriptive and exploratory research questions. Qualitative research is not appropriate for answering correlational and causal (cause and effect) questions. As pointed out in Chapter 4 descriptive questions can be answered by qualitative as well as quantitative methods, depending on the type of data that researchers want to collect. To illustrate this point, we can look at and compare two 'descriptive' studies.

Cengiz and Budak (2019) carried out a descriptive study on 'the use of complementary medicine among people with diabetes in eastern Turkey'. Their aim was to 'measure the frequency, type and purpose of complementary medicine (CM) use among people with diabetes mellitus (p. 120). They wanted to know the prevalence of the use of CM as well as the most frequently used CM method among this population. They collected data, using a questionnaire, from a random sample of 316 patients and carried out descriptive statistical analysis. Clearly, Cengiz and Budak (2019) wanted measurable data that could be generalised to this population. In this example, a quantitative, descriptive study was appropriate to answer descriptive research questions.

On the other hand, Bowden et al. (2018) carried out a qualitative descriptive study of the 'contribution of occupation to children's experience of resilience'. This was a qualitative exploratory study because 'little is known about how occupations contribute to resilience, and less is known from children's perspectives' (p. 268). The 'qualitative descriptive method was selected to ensure that participants' perspectives were grounded in their personal experiences of occupation and resilience, and an individual real account of their subjective experience was gained' (p. 269). The authors wanted to 'understand complex perspectives from children themselves, given their developmental vulnerability and the significance that resilience in childhood has on the trajectory of adulthood' (p. 269). Data were collected from 'eight face-to-face interviews and one focus group' (p. 270). Bowden et al. (2018) chose a 'thematic analysis' because this method 'reports the experiences and reality of the participants and offers a rich description of the data' (p. 271). The authors explained that the 'intent was not to make the findings generalisable' (p. 274). Their aim was to understand how occupation contributes to children's experience of resilience. These two examples show that the choice of qualitative or quantitative approaches (or mixed methods) depends on what researchers want to find out and the type of data (qualitative or quantitative) that they seek to collect.

A topic in itself does not indicate whether the study should be qualitative or quantitative. For example, Zhou et al. (2015) conducted a study on 'barriers to research utilization among registered nurses in traditional Chinese medicine hospitals' in China. They wanted to correlate demographic variables (e.g. educational attainment) with other variables such as work pressure, attitudes to nursing, job satisfaction, etc. To do so they had to measure these variables and carry out statistical tests. This study provided an overview of the barriers to research utilisation in the hospitals where the study was carried out. The authors were able to compare their findings with those of studies in other countries such as Sweden and Taiwan.

On the other hand, Gifford et al. (2018) carried out a qualitative study of barriers and facilitators to evidence-based practice in Hunan, China. The authors believed that while barriers to research utilisation have been extensively studied, many of these barriers do not apply to the Chinese context and that barriers not commonly documented in western countries may not exist in China. They cited factors such as the influence of traditional Chinese medicine, 'reverence for authority' and 'obedience to superiors' on Chinese nurses' motivation and autonomous practice. Gifford et al. (2018) wanted to find out from nurses themselves what the barriers were and not give them a list of barriers to rate (as in Zhou's study). Gifford et al. (2018) conducted individual, face-to-face semi-structured interviews to explore nurses' perspectives of 'barriers and supports' to evidence-based practice.

We can see that although the topic is the same in both studies (barriers to the use of research or evidence), the purpose of the study and the type of data required determine whether a study is qualitative or quantitative. Qualitative descriptive questions are asked when researchers know very little about the phenomena (e.g. beliefs, attitudes, experience, concepts, etc.) they want to study. They rely on participants to *describe* and explain these phenomena, in their own words and from their own perspectives.

MAIN REASONS FOR UNDERTAKING QUALITATIVE STUDIES

Qualitative studies are appropriate when we need to know participants' perspectives on a range of issues. At a descriptive level, we may want to know clients' views and experience of the services they receive. These data can be used to improve care organisation, delivery and outcome. If we want to know if clients are generally satisfied with the care they receive, a quantitative approach is appropriate because researchers want to know the percentages of clients who are or are not satisfied. If the aim is to find out what aspect of services patients value most, from their own perspectives, then qualitative research is better suited to answer this question.

As explained earlier, qualitative research is not appropriate for answering correlational or causative questions, although it can explore, qualitatively, the relationships and differences between people's perspectives. For example, qualitative research may uncover differences in beliefs or attitudes in men and women in the sample. However, one cannot make generalisations from these findings. Such differences should be tested further in quantitative studies if the aim is make generalisations about the population being studied.

An example of a descriptive qualitative study is Sun et al.'s (2019): 'exploration of home care nurse's experiences in deprescribing of medications'. Their aim was 'to explore the barriers and enablers of deprescribing from the perspectives of home care nurses, as well as to conduct a scalability assessment of an educational plan to address the learning needs of home care nurses about deprescribing' (p. 1). The authors explained that they used 'an exploratory qualitative descriptive design' because they wanted to 'provide a comprehensive summary of descriptions of the phenomenon of interest: deprescribing in the context of home care. They carried out two focus groups with five and six nurses and this 'allowed the researchers to gain valuable insight into a wide range of perceptions and beliefs that home care nurses hold in relation to medication optimisation for older adults' (p. 8). Clearly, the aim was to gain as many perspectives and beliefs as possible of the phenomenon of deprescribing. The aim was not to find out how many nurses held these. Finally, the authors concluded that their study findings 'highlighted the complexity of managing polypharmacy among older adults in home care, as well as the facilitators and challenges that home care nurses face when undertaking deprescribing approaches' (p. 7).

Qualitative studies are also appropriate for developing conceptual frameworks, models or theories (from participants' perspectives). Sometimes qualitative descriptions can be built upon to provide a conceptual understanding of the phenomenon. Such qualitative studies are referred to as theory generating research. For example, Bogosian et al. (2017) carried out a qualitative study to examine cognitive and behavioural challenges and adaptations for people with progressive multiple sclerosis. Their aim was to develop 'a preliminary conceptual model of changes in adjustment over time' (p. 343). They explained that the focus of previous descriptive studies was to identify factors that influence changes in the process of adjustment. Bogosian et al. (2017) aimed to move beyond the 'identification of specific influences' by bringing 'various adjustment factors under a conceptual model using grounded theory.' (p. 345) They developed a model of adjustment to progressive multiple sclerosis that showed how the different factors or influences interact in the process of adaption. Descriptive qualitative studies tend to identify a number of themes; conceptual qualitative studies show how these themes are related to one another to produce a conceptual understanding of phenomena.

Another example is Ledoux et al.'s (2020) study that explored determinants of parent behaviours during eating episodes. The aim of this study was to develop a preliminary conceptual model of the determinants of parent feeding behaviours with children aged 2–5 years. The authors pointed out that 'little is known about how and why parents decide to use particular feeding practices during eating episodes' (p. 240). They chose qualitative research methods because they 'allow investigators to explore a phenomenon openly from the perspective of the target audience' (p. 241). The key word here is 'explore', not 'measure' or 'correlate'. Using qualitative semi-structured interviews, the researchers used 'probes' and 'prompts' to encourage an in-depth description of parent's behaviours, thoughts and feelings, and children's behaviours, as well as environmental conditions. Data analysis revealed five themes that were then used to construct the conceptual model of determinants of parent behaviours during eating episodes (see below). Ledoux et al. (2020) gave this overview of the conceptual model and 'emergent' themes:

> *Themes included behaviors of parents and children during mealtime interactions, contextual factors, and parent beliefs. There were 2 types of parent behaviors at meals: proactive, aimed at preventing or promoting certain child behaviors; and reactive, which were responses to children's behaviors. The model centered on parent beliefs, which influenced both types of eating behaviors and were directly influenced by contextual factors and child behaviors.*

> *(p. 242)*

The authors also recommended that this model is tested quantitatively 'among a large, nationally representative' sample of parents of pre-schoolers.

USE OF THEORIES AND CONCEPTUAL FRAMEWORKS TO UNDERPIN QUALITATIVE STUDIES

Generally, the aim of qualitative research is to generate descriptive accounts and conceptual and theoretical understandings from participants' perspectives, not to test theories. Qualitative researchers tend to 'bracket' known assumptions about the phenomena they study. It is highly likely that there are prior knowledge or even theories for nearly every concept or phenomenon they explore. Qualitative research is flexible enough to accommodate known conceptual frameworks and theories, and the literature is full of examples of qualitative researchers doing just that. For example, White and Palmieri (2022), in their proposal for a descriptive phenomenological study of the lived experience of women caregivers of husbands living with Parkinson's disease, draw upon three theories to underpin their methodology: 'caregiver identity theory', 'self-determination theory' and the 'theory of human caring'.

For an example of the use of theories in a qualitative study, see Proposal Example 6.1.

PROPOSAL EXAMPLE 6.1
USE OF THEORIES IN QUALITATIVE STUDY DESIGN

Creaven et al. (2021), 'Protocol for a qualitative study: Exploring loneliness and social isolation in emerging adulthood (ELSIE)'.

COMMENTS

1. The aims of the study are to explore the 'experience of loneliness from the perspective of young adults' and to 'identify what young adults believe precipitates and maintains feelings of loneliness' (p. 2). In the aims, there are two key concepts ('loneliness' and 'young adults') about which theories have already been developed. In this study the authors will draw on 'macro-theories of development that describe "emerging" adulthood as a life stage that is theoretically and empirically distinct from adolescence and fully-fledged adulthood' (Arnett, 2000, p. 2). They will also 'tap' into a number of existing theories of loneliness, rather than 'ground' the study in 'one theoretical perspective'.

2. As this is a qualitative study, the aim is not to test theories but to develop an understanding of the phenomenon (loneliness in young adults). The authors will 'prioritize young adults' descriptions and narration on this topic, regardless of whether their perspectives align with a particular theory, or not' (p. 2).

3. This proposal does not mention any particular approach, such as grounded theory, phenomenology or ethnography. However, the researchers will use 'framework analysis' to analyse the data. They explain that 'framework analysis is not bound by a particular epistemological position'. After careful consideration, they reject 'interpretive phenomenological analysis' and 'thematic analysis' in favour of framework analysis and give the reasons for doing so.

4. This is a good example of how researchers make use of existing theories in qualitative research but still aim to develop a new understanding of phenomena. It is also a good example of the thought process that they follow when selecting frameworks to analyse their data.

THE USE OF THE TERM 'DESIGN' IN QUALITATIVE STUDIES

A quick read of a sample of qualitative studies will show that researchers use different terms to 'label' their design. Sometimes the term 'design' is not used at all. For example, Nyanchoka et al. (2022), in their study of 'facilitators and barriers to cervical cancer screening follow-up after an abnormal cervical cancer screening examination among underserved women living in remote areas of Romania', stated (in the design section of their proposal) that they will 'conduct an exploratory qualitative study using semi-structured interviews' (p. 1).

There is no single agreed term that qualitative researchers use to describe their design. Qualitative researchers are more familiar with the term 'approach' or 'methodology' than 'design'. Some of the common approaches used in nursing, health and social care research are grounded theory, phenomenology and ethnography. These approaches are often used to underpin or describe the ontological, philosophical and epistemological assumptions on which the whole study is based. None of these three approaches (above) can be described as research designs. However researchers can explain how the selection of participants and the collection and analysis of data are guided by one or more of these approaches.

Grounded theory is perhaps the most well known of the qualitative approaches. Glaser and Strauss (1967) pioneered the grounded theory movement with their seminal book *The Discovery of Grounded Theory*. Since then, much has been written about grounded theory, in its different versions, and the literature is full of examples of grounded theory studies.

Grounded theory is a research methodology whereby hypotheses and theories are developed from data collected from participants (through interviews, observations, etc.). Grounded theory, as a methodology, seems to be more suited to phenomena that involve processes (e.g. 'learning to live with a hand nerve disorder' [Ashwood et al., 2019] and 'transitions in the embodied experience after stroke' [Timothy et al., 2016]). This is because it has its roots in symbolic interactionism, a social psychological theory that explains such concepts as interactions and meanings. For an introduction to, and a summary of grounded theory, see Parahoo (2014). See Proposal Example 6.2 for the use of a grounded theory approach in a study.

Phenomenology, in its different versions (Husserl, 1931), provides the philosophical background to qualitative studies where the focus is on how participants experience phenomena. Phenomenologists are interested in how events, actions, ideas and so on appear to us, not on whether or not they exist in reality (Parahoo, 2014). As a methodology, it is particularly attractive to nurses and other health professionals as they care for people with a wide range of experiences

---

PROPOSAL EXAMPLE 6.2
SELECTING A GROUNDED THEORY DESIGN

Palmquist et al. (2017), 'Protocol: A grounded theory of 'recovery'-perspectives of adolescent users of mental health services'.

COMMENTS

1. The overall aim of this study is 'to develop a comprehensive contextualised explanation of adolescents' experiences as they encounter onset and progression of mental disorder and transition into and through mental health services (hereafter their 'journey')' (p. 2). One of the objectives of this study is to 'conceptually model the journey and "recovery" including the core process and critical moments involved in the journey' (p. 2). Their choice of grounded theory is justified because this approach is appropriate for the study of process and the development of theory and conceptual frameworks and models. As the authors explain, grounded theory is 'appropriate when research aims to explain a process where the concerns of those involved are central to its understanding and cannot be predetermined' (p. 2).

2. The choice of a qualitative approach is justified in the proposal. According to the authors, 'little is known, however, about adolescents' expectations or experience of services' (p. 2). They explained that adolescents' 'views about "recovery" remain uncertain but the limited evidence available suggests that they may be inconsistent with the prevailing recovery paradigm' (p. 2).

3. The choice of grounded theory is also justified on the basis that this approach 'is flexible' and can accommodate the use of quantitative and qualitative data. In this study, the authors aim to carry out semi-structured interviews and administer two self-report questionnaires on mental health.

that impact on how they perceive, access and use services and how they react to, and cope with, illness (Parahoo, 2014). Two examples of phenomenological studies are:

- Žiaková et al. (2020), 'An interpretative phenomenological analysis of dignity in people with multiple sclerosis'.
- Rodriguez-Vasquez et al. (2020), 'Intergenerational transmissible meanings in breastfeeding in Spain: a phenomenological study'.

For an example of a phenomenological design in a proposal, see Proposal Example 6.3.

Ethnography, with its origin in anthropology, involves researchers interacting with participants in such a way that they can begin to experience, feel and think like the participants themselves. By immersing themselves in the participants' environment and culture, researchers seek to be able to understand why participants perceive things the way they (the participants) do. They can potentially obtain an 'insider' view of participants' thinking, attitudes and behaviour.

PROPOSAL EXAMPLE 6.3
SELECTING A PHENOMENOLOGICAL DESIGN

White and Palmieri (2022), 'Women caring for husbands living with Parkinson's disease: a phenomenological study protocol'.

According to the authors, 'the purpose of this descriptive phenomenological study is to understand the lived experience of women caregivers of husbands living with Parkinson's disease'.

COMMENTS

1. The reason given for using a qualitative approach is that 'few studies provide insights about the lived experiences of wife caregivers' and that 'the daily activities of caregivers are poorly understood, including how they negotiate daily activities, manage medications, and assist with physical therapy' (p. 6).
2. The design selected for this study is the Husserlian version of 'descriptive phenomenology'. The authors chose this design because 'phenomenology guides this inquiry to capture the lived experiences of participants within the context of a phenomenon, in this case caregiving, by probing their subjective consciousness'. They go on to say that 'because the experience is lived daily by the caregiver and evolves contextually with caring longevity, the caregiver can provide clarity and depth about the phenomenon to reveal deep hidden meanings' (p. 6).
3. The authors explain that they will use the seven-step process of Colaizzi (1973) to analyse the data because this process is designed for descriptive phenomenological studies and it aligns with their study design.
4. In this study, the authors draw upon the following three theories to underpin their methodology: 'caregiver identity theory', 'self-determination theory' and the 'theory of human caring'. They explain in detail how these theories are used and provide a figure to illustrate how the interaction of these theories is conceptualised into a model of caregiving.
5. Two guidelines for 'reporting' qualitative studies are used by the authors to develop their proposal: the Standards for Reporting Qualitative Research (SRQR) 'guided development of the protocol', and the Consolidated Criteria for Reporting Qualitative Research (COREQ) 'guided the development of the interview process' (p. 14).

However, it is not always possible or practical to 'live' among participants to study their behaviour or culture. The COVID-19 pandemic has provided alternative ways in which qualitative research can be conducted. For a useful discussion of this topic, see Howlett (2022), who explored the methodological and epistemological questions and challenges of conducting online qualitative research, including ethnographic studies, in her paper 'Looking at the "field" through a Zoom lens'. Two examples of ethnographic studies are:

- Kjær et al. (2022), ' "Making room for student autonomy" – an ethnographic study of student participation in clinical work'.
- Skyberg (2022), 'Diversity, friction, and harmonisation: an ethnographic study of interprofessional teamwork dynamics'.

For an example of an ethnographic design in a proposal, see Proposal Example 6.4.

In research proposals, it is important to show that you have a good understanding of the qualitative approach that you have selected. You should justify this choice and show how you intend to use the approach in your study. The National Institute for Health Research (now the National Institute for Health and Care Research; NIHR, 2022) explained that qualitative panel members reviewing your proposal 'are likely to be experts in only one or a few methodologies'

PROPOSAL EXAMPLE 6.4
SELECTING AN ETHNOGRAPHIC DESIGN

Shrestha et al. (2022), 'Kidney sellers from a village in Nepal: protocol for an ethnographic study'.
 The main objective of this study is to 'explore the drivers of kidney selling and its consequences' (p. 1) in a village in central Nepal.

COMMENTS

1. The authors explain that 'a qualitative research design is deemed to be the most appropriate for exploring and understanding the concept of kidney selling, the meaning of the kidney, and the interplay of myriad factors affecting the kidney trade' (p. 2). In order to do so, they believe that the researcher 'will have to familiarize with the villagers by living in the villages, and will observe and note down the life, culture, and traditions in the village' (p. 3). This is expected to last at least 3 months. The ethnographic approach, which requires researchers to immerse themselves in the participants' setting in order to get close to the phenomenon (kidney selling) they are focused on, is the design of choice for this study.
2. The ethnographic approach relies heavily on observations and 'conversations' with participants. In this study, these observations will include 'nonverbal communication, including the personal presentation of the participant, body expressions, gestures, facial expressions, style, and alterations in speech (e.g., silences, choking speech, blatant speech, fading speech, cringing and tremors in the speech), laughter, and other manifestations' (p. 3).
3. One of the strengths of this proposal is that the team comprises an expert medical anthropologist, a public health specialist with expertise and experience around community engagement and a researcher who has experience in gender-related issues. Such information can give the impression that the team has the necessary requisites to successfully complete the study.

and 'may need convincing of the merits and quality' (p. 1) of the approach you are proposing to use in your study. The research questions or aims of the study should also be compatible with the selected approach.

THE FLEXIBLE AND EMERGING NATURE OF 'DESIGN' IN QUALITATIVE STUDIES

In research proposals, the aim is to decide and plan ahead, as far as possible, every step and action that will be taken to undertake and complete the study. Deviations from the original plan can compromise not only the aim of the study, but also the validity and reliability of the findings. For example, if the aim is to recruit a random sample of 125 participants for a survey but only 50 volunteers have been recruited, this will have implications for the generalisability of the findings. The nature of qualitative research is such that not every detail can be planned in advance and implemented as intended. The design in qualitative studies has been described as 'emergent'. Sandelowski and Barroso (2003) explained what this means: 'Designing studies by conducting them – as opposed to conducting studies by design – proposal writers can only anticipate how their studies will proceed (p. 781). 'Qualitative research proposals are thus exercises in imaginative rehearsal' (p. 781).

In quantitative studies, data collection tools (see Chapter 8) are constructed and tested in advance of the study (unless the aim of the study is to develop tools). In qualitative studies, researchers can only speculate on how, for example, interviews will evolve. While the interviewer may have some questions to start with, the rest will be 'thought of' during the interview. In quantitative studies the validity and reliability of a tool (e.g. questionnaire or scale) are determined prior to administering them. In qualitative studies, the process of ensuring rigour is normally described after the study is completed. For example, an audit trail is maintained as the study proceeds. An audit is a record of how, what and why decisions were taken during the study. It includes how the data were collected, analysed and reported.

Despite the differences between the quantitative and qualitative approaches to writing research proposals, there are a number of 'guides' in the literature for developing qualitative research proposals (see e.g. Sandelowski and Barroso, 2003; Klopper, 2008; Kaba et al., 2021; NIHR, 2022) and examples of qualitative research proposals on the internet.

In qualitative proposals, the authors should describe, explain and justify how they intend to conduct the study, even if not everything can be decided in advance. The proposals have to show that much thought has gone into planning them. There should be evidence that the authors have the knowledge of, and skills in, qualitative research to undertake the research. In particular, they should demonstrate sufficient insight into their choice of the qualitative approach they propose to use in their study.

Some examples of qualitative proposals are:

■ Willett et al. (2019), 'Barriers and facilitators to recommended physical activity in lower-limb osteoarthritis: protocol for a qualitative study exploring patients and physiotherapist perspectives using the theoretical domains framework and behaviour change taxonomy'. This proposal uses a phenomenological framework.

- Georgiadis et al. (2018), 'Coproducing healthcare service improvement for people with common mental health disorders including psychotic experiences: a study protocol of a multiperspective qualitative study'. The authors state that 'this study is located within the interpretivist tradition of scientific enquiry' (p. 2).
- Mueller et al. (2015), 'Interprofessional collaboration and communication in nursing homes: a qualitative exploration of problems in medical care for nursing home residents – study protocol'. Mueller et al. state that 'the overarching approach to our study, which encompasses philosophy and methods, is the grounded theory methodology' (p. 453).
- Peart et al. (2019), 'Providing person-centred care for people with multiple chronic conditions: protocol for a qualitative study incorporating client and staff perspectives; this proposal uses a hermeneutic phenomenological perspective'.
- Kloss et al. (2019), 'Factors influencing access to kidney transplantation: a research protocol of a qualitative study on stakeholders' perspectives'. This proposal uses grounded theory as the qualitative research method.
- Merry et al. (2019), 'Migrant families with children in Montreal, Canada and transnational family support: a protocol for a focused ethnography'.

Note that these proposals were written for academic journals and aimed at their readership. Proposals written as academic assignments or for funders have their own requirements. Proposals in journals do not normally provide detailed information on the time scale of the proposed study or on the resources required to complete it. However, proposals published in journals provide an insight into study designs and the rationale for the choice of design. For a helpful guide, see Kaba et al. (2021), 'Ten key steps to writing a protocol for a qualitative research study: a guide for nurses and health professionals'.

Checklist for the design section in qualitative proposals:
This checklist relates only to the introduction in the design section of a proposal. Checklists for research questions, data collection, sampling, ethical approval, etc. are dealt with in other chapters.
1. Is qualitative research appropriate to answer your research questions? Has a justification been provided?
2. Is a specific approach (e.g. grounded theory) selected for this study?
3. What is the rationale for the choice of this design/approach?
4. How is the selected approach used to underpin the study (e.g. data collection, data analysis etc.)?

SUMMARY AND CONCLUSIONS

In this chapter, we have explored the meaning of design, and the different types of design that qualitative researchers can choose from to suit their research questions. Although the aim of qualitative research is to produce a new understanding of phenomena, theories and conceptual frameworks can also be used to underpin these studies.

The flexible and emergent nature of qualitative research may provide a challenge to researchers when developing research proposals. However, as much information as possible should be provided. The selection of the research approach or design should be fully justified. Researchers should also explain, in the proposal, how the selected approach will be used to inform the research process, including data collection and analysis.

REFERENCES

Arnett, J. J. (2000). Emerging adulthood: A theory of development from the late teens through the twenties. *American Psychologist, 55*(5), 469.

Ashwood, M., Jerosch-Herold, C., & Shepstone, L. (2019). Learning to live with a hand nerve disorder: A constructed grounded theory. *Journal of Hand Therapy: official journal of the American Society of Hand Therapists, 32*(3), 334–344.e1.

Bogosian, A., Morgan, M., Bishop, F. L., Day, F., & Moss-Morris, R. (2017). Adjustment modes in the trajectory of progressive multiple sclerosis: A qualitative study and conceptual model. *Psychology and Health, 32*(3), 343–360.

Bowden, L., Reed, K., & Nicholson, E. (2018). The contribution of occupation to children's experience of resilience: A qualitative descriptive study. *Australian Occupational Therapy Journal, 65*(4), 268–275.

Cengiz, Z., & Budak, F. (2019). Use of complementary medicine among people with diabetes in eastern Turkey: A descriptive study. *Complementary Therapies in Clinical Practice, 36*, 120–124.

Colaizzi, P. F. (1973). *Reflection and research in psychology.* Dubuque, IA, USA: Kendall Hunt.

Creaven, A. M., Kirwan, E., Burns, A., & O'Súilleabháin, P. S. (2021). Protocol for a qualitative Study: Exploring loneliness and social isolation in emerging adulthood (ELSIE). *International Journal of Qualitative Methods, 20.* https://doi.org/10.1177/16094069211028682

Georgiadis, A., Duschinsky, R., Perez, J., Jones, P. B., Russo, D., Knight, C., Soneson, E., & Dixon-Woods, M. (2018). Coproducing healthcare service improvement for people with common mental health disorders including psychotic experiences: A study protocol of a multiperspective qualitative study. *BMJ Open, 8*(11), e026064. https://doi.org/10.1136/bmjopen-2018-026064

Gifford, W., Zhang, Q., Chen, S., Davies, B., Xie, R., Wen, S. W., & Harvey, G. (2018). When east meets west: A qualitative study of barriers and facilitators to evidence-based practice in Hunan China. *BMC Nursing, 17*, 26. https://doi.org/10.1186/s12912-018-0295-x

Glaser, B. G., & Strauss, A. L. (1967). *The discovery of grounded theory. Strategies for qualitative research.* Chicago: Aldine.

Howlett, M. (2022). Looking at the 'field' through a Zoom lens: Methodological reflections on conducting online research during a global pandemic. *Qualitative Research: QR, 22*(3), 387–402.

Husserl, E. (1931). *Ideas: General introduction to pure phenomenology.* [Trans. by W. R. B. Gibson]. New York: Macmillan.

Kaba, E., Stavropoulou, A., Kelesi, M., Triantafyllou, A., Goula, A., & Fasoi, G. (2021). Ten Key Steps to Writing a Protocol for a Qualitative Research Study: A Guide for Nurses and Health Professionals. *Global Journal of Health Science, 13*, 58. https://doi.org/10.5539/gjhs.v13n6p58.

Kjær, L. B., Strand, P., & Christensen, M. K. (2022). 'Making room for student autonomy' – an ethnographic study of student participation in clinical work. *Advances in Health Sciences Education: Theory and Practice, 27*(4), 1067–1094.

Klopper, H. C. (2008). The qualitative research proposal. *Curationis, 31*(4), 62–72.

Kloss, K., Ismail, S., Redeker, S., van Hoogdalem, L., Luchtenburg, A., Busschbach, J., & van de Wetering, J. (2019). Factors influencing access to kidney transplantation: A research protocol of a qualitative study on stakeholders' perspectives. *BMJ Open, 9*(9), e032694. https://doi.org/10.1136/bmjopen-2019-032694

Ledoux, T., Robinson, J., Thompson, D., & Baranowski, T. (2020). Exploring determinants of parent behaviors during eating episodes. *Journal of Nutrition Education and Behavior, 52*(3), 240–248.

Merry, L., Hanley, J., Ruiz-Casares, M., Archambault, I., & Mogere, D. (2019). Migrant families with children in Montreal, Canada and transnational family support: A protocol for a focused ethnography. *BMJ Open*, *9*(9), e029074. https://doi.org/10.1136/bmjopen-2019-029074

Mueller, C. A., Tetzlaff, B., Theile, G., Fleischmann, N., Cavazzini, C., Geister, C., Scherer, M., Weyerer, S., van den Bussche, H., & Hummers-Pradier, E. (2015). Interprofessional collaboration and communication in nursing homes: A qualitative exploration of problems in medical care for nursing home residents – study protocol. *Journal of Advanced Nursing*, *71*(2), 451–457.

NIHR. (2022). Writing a qualitative research proposal. https://www.rds-london.nihr.ac.uk (written by Rivas C).

Nyanchoka, L., Damian, A., & Nygård, M. (2022). Understanding facilitators and barriers to follow-up after abnormal cervical cancer screening examination among women living in remote areas of Romania: A qualitative study protocol. *BMJ Open*, *12*(2), e053954. https://doi.org/10.1136/bmjopen-2021-053954

Palmquist, L., Patterson, S., O'Donovan, A., & Bradley, G. (2017). Protocol: A grounded theory of 'recovery'-perspectives of adolescent users of mental health services. *BMJ Open*, *7*(7), e015161. https://doi.org/10.1136/bmjopen-2016-015161

Parahoo, K. (2014). *Nursing research: Principles, process and issues* (3rd ed.). London: Palgrave Macmillan.

Peart, A., Lewis, V., Barton, C., Brown, T., White, J., Gascard, D., & Russell, G. (2019). Providing person-centred care for people with multiple chronic conditions: Protocol for a qualitative study incorporating client and staff perspectives. *BMJ Open*, *9*(10), e030581. https://doi.org/10.1136/bmjopen-2019-030581

Rodriguez-Vazquez, R., Jiménez-Fernández, R., Corral-Liria, I., Cabrera-Fernandez, S., Losa-Iglesias, M. E., & Becerro-de-Bengoa-Vallejo, R. (2020). Intergenerational Transmissible Meanings in Breastfeeding in Spain: A Phenomenological Study. *Journal of Pediatric Nursing*, *51*, e108–e114. https://doi.org/10.1016/j.pedn.2019.12.017

Sandelowski, M., & Barroso, J. (2003). Writing the proposal for a qualitative research methodology project. *Qualitative Health Research*, *13*(6), 781–820.

Shrestha, B., Adhikari, B., Shrestha, M., & Sringernyuang, L. (2022). Kidney sellers from a village in Nepal: Protocol for an Ethnographic Study. *JMIR Research Protocols*, *11*(2), e29364. https://doi.org/10.2196/29364

Skyberg, H. L. (2022). Diversity, friction, and harmonisation: An ethnographic study of interprofessional teamwork dynamics. *BMC Health Services Research*, *22*(1), 227. https://doi.org/10.1186/s12913-022-07596-0

Sun, W., Tahsin, F., Barakat-Haddad, C., Turner, J. P., Haughian, C. R., & Abbass-Dick, J. (2019). Exploration of home care nurses' experiences in deprescribing of medications: A qualitative descriptive study. *BMJ Open*, *9*(5), e025606. https://doi.org/10.1136/bmjopen-2018-025606

Timothy, E. K., Graham, F. P., & Levack, W. M. (2016). Transitions in the embodied experience after stroke: Grounded theory study. *Physical Therapy*, *96*(10), 1565–1575.

White, D. R., & Palmieri, P. A. (2022). Women Caring for husbands living with Parkinson's disease: A phenomenological study protocol. *Journal of Personalized Medicine*, *12*(5), 659. https://doi.org/10.3390/jpm12050659

Willett, M. J., Greig, C., Rogers, D., Fenton, S., Duda, J., & Rushton, A. (2019). Barriers and facilitators to recommended physical activity in lower-limb osteoarthritis: Protocol for a qualitative study exploring patients and physiotherapist perspectives using the theoretical domains framework and behaviour change taxonomy. *BMJ Open*, *9*(10), e029199. https://doi.org/10.1136/bmjopen-2019-029199

Zhou, F., Maier, M., Hao, Y., Tang, L., Guo, H., Liu, H., & Liu, Y. (2015). Barriers to research utilization among registered nurses in traditional Chinese medicine hospitals: A Cross-Sectional Survey in China. *Evidence-Based Complementary and Alternative Medicine: eCAM*, *2015*, 475340.

Žiaková, K., Čáp, J., Miertová, M., Gurková, E., & Kurucová, R. (2020). An interpretative phenomenological analysis of dignity in people with multiple sclerosis. *Nursing Ethics*, *27*(3), 686–700.

7 SELECTING MIXED METHODS DESIGNS

INTRODUCTION

The use of mixed methods designs in nursing, health and social care research has increased over the last decade. It has almost become 'fashionable' to combine qualitative and quantitative methods in the same study. However, careful consideration should be given when selecting a mixed methods design, not least to how it aligns with the research questions and how the different methods will be used and for what purpose.

In proposals, researchers should provide a strong justification for more than one method in the same study and their choice of data collection methods. They should explain how the different methods are integrated in the design and demonstrate the potential added value of mixed methods in answering their research questions. The expertise of the research team in each of the different methods should also be evident in the research proposal.

MIXED METHOD DESIGNS

Mixed methods studies have been described as 'mixed methods designs', 'mixed methods frameworks' or 'mixed methods approaches'. A number of labels, such as 'concurrent', 'embedded' or 'sequential', have also been used to describe mixed methods studies. It is not uncommon for researchers to be confused when describing the design of their mixed methods studies. Below is an example, taken from an internet blog, showing the dilemma, agony and confusion that some researchers can face:

> *I collected my data from three medical settings in one phase time where I conducted non-participant observation (i.e., medical consultation was recorded), then a questionnaire that patients had to fill. In the questionnaire, there are qualitative or embedded open-ended questions. I collected documents by the end of my fieldwork. My question is that:*
>
> *Can I say that I used two mixed methods, namely convergent parallel and embedded design? I want to make sure that I am using the correct designs. I would be so grateful if any expert in mixed method research can help in this regard? Am I using the correct design? Or are there*

other designs better than the ones I have used? From my readings, I found these might be the best designs to be used? What do you think?

The consensus among researchers is that a mixed methods study is one that uses qualitative and quantitative approaches (and methods of data collection and analysis aligned with them) in the same study. According to Creswell and Plano Clark (2011), the central premise of mixed methods studies is that 'the use of quantitative and qualitative approaches in combination provides a better understanding of research problems than one approach alone' (p. 5).

The term 'mixed methods' is unfortunate when researchers are in reality combining different approaches (qualitative and quantitative) in the same study. The terms 'multimethod' or 'combination of methods' are sometimes used to refer to studies in which two or more methods from the same approach are used in the same study. For example, we can use focus groups and one-to-one semi-structured interviews in one qualitative study, or questionnaires and structured observations in a quantitative study.

The term 'mixed methods' is credited to Campbell and Fiske (1959). However, it was not until 2006 that mixed methods studies began to increase rapidly in the health and social sciences (Timans et al., 2019). Academic journals have grown accustomed to mixed methods studies and, indeed, some of them welcome such studies. The *Journal of Mixed Methods Research* was established in 2007. The Medical Research Council guidance on developing and evaluating complex interventions (Moore et al., 2015) highlighted the benefits of using qualitative and quantitative approaches, including to provide a better understanding of the barriers to participation (in interventions) and to estimate response rates. The guidance gives a number of examples of how qualitative and quantitative approaches have been used to develop and evaluate interventions. Whitley et al. (2020) have pointed out that 'mixed methods research, where quantitative and qualitative methods are integrated, is an ideal solution to comprehensively understand complex clinical problems in the pre-hospital setting' (p. 44).

TYPES OF MIXED METHODS DESIGN

There are a number of mixed methods designs as well as variants of these. Creswell and Plano Clark (2011) identified four major types of mixed methods design: triangulation, embedded, explanatory and exploratory.

The Triangulation Design

The triangulation design is appropriate when researchers want to answer the same research question by collecting data from different methods. The aim is to find out if there is agreement (convergence) or contradiction (divergence) between the findings of the different data collection methods. There are variants of the triangulation designs, but a detailed discussion of these is outside the scope of this chapter. For a debate on triangulation, see Maxwell (2022) and Morgan (2022).

Heale and Forbes (2013) reminded us that 'triangulation originates in the field of navigation where a location is determined by using the angles from two known points' (p. 98). They explained that triangulation in research 'is the use of more than one approach to researching a question' (p. 98), with the aim of 'increasing confidence in the findings through the confirmation of a proposition using two or more independent measures' (p. 98). When the findings are similar, researchers tend to have more confidence that they are valid and reliable. However, researchers may find that the findings are contradictory. For example, if a questionnaire and qualitative interviews were used to find out if patients are satisfied with the information they received prior to receiving a particular therapy, the findings may show that one method shows that they are satisfied and the other may show the opposite. Researchers in this case would be faced with the challenge of how to interpret these findings. They would need to reflect on the questions asked, the validity and reliability of the two methods, the composition and size of the samples and the context in which data were collected and by whom.

It is not simply a question of choosing to believe the findings of one method rather than the other. Sometimes, the two methods can reveal different or contradictory realities. Take the example of a number of drivers caught speeding along a particular road with the use of a speeding radar gun. All those caught speeding in interviews afterwards stated that they did not think that they were driving over the speed limit. In law, the readings taken by the gun has primacy over the perceptions of the drivers. If this was a research study, one would question whether the radar gun was defective (in terms of calibration) or whether the policeman used it in an appropriate way (in terms of distance and ability to use it). Therefore, the method used to get the readings can be questioned.

On the other hand, the drivers who said they were not speeding may have been talking about their 'impression' or 'perception' of the speed at which they were driving. Sometimes one may get the impression that the car is not going as fast as it is. This information is useful because it forms part of the phenomenon of driving over the speed limit. If one assumes that the radar gun was not defective and that it was used appropriately, the researcher can assume that these drivers were talking about their perceptions of the speed, not the exact speed they were travelling. A subsequent health promotion campaign to reduce speeding can use the interview findings to inform the drivers that when in a car, speed may not seem what it actually is; therefore, they should check their speedometers to make sure they stay within speeding limits.

Triangulation of findings is often used in the evaluation of interventions. For example, Gentry et al. (2018) administered a questionnaire, conducted qualitative interviews and analysed routine data in their evaluation of a 'voluntary family befriending service' (the Home-Start Suffolk [HSS]). They reported, among other things, that the 'triangulation of data from each component revealed that HSS was perceived by diverse stakeholders to successfully support families in need of additional help' (p. 87). Koorts and Gillison (2015) also used triangulation in their evaluation of a community-based physical activity programme. Their rationale was that triangulation strengthens the validity of interpretations through the use of multiple data sources. They explained that integrating findings from different methodologies can improve the study's validity, and overcome the biases inherent in using quantitative and qualitative methodologies alone. Koorts and Gillison (2015) concluded that 'triangulation of the evidence enabled conflicts and consistencies to emerge and be addressed in a transparent and systematic fashion' (p. 7).

Sometimes the two terms 'triangulation' and 'mixed methods' are used interchangeably when different methods are used to study the same phenomenon. However, for purists, triangulation is aimed at answering the same research question about a phenomenon. Apart from methodological triangulation, there are other types such as 'investigator' (two or more researchers), 'theory' (two or more theories) or 'data sources' (several sources). For more detail of the different types of triangulation and their uses see Adams et al. (2015).

Triangulation can also be used within solely qualitative studies or within quantitative studies. Carter et al. (2014) and Fusch et al. (2018) provided helpful insights into the use of triangulation in qualitative studies. Noble and Heale (2019) provided examples of how triangulation was used in two studies. Fisher et al. (2021) published a protocol for a study on the impact of the large-scale implementation of early supported discharge for stroke, with the protocol including triangulation. Proposal Example 7.1 shows how a triangulation design will be used in a mixed methods study.

The Embedded Design

In some ways the embedded design is similar to the triangulation as used by Gentry et al. (2018) and Koorts and Gillison (2015) in their evaluation studies. The difference between the two (triangulation and embedded) is that an embedded design is mainly quantitative or qualitative. To 'embed' is, according to the Longman dictionary, to 'put something firmly and deeply into something else'. Creswell and Plano Clark (2011) described the embedded design as 'one in

---

PROPOSAL EXAMPLE 7.1
A TRIANGULATION DESIGN IN A MIXED METHODS STUDY

Liu et al. (2022), 'Multilevel determinants of racial/ethnic disparities in severe maternal morbidity and mortality in the context of the COVID-19 pandemic in the USA: protocol for a concurrent triangulation, mixed-methods study'.

COMMENTS

1. In this study, the authors 'hypothesise that social contexts might hinder maternity care and worsen mental health conditions among black and Hispanic women during the pandemic and exacerbate racial/ethnic disparities' (p. 6) in maternal morbidity and mortality.

2. They will use a convergent, parallel, triangulation design to collect quantitative and qualitative data to answer their research questions. According to Liu et al. (2022), this will allow them to 'comprehensively examine the impacts of structural racism and discrimination on maternal health and the complex pathways between multilevel determinants' (p. 8). Quantitative data retrieved from a number of national and local databases and records, and qualitative data, will be collected via in-depth interviews with pregnant and postpartum women (20 African American and 20 Hispanic) and 10 maternity care providers.

3. It is rare that a triangulation mixed methods study will aim narrowly at comparing the findings of two or more methods to answer the same question. It is more likely that the triangulation design will be used for multiple purposes. For example, in this study, the authors will propose using quantitative and qualitative methods to look for congruence as well as complementarity, by comparing and contrasting the data from the two methods.

4. To help readers understand how data from the different methods will be integrated, Lui et al. (2022) provide a visual display.

which one data set provides a supportive, secondary role in a study based primarily on the other data type' (p. 67).

A common type of embedded design is the randomised controlled trial that includes some qualitative methods to explore the process of the implementation of an intervention and/or participants' perceptions of the intervention. In a randomised controlled trial evaluating a psychosocial intervention for men with prostate cancer and their partners, McCaughan et al. (2015) wanted to explore the experience and perceptions of these men and their partners of the intervention through qualitative interviews with participants. They also interviewed and observed the facilitators to find out how they delivered the intervention and their views on its implementation. In this project, the main design was the controlled trial, because without the trial there would be no need for the qualitative phase. The primary focus of the study was on the outcomes of the intervention. The qualitative element added value to the study by providing insight into the process of implementating the intervention. Together the quantitative and qualitative data provided a more rounded evaluation of the intervention and helped to put the findings of the quantitative part of the study in context. In this study, the qualitative methods were firmly and deeply embedded in the trial (quantitative).

Embedded mixed methods designs normally consist of one large study using one approach (e.g. quantitative) with smaller components of another approach (e.g. qualitative). This could also be the other way around. For example, in a study of patients' perspectives on handling multidrug-resistant bacterial microorganisms and hygiene measures in end-of-life care, Heckel et al. (2020) used a mixed methods design where a qualitative approach was the larger study into which a smaller quantitative approach was embedded. As Heckel et al. (2020) explained, 'a quantitative component was embedded in qualitative data collection and analysis with the qualitative component being dominant in the mixed-methods study design' (p. 220). Their choice of an exploratory design (qualitative) supported by a smaller quantitative component was based on the lack of studies on this topic.

One rule of thumb in deciding when to use an embedded mixed-methods design is to identify which of the two components (qualitative or quantitative) is the main part, without which the other is not required or necessary. For example, in the above study by McCaughan et al. (2015), the primary or main study is the randomised controlled trial, without which there would be no need to explore patients' views of the intervention or the facilitators' experience of implementing the intervention. Terms such as 'dominant', 'core', 'main', 'primary' and 'larger' study have been used to describe the part of an embedded mixed methods study into which the smaller part fits. However, using terms such as 'dominant' or 'core' should not give the impression that the smaller component is subordinate and therefore 'less important'. In a proposal, it is crucial that the two components (quantitative and qualitative) are fully described and justified. Reviewers are likely to scrutinise every aspect of the design and will expect all the necessary detail to be provided when assessing proposals.

Two examples of proposals for studies using an embedded mixed methods design in proposals are:

- Wiangkham et al. (2019), 'Pragmatic cluster randomised double-blind pilot and feasibility trial of an active behavioural physiotherapy intervention for acute non-specific neck pain: a mixed-methods protocol'.

- Salomon-Gimmon et al. (2019), 'Process and outcomes evaluation of a pre-academic arts program for individuals with mental health conditions: a mixed methods study protocol.

Proposal Example 7.2 shows how a qualitative component was embedded in a feasibility trial of a 'telerehabilitation combined with exergames' intervention.

The Explanatory Design

As the term 'explanatory' suggests, this is used when one method/approach is used to explain the findings and issues arising from the use of another. In particular, it is a design selected when quantitative findings require further exploration by qualitative methods. For example, if the results of a quantitative study are not what the researchers expected, they can go back to some of the participants and find out why this may be the case. It may be that they did not understand some terms or questions in the questionnaire or that the sample was not broadly representative of the population (i.e. there was an over-representation of certain groups). Researchers may also want to explore some of the quantitative findings in more depth.

The key to using this design is that the questions explored by the qualitative methods (interviews or focus groups) must come from, or be based on, the findings of the first (quantitative) phase. This is a rather tricky issue for researchers developing a proposal for a study based on an

---

PROPOSAL EXAMPLE 7.2
AN EMBEDDED DESIGN IN A MIXED METHODS STUDY

Allegue et al. (2019), 'Optimization of upper extremity rehabilitation by combining telerehabilitation with an exergame in people with chronic stroke: protocol for a mixed methods study'.

This is a mixed methods study, including a randomised, blinded feasibility trial (quantitative component) with an 'embedded multiple case study' (qualitative component).

COMMENTS

1. It is clear that the trial is the main component without which the qualitative phase would not be required. However, the authors recognise that combining quantitative and qualitative approaches 'makes it possible to construct a more complete image of the studied phenomenon' (p. 8) and that 'the combination of the two methodologies should be approached not from the point of view of their differences but from the complementarities they can bring to the study'(p. 8).

2. The outcomes measured in the trial include 'upper extremity motor recovery, function, quality of life, and motivation in participants with chronic stroke' (p. 1). These outcomes will be measured quantitatively. The qualitative component will consist of semistructured interviews with some participants and with therapists delivering the intervention. Therefore, 'the feasibility trial examines the content of the intervention to see if it is effective and feasible' (p. 8) and the qualitative approach 'examines the context of the intervention to see if it can be accepted and applied in clinical practice and explain some of the quantitative findings' (p. 8). One can see how the two approaches (quantitative and qualitative) are integrated into one study.

3. Of note in this proposal is the equal amount of detail provided by the authors to describe and justify each of the two components. It is clear that the authors do not believe that one component is more important than the other.

explanatory mixed methods design. The reason for this is that researchers do not know in advance the questions to be explored by the qualitative methods in the second phase. In the proposal for a study exploring 'symptom burden and its management, in Saudi Arabian patients receiving haemodialysis, and their caregivers', Alshammari et al. (2019) chose a sequential explanatory design. They explain that the main focus of qualitative interviews will be 'to provide an in-depth understanding of the significant, unexpected or unexplained results which may arise during the quantitative phase, such as individuals who reported extreme symptom burden scores, either low or high' (p. 3). They go on to say that qualitative interviews will also explore the impact of living with symptoms in patients receiving haemodialysis and their caregivers as well as to discuss self-management strategies. This example from Alshammari et al. (2019) shows that research designs in practice do not always follow the 'ideal type' described in articles or textbooks. Apart from using qualitative interviews to explain unexpected questions from the quantitative phase, the authors aim to explore additional, pre-selected questions that would normally fit into an embedded mixed methods design.

In a proposal for a study on recreational cannabis usage among young adults living with diabetes', Ibrahim et al. (2020) propose to 'use a sequential, explanatory mixed (quantitative followed by qualitative) methods design' (p. 1409). In phase 1, a quantitative online survey will be completed. Phase 2 will involve semi-structured, one-to-one telephone interviews 'to attain a more comprehensive understanding of the motivations for cannabis use and the management of diabetes' (p. 1409). On the face of it, one could say that this is more of an embedded than explanatory design, since the focus of the qualitative interviews is pre-selected and does not seem to aim to explain the results of phase 1. This example shows that researchers sometimes use these terms loosely and subjectively. This, of course, does not affect the rigour of the study, or the findings. When in doubt, it is always better to explain what is to be done and why, without applying labels that may confuse rather than clarify.

Meixner et al. (2013) carried out a mixed methods study to understand the perceived barriers to accessing crisis intervention services for individuals with acquired brain injury. In phase 1, they carried out a survey of 226 providers. Phase 2 consisted of seven focus group interviews with 25 participants, the purpose of which was to 'add explanatory power to phase one results' (p. 377). The focus group interview questions were developed after a preliminary analysis of phase one data. The aim was 'to explain quantitative findings and add depth to the analysts' understanding of the research phenomenon' (p. 379). The qualitative phase was also useful in adding depth to the researchers' understanding of the barriers to accessing general mental health services. According to the authors, 'this design added rigor to the study – allowing the research team to expand, explore, and understand descriptive survey findings' (p. 384). Meixner et al. (2013) did not actually use the label 'explanatory mixed methods' in this paper. However, what they described and the reasons they gave for their decisions were clear enough for readers to understand the way in which they were using a qualitative phase to explain the findings of the survey.

Some examples of research proposals of studies using explanatory mixed methods design are:

- Steen et al. (2022), 'Self-compassion education for health professionals (nurses and midwives): protocol for a sequential explanatory mixed methods study'.

- Sridhar et al. (2022), 'Implementation strategy mapping methods to improve autism intervention use in community settings: a study protocol'.
- Brockway et al. (2018), 'Breastfeeding self-efficacy and breastmilk feeding for moderate and late preterm infants in the family integrated care trial: a mixed methods protocol'.

Proposal Example 7.3 shows how an explanatory mixed methods design was used in a study.

The Exploratory Design

While the aim of the explanatory design is to use one method (e.g. qualitative) to explain issues arising out of the other (e.g. quantitative), the aim of the exploratory design in mixed methods studies is for one method (e.g. qualitative) to inform the use of another method (e.g. quantitative). The most common example is when qualitative methods (e.g. interviews, focus groups or observations) are used to develop and reinforce quantitative methods (questionnaires, scales or instruments).

PROPOSAL EXAMPLE 7.3
AN EXPLANATORY DESIGN IN A MIXED METHODS STUDY

Keys et al. (2018), 'Using play to improve infant sleep: a mixed methods protocol to evaluate the effectiveness of the Play2Sleep intervention'.

The overall research question in this study is 'how do parental perceptions of family experiences, processes, and contexts related to infant sleep explain the effectiveness of Play2Sleep?' (p. 1).

COMMENTS

1. This study is in three phases. Phase 1 will be a randomised controlled trial. Phase 2 will consist of qualitative interviews with participating families about their perceptions and experiences related to their infant's sleep. Phase 3 will focus on explaining the quantitative results from phase 1 using the qualitative findings from phase 2. Therefore, the explanatory design is operational in phase 3, where 'mixed methods integration will use qualitative findings to explain quantitative results' (p. 3).

2. The authors explained that:

   in Phase 3, the researchers will use the themes from the qualitative data to explain the quantitative results. During this phase, the researchers will explore how themes relate not only to the quantitative results but also how they relate to the theoretical research framework from which the Play2Sleep intervention was developed.

   (p. 10)

   They went on to explain how 'understanding the explanatory mechanisms that contribute to the effectiveness of infant sleep interventions may help researchers and practitioners design and tailor future infant sleep interventions that are meaningful and effective for families' (p. 10). According to them 'this approach will maximize the value of using a mixed methods approach to evaluate Play2Sleep' (p. 10).

3. This proposal is a good example of how the different methods and phases are well described and justified.

The strength of qualitative research is in exploring phenomena. Therefore, it is not surprising that it is used, in particular, to provide understanding and insight into issues that we know little about. Scales and other quantitative instruments are often developed for a specific population. They may not be wholly appropriate for use with populations in other cultures. For example, Shiyanbola et al. (2021) conducted an exploratory sequential mixed methods study to 'culturally adapt' the Illness Perception Questionnaire-Revised (IPQ-R) to address the sociocultural contexts of African American individuals with type 2 diabetes because the tool does not take into account 'the underlying sociocultural factors that might influence the illness beliefs of African Americans' (p. 797). According to Shiyanbola et al. (2021) 'mixed method approaches offer opportunities to study contextual factors such as culture, perceptions, beliefs qualitatively and develop quantitative measures' (p. 798). They used the 'building approach to systematically develop quantitative items' (p. 798) for the questionnaire based on qualitative data. They also concluded that 'the exploratory sequential mixed methods study design was needed in this study for increasing the validity and reliability of the adapted instrument' (p. 799).

Exploratory mixed methods have the potential to make questionnaires or instruments more 'participant' and 'setting' centred. In a study of 'Trauma coping of mothers and children among poor people in Haiti', Roysircar et al. (2019) used a mixed method exploratory design. They explained that 'The goal of the mixed methods was to use both types of evidence: the qualitative to develop a model and to identify some hypotheses based on the model, and the quantitative to test that model' (p. 1192). They conducted focus groups 'to develop a conceptual model of Haitian mothers' ways of coping and beliefs' (p. 1192). In the quantitative phase they tested 'children's trauma adjustment scores based upon the qualitative conceptual model' (p. 1192). Roysircar et al. (2019) explained that 'their strategy was an appropriate methodology to understand coping with continuous trauma from the perspective of Haitian mothers, especially when the mothers were of different cultural groups than the investigators' (p. 1192).

The value of exploratory mixed methods designs has been well articulated by Berman (2017) in their study of researchers' data management practices at the University of Vermont, USA. The author gave a broad rationale for combining both qualitative and quantitative approaches and went on to explain how the data from phase 1 (qualitative) were used to develop a survey instrument for the second, quantitative phase. This study has a third phase in which Berman (2017) showed how data from the first two phases were integrated. The author explained that the use of qualitative and quantitative data collection methods in a single study is not enough to categorise a study as mixed methods; 'it is in the integration or linking of the two strands of data that defines mixed methods research and highlights its value' (Berman, 2017, p. 7). According to Berman (2017), the 'strength of the mixed methods approach allowed for a deep dive into understanding the lived experiences of researchers' data management practices via qualitative methods, while using the results of the qualitative analysis to build a survey instrument to more accurately measure data management activities', including 'behaviours and attitudes towards data management planning' (p. 19).

For examples of protocols of exploratory mixed methods, see:

■ Salvador et al. (2019), 'Development of Filipino nurse educator's wellbeing survey (FNEWS): an exploratory sequential mixed methods study'.

- Taylor et al. (2019), " 'Your Tube': the role of different diets in children who are gastrostomy fed: protocol for a mixed methods exploratory sequential study'.
- Halim et al. (2021), 'Compliance of Malaysian healthcare workers towards tuberculosis prevention programmes in workplace: An exploratory sequential mixed method study protocol'.

Proposal Example 7.4 shows how qualitative and quantitative methods complement each other in an exploratory mixed methods study.

Concurrent and Sequential Designs

Another aspect of mixed methods design that some researchers agonise about is whether the methods should be concurrent or sequential. Concurrent, or parallel, data collection and analysis means that the quantitative and qualitative parts of the study are carried out at the same time; there are no phases. Sequential means that there are at least two phases, one followed by the other. A mixed methods is sequential when one component (e.g. quantitative) has to be completed before the other (qualitative) can start, because one depends on the other (for more explanation see, for example, Schoonenboom and Johnson, 2017).

PROPOSAL EXAMPLE 7.4
AN EXPLORATORY DESIGN IN A MIXED METHODS STUDY

Diaz et al. (2021), 'Female genital mutilation/cutting education for midwives and nurses as informed by women's experiences: protocol for an exploratory sequential mixed methods study'.

COMMENTS

1. This study is in three phases. In phase 1, semistructured interviews will be carried out to explore the views and experiences of women with female genital mutilation/cutting (FGM/C) accessing maternity and gynecological (including sexual health) services in South Australia. The aim of phase 1 is to produce findings 'to develop an educational program for midwives and nurses on the health and cultural needs of women with FGM/C' (p. 1).

2. The authors explained that 'exploratory designs are data driven and enable researchers to explore the topic first where there is limited understanding of it or no prior conceptual frameworks' (p. 3). FGM/C is not likely to be a topic that midwives and nurses will know a lot about since it is an illegal activity in Australia and in many other countries. The qualitative phase is therefore crucial to the development of this educational programme to 'improve midwives' and nurses' clinical skills, cultural competence, confidence, and awareness of legal responsibilities to effectively support the needs of women with FGM/C' (p. 2). The program will be evaluated in phase 3.

3. The findings of the qualitative, exploratory phase will enable the development in a programme that will be tested quantitatively in the third phase. This shows how, according to the authors, 'integrating qualitative and quantitative data in mixed methods allows each approach to complement each other' (p. 3).

MIXED METHODS DESIGNS AS IDEAL TYPES

The aim of describing and differentiating between these four mixed methods designs (triangulation, embedded, explanatory and exploratory) was to show the many ways in which mixed designs can be used in the same study. It was not an exercise in how to label mixed methods designs 'correctly'. This is because these four designs are 'ideal types' or how 'purists' would perceive them. The term 'ideal type' was developed by the German sociologist Max Weber, who used the term for sociological analysis. These ideal type descriptions or definitions rarely exist in real life. They overlap in that they have elements of complementarity, exploration, triangulation and explanation. This is why it is difficult to find research examples in the literature that fit neatly into these four types of design. Researchers should understand that selecting designs depends on the aim of the study. They should explain why and how combining quantitative and qualitative methods would be more enlightening for the phenomenon under investigation than a single method or approach. Above all they should show how the different methods or approaches will be integrated.

Some useful articles on designing mixed methods studies are:

- Schoonenboom and Johnson (2017), 'How to construct a mixed methods research design'.
- Vedel et al. (2019), 'Why and how to use mixed methods in primary health care research'.
- Kajamaa et al. (2020), 'How to ... do mixed-methods research'.
- Fetters et al. (2013), 'Achieving integration in mixed methods designs – principles and practices'.

DESCRIBING MIXED METHODS STUDIES IN RESEARCH PROPOSALS

As the number of mixed methods studies increases, attention turns to how to conduct high-quality mixed methods studies. Reviewers are also getting more experience in evaluating mixed methods research proposals. It is not surprising to find more and more papers on how to appraise mixed methods studies' papers and proposals. Examples of publications on the appraisal of mixed methods studies and how to report these studies, include:

- Heyvaert et al. (2013), 'Critical appraisal of mixed methods studies'.
- Cameron et al. (2013), 'Lessons from the field: applying the good reporting of a mixed methods study (GRAMMS) framework'.
- Creswell and Hirose (2019), 'Mixed methods and survey research in family medicine and community health'.
- Moorley and Cathala (2019), 'How to appraise mixed methods research'.

These appraisals are also useful for those developing proposals as they identify areas or aspects of mixed methods studies that are missing or not presented when they are reported in journals. For example, Huynh et al. (2019), who reviewed mixed methods in 'mindful research', found a number of gaps in reporting, including the rationale for mixing methods. Younas et al. (2019) reviewed 175 mixed method studies in nursing and reported, among other things, that 31% of the studies did not justify using mixed methods, 95% did not identify the research paradigm, and 78% did not state the weight given to individual phases.

Mixed methods research proposals seem to have some of the same limitations. Mabila (2017) reviewed the mixed methods research proposals of 67 postgraduate students in one university. The author reported that there were 'conflicting and divergent interpretations' (p. 136) of mixed methods research. Most of these proposals 'give no philosophical foundation' (p. 136) for combining methods and were unclear about their selected design and justification for their choice of design.

Guetterman et al. (2019) analysed comments of panel members, for grant applications submitted to the National Institutes of Health (NIH) in the USA. The proposals that were favourably appraised showed 'coherence among aims and research designs/elements, detailed methods, plans for mixed methods integration and the use of theoretical models' (p. 1). The identified weaknesses in these proposals were: 'lack of methodological details, high 'participant burden', failure to show integration between the qualitative and quantitative components and a lack of detail regarding investigator roles. Some of these comments (such as on the use of conceptual frameworks or models) would apply to any proposal. However, mixed methods proposals are different in that they involve two methodologies (quantitative and qualitative), both requiring equal treatment and equal attention to detail, even if one method forms the larger or core part of the study. Therefore, researchers should be twice as vigilant when developing mixed methods proposals.

Perhaps the first thing reviewers look for in such proposals is the rationale for mixing methods. Broad statements that qualitative methods will provide a deeper understanding of the topic or phenomenon under investigation are not sufficient. Authors of proposals should show the gap in knowledge on the topic and how the methods, together, will address it. Similarly, it is not enough to say that the qualitative methods and their findings will be used to inform the development of interventions or instruments. It is crucial to explain, in some detail, how this will be done.

Comments from one of the panel reviewers in Guetterman et al.'s (2019) study related to the integration of the two methods in mixed methods studies. Fetters et al. (2013) have outlined the principles and practices for achieving integration in mixed methods designs. They gave examples of how integration occurs at the 'study design level', at the 'method level' and at the 'interpretation and reporting level' (p. 2134). One of the ways in which these types of integration can be presented is through visual displays. For examples and discussion of visual displays in mixed methods articles and proposals, see Guetterman et al. (2020).

Based on their review of the NIH panel's comments, Guetterman et al. (2019) made a series of recommendations that can be used as a checklist for mixed methods proposals to any funding panel or simply for writing good quality proposals.

Checklist for the design section of mixed methods proposals:
  This checklist is only for the design section of mixed methods studies in proposals.
  1. What is the rationale for choosing a mixed methods design? (e.g. What will the different methods, as opposed to a single method, add to the study?)
  2. What type of mixed methods design is selected for this study?
  3. Is there evidence that the different methods are carefully selected? (e.g. Why choose a survey, case study or ethnography?)
  4. Is there a clear plan of how the different methods relate to one another and are integrated?
  5. Are all the different methods (and phases) sufficiently described?
  6. Is there evidence in the proposal that the team includes researchers experienced in quantitative and qualitative methods?

SUMMARY AND CONCLUSIONS

While the popularity of mixed methods studies is increasing, it is important to show that the proposed study would really benefit from the use of different methods. The gap that the study fills and the added value of combining methods should be clearly articulated. The research questions that each method seeks to answer, and the conceptual framework underpinning the questions should also be clear.

Although one method may be dominant, the methodological details of the smaller component of the study should, nevertheless, be adequately described. Each method's contribution should be equally recognised. Clear pathways with data for each method should be shown, if possible, in the form of visual displays.

REFERENCES

Adams, J., Bateman, B., Becker, F., Cresswell, T., Flynn, D., McNaughton, R., Oluboyede, Y., Robalino, S., Ternent, L., Sood, B. G., Michie, S., Shucksmith, J., Sniehotta, F. F., & Wigham, S. (2015). Effectiveness and acceptability of parental financial incentives and quasi-mandatory schemes for increasing uptake of vaccinations in pre-school children: Systematic review, qualitative study and discrete choice experiment. *Health Technology Assessment (Winchester, England)*, *19*(94), 1–176.

Allegue, D. R., Kairy, D., Higgins, J., Archambault, P., Michaud, F., Miller, W., Sweet, S. N., & Tousignant, M. (2020). Optimization of upper extremity rehabilitation by combining telerehabilitation with an exergame in people with chronic stroke: Protocol for a Mixed Methods Study. *JMIR Research Protocols*, *9*(5), e14629. https://doi.org/10.2196/14629

Alshammari, B., Noble, H., McAneney, H., & O'Halloran, P. (2019). An exploration of symptom burden and its management, in Saudi Arabian patients receiving haemodialysis, and their caregivers: A mixed methods study protocol. *BMC Nephrology*, *20*(1), 250. https://doi.org/10.1186/s12882-019-1424-9

Berman, E. A. (2017). An exploratory sequential mixed methods approach to understanding researchers' Data Management Practices at UVM: Integrated findings to develop research data services. *Journal of eScience Librarianship*, *6*(1), e1104. https://doi.org/10.7191/jeslib.2017.1104; https://escholarship.umassmed.edu/jeslib/vol6/iss1/7

Brockway, M., Benzies, K. M., Carr, E., & Aziz, K. (2018). Breastfeeding self-efficacy and breastmilk feeding for moderate and late preterm infants in the family integrated care trial: A mixed methods protocol. *International Breastfeeding Journal*, *13*, 29. https://dx.doi.org/10.1186/s13006-018-0168-7

Cameron, R., & Dwyer, T., Richardson, S., Ahmed, E., & Sukumaran, A. (2013). Lessons from the Field: Applying the Good Reporting of a Mixed Methods Study (GRAMMS) Framework. *Electronic Journal of Business Research Methods*, *11*(2), 53–66.

Campbell, D., & Fiske, D. (1959). Convergent and discriminant validation by the multitrait-multimethod matrix. *Psychological Bulletin*, *56*(2), 81–105.

Carter, N., Bryant-Lukosius, D., DiCenso, A., Blythe, J., & Neville, A. J. (2014). The use of triangulation in qualitative research. *Oncology Nursing Forum*, *41*(5), 545–547.

Creswell, J. W., & Hirose, M. (2019). Mixed methods and survey research in family medicine and community health. *Family Medicine and Community Health*, *7*(2), e000086. https://doi.org/10.1136/fmch-2018-000086

Creswell, J. W., & Plano Clark, V. L. (2011). *Designing and conducting mixed methods research*. Los Angeles, Calif: SAGE Publications.

Diaz, M. P., Steen, M., Brown, A., Fleet, J., & Williams, J. (2021). Female genital mutilation/cutting education for midwives and nurses as informed by women's experiences: Protocol for an exploratory sequential mixed methods study. *JMIR Research Protocols, 10*(10), e32911 https://doi.org/10.2196/32911

Fetters, M. D., Curry, L. A., & Creswell, J. W. (2013). Achieving integration in mixed methods designs – principles and practices. *Health Services Research, 48*(6 Pt 2), 2134–2156.

Fisher, R. J., Chouliara, N., Byrne, A., Cameron, T., Lewis, S., Langhorne, P., Robinson, T., Waring, J., Geue, C., Paley, L., Rudd, A., & Walker, M. F. (2021). *Large-scale implementation of stroke early supported discharge: The WISE realist mixed-methods study.* Health Services and Delivery Research, No. 9.22. Southampton, UK: NIHR Journals Library. https://www.ncbi.nlm.nih.gov/books/NBK575455.

Fusch, P., Fusch, G. E., & Ness, L. R. (2018). Denzin's paradigm shift: Revisiting triangulation in qualitative research. *Journal of Social Change, 10*(1), 19–32.

Gentry, S. V., Powers, E. F. J., Azim, N., & Maidrag, M. (2018). Effectiveness of a voluntary family befriending service: A mixed methods evaluation using the Donabedian model. *Public Health, 160*, 87–93.

Guetterman, T. C., Molina-Azorin, J. F., & Fetters, M. D. (2020). Virtual Special Issue on 'Integration in Mixed Methods Research.' *Journal of Mixed Methods Research, 14*(4), 430–435.

Guetterman, T. C., Sakakibara, R. V., Plano Clark, V. L., Luborsky, M., Murray, S. M., Castro, F. G., Creswell, J. W., Deutsch, C., & Gallo, J. J. (2019). Mixed methods grant applications in the health sciences: An analysis of reviewer comments. *PLoS One, 14*(11), e0225308. https://doi.org/10.1371/journal.pone.0225308

Halim, I., Reffin, N., Sharifa Ezat, W. P., Muhamad, N. A., & Harith, A. A. (2021). Compliance of Malaysian healthcare workers towards tuberculosis prevention programmes in workplace: An exploratory sequential mixed method study protocol. *Medical Journal of Malaysia, 76*(6), 857–864.

Heale, R., & Forbes, D. (2013). Understanding triangulation in research. *Evidence-Based Nursing, 16*(4), 98.

Heckel, M., Sturm, A., Stiel, S., Ostgathe, C., Herbst, F. A., Tiedtke, J., Adelhardt, T., Reichert, K., & Sieber, C. (2020). '. . . and then no more kisses!' Exploring patients' experiences on multidrug-resistant bacterial microorganisms and hygiene measures in end-of-life care A mixed-methods study. *Palliative Medicine, 34*(2), 219–230.

Heyvaert, M., Hannes, K., Maes, B., & Onghena, P. (2013). Critical appraisal of mixed methods studies. *Journal of Mixed Methods Research, 7*(4), 302–327.

Huynh, T., Hatton-Bowers, H., & Howell Smith, M. (2019). A critical methodological review of mixed methods designs used in mindfulness research. *Mindfulness, 10*, 786–798.

Ibrahim, S., Sidani, S., Lok, J., Mukerji, G., & Sherifali, D. (2020). Recreational cannabis usage among young adults living with diabetes: Protocol for a mixed methods study. *Diabetes Therapy: Research, Treatment and Education of Diabetes and Related Disorders, 11*(6), 1407–1417. https://doi.org/10.1007/s13300-020-00818-w

Kajamaa, A., Mattick, K., & de la Croix, A. (2020). How to ... do mixed-methods research. *The Clinical Teacher, 17*(3), 267–271.

Keys, E., Benzies, K. M., Kirk, V., & Duffett-Leger, L. (2018). Using play to improve infant sleep: A mixed methods protocol to evaluate the effectiveness of the Play2Sleep intervention. *Frontiers in Psychiatry Frontiers Research Foundation, 9*, 109. https://dx.doi.org/10.3389/fpsyt.2018.00109

Koorts, H., & Gillison, F. (2015). Mixed method evaluation of a community-based physical activity program using the RE-AIM framework: Practical application in a real-world setting. *BMC Public Health, 15*, 1102. https://doi.org/10.1186/s12889-015-2466-y

Liu, J., Hung, P., Liang, C., Zhang, J., Qiao, S., Campbell, B. A., Olatosi, B., Torres, M. E., Hikmet, N., & Li, X. (2022). Multilevel determinants of racial/ethnic disparities in severe maternal morbidity and mortality in the context of the COVID-19 pandemic in the USA: Protocol for a concurrent triangulation, mixed-methods study. *BMJ Open, 12*(6), e062294. https://doi.org/10.1136/bmjopen-2022-062294

Mabila, T. E. (2017). Postgraduate students' understanding of mixed methods research design at the proposal stage. *South African Journal of Higher Education, 31*, 136–153.

Maxwell, J. A. (2022). Response to David Morgan on Triangulation. *Journal of Mixed Methods Research*, *16*(4), 412–414.

McCaughan, E., McKenna, S., McSorley, O., & Parahoo, K. (2015). The experience and perceptions of men with prostate cancer and their partners of the CONNECT psychosocial intervention: A qualitative exploration. *Journal of Advanced Nursing*, *71*(8), 1871–1882.

Meixner, C., O'Donoghue, C. R., & Witt, M. (2013). Accessing crisis intervention services after brain injury: A mixed methods study. *Rehabilitation Psychology*, *58*(4), 377–385. https://doi.org/10.1037/a0033892

Moore, G. F., Audrey, S., Barker, M., Bond, L., Bonell, C., & Hardeman, W. (2015). Process evaluation of complex interventions: Medical Research Council guidance. *BMJ*, *350*, h1258. https://doi.org/10.1136/bmj.h1258

Moorley, C., & Cathala, X. (2019). How to appraise mixed methods research. *Evidence-Based Nursing*, *22*(2), 38–41.

Morgan, D. L. (2022). Reply to Maxwell. *Journal of Mixed Methods Research*, *16*(4), 415–417.

Noble, H., & Heale, R. (2019). Triangulation in research, with examples. *Evidence-Based Nursing*, *22*(3), 67–68.

Roysircar, G., Thompson, A., & Geisinger, K. F. (2019). Trauma coping of mothers and children among poor people in Haiti: Mixed methods study of community-level research. *American Psychologist*, *74*(9), 1189–1206.

Salomon-Gimmon, M., Orkibi, H., & Elefant, C. (2019). Process and outcomes evaluation of a pre-academic arts program for individuals with mental health conditions: A mixed methods study protocol. *BMJ Open*, *9*, e025604. https://doi.org/10.1136/bmjopen-2018-025604

Salvador, J. T., Alqahtani, F. M., Al-Garni, R. S. S. (2019). Development of Filipino Nurse Educator's Wellbeing Survey (FNEWS): An Exploratory Sequential Mixed Methods Study. *Open Nursing Journal*, *13*, 139–152.

Schoonenboom, J., & Johnson, R. B. (2017). How to construct a mixed methods research design. *Kolner Zeitschrift fur Soziologie und Sozialpsychologie*, *69*(Suppl. 2), 107–131.

Shiyanbola, O. O., Rao, D., Bolt, D., Brown, C., Zhang, M., & Ward, E. (2021). Using an exploratory sequential mixed methods design to adapt an Illness Perception Questionnaire for African Americans with diabetes: The mixed data integration process. *Health Psychology and Behavioral Medicine*, *9*(1), 796–817.

Sridhar, A., Drahota, A., & Tschida, J. E. (2022). Implementation strategy mapping methods to improve autism intervention use in community settings: A study protocol. *Implementation Science Communications*, *3*, 92. https://dx.doi.org/10.1186/s43058-022-00339-6

Steen, M., Othman, S. M. E., Briley, A., Vernon, R., Hutchinson, S., & Dyer, S. (2022). Self-compassion Education for Health Professionals (Nurses and Midwives): Protocol for a Sequential Explanatory Mixed Methods Study. *JMIR Research Protocols*, *11*(1), e34372. https://dx.doi.org/10.2196/34372PMID: 34848389

Taylor, J., O'Neill, M., Maddison, J., Richardson, G., Hewitt, C., Horridge, K., Cade, J., McCarter, A., Beresford, B., & Fraser, L. K. (2019). 'Your Tube': The role of different diets in children who are gastrostomy fed: Protocol for a mixed methods exploratory sequential study. *BMJ Open*, *9*(10), e033831. https://doi.org/10.1136/bmjopen-2019-033831

Timans, R., Wouters, P., & Heilbron, J. (2019). Mixed methods research: What it is and what it could be. *Theory and Society*, *48*, 193–216.

Vedel, I., Kaur, N., Hong, Q. N., El Sherif, R., Khanassov, V., Godard-Sebillotte, C., Sourial, N., Whitley, G. A., Munro, S., Hemingway, P., Law, G. R., Siriwardena, A. N., Cooke, D., & Quinn, T. (2020). Mixed methods in pre-hospital research: Understanding complex clinical problems. *British Paramedic Journal*, *5*(3), 44–51.

Wiangkham, T., Uthaikhup, S., & Rushton, A. B. (2019). Pragmatic cluster randomised double-blind pilot and feasibility trial of an active behavioural physiotherapy intervention for acute non-specific neck pain: A mixed-methods protocol. *BMJ Open*, *9*(9), e029795. https://doi.org/10.1136/bmjopen-2019-029795

Younas, A., Pedersen, M., & Tayaben, J. L. (2019). Review of mixed-methods research in nursing. *Nursing Research*, *68*(6), 464–472.

8 QUANTITATIVE DATA COLLECTION AND ANALYSIS

■ ■

INTRODUCTION

If the research questions are at the heart of a study and the design describes its overall plan, then the data collection and analysis are the practical sections of the proposal. This is the part that shows 'how' data will be collected and analysed. Therefore, it should, within word limits, give all the important information to show that the methods of data collection and analysis are appropriate, feasible, rigorous and well thought out.

In this chapter, we will explore the main quantitative data collection and analysis methods that researchers designing a study can select from. We will also highlight the key information regarding these methods that should be provided in research proposals. Chapter 9 will examine qualitative data collection and analysis methods. Structured and unstructured observations will be discussed in Chapter 10.

SELECTING METHODS OF DATA COLLECTION

Data collection methods are the tools or strategies used to collect data. Some of these tools are more suited to certain types of design than others. As in previous chapters, we will use the three main types of design to show which data collection methods are appropriate for each of them. For quantitative descriptive and correlational studies, a range of data collection methods are available to collect and analyse data. The choice of method depends on the research questions to be answered.

Quantitative descriptive and correlational studies use measurements to answer questions related to prevalence, incidence and correlations. The most appropriate methods for these types of questions are questionnaires and scales/tools/instruments. These types of data collection methods are structured (a questionnaire/scale is organised into parts or sections), standardised (e.g. everyone receives the same questionnaire/scale), predetermined (the questionnaire/scale is developed prior to being administered) and objective (researchers' views or preferences should not influence the way the data are collected). These questionnaires or scales are administered in the same way to all participants and data obtained from them are statistically analysed using software such as SPSS (Statistical Package for the Social Sciences). For causal questions (in trials), outcomes are measured by instruments or scales and the data are also analysed statistically.

In research proposals, the link between research questions and the methods of data collection should be made clear. Reviewers should not have to search for this information by reading large chunks of the text. If a number of outcomes are to be measured, each of these should be linked to the outcome measures (scales) that will be used. Sometimes, it is helpful to reviewers if a visual display (e.g. in the form of a table) to show these links is provided. For an example of this, see a protocol by Nishi et al. (2020) on a trial on 'an internet-based cognitive-behavioural therapy for prevention of depression during pregnancy and in the postpartum'. The authors provide a table listing all the outcomes (e.g. quality of life) and align them to the outcome measures (e.g. EQ-5D-5L scale). They also provide information about the timings of these measurements (e.g. at 32 weeks' gestation, etc.).

DATA COLLECTION AND ANALYSIS METHODS

The main data collection methods discussed below are questionnaires and scales. For each of these methods, we will highlight the type of information that should be provided in the relevant section of the proposal and an indication of how appropriate, feasible and rigorous the methods are. Sampling and recruitment, although linked to methods, will be discussed in Chapters 11 and 12.

Questionnaires and Scales

The terms 'questionnaire' and 'scale' are sometimes used interchangeably. While they are both measuring tools, they are different in terms of their purpose, scope and precision. Questionnaires are used mostly to collect broad data on a particular topic. They usually consist of open-ended and closed-ended questions. They are structured into sections, one of which normally collects demographic data such as occupation, age, education, gender, etc. The other sections cover different aspects of the topic being studied. In their study of 'patient's satisfaction with health care', Spasojevic et al. (2015) used a questionnaire that consisted of 44 questions. Apart from demographic questions, there were questions on different aspects of care such as:

> the quality of physical examinations and medical treatment conducted by physician; professional conduct of hospital staff at admission and during hospital stay; conduct of health care professionals in dealing with the patient and satisfaction with primary, secondary and tertiary health care practices.

> *Spasojevic et al. (2015, p. 221)*

Sometimes questionnaires can also include scale-type questions to measure the frequency or intensity of particular feelings or behaviours. For example, in their study, Spasojevic et al. (2015) asked respondents to rate their satisfaction on a 5-point scale of 'poor, fair, good, very good and excellent'.

Scales, on the other hand, are measuring instruments typically designed to measure concepts, variables or outcomes such as resilience, stress, quality of life or self-esteem. They are similar to the scales or instruments that measure temperature, blood pressure, height, weight or body mass. The difference is that scales in nursing, health and social research tend to measure concepts that are not physical or material and are based on participants' responses to particular questions. These scales are carefully developed to represent all important aspects of the concept to be measured and they are tested for validity and reliability.

An example of a scale is the Short Assessment of Patient Satisfaction (SAPS), which was developed by Hawthorne et al. (2006). The SAPS consists of seven items assessing patients' satisfaction with their treatment. The seven 'core domains' are 'treatment satisfaction', 'explanation of treatment results', 'clinician care', 'participation in medical decision-making', 'respect by the clinician', 'time with clinician' and 'satisfaction with hospital/clinic care' (Hawthorne et al., 2006). Each of these items is scored from 0 to 4. These scales have a scoring system and guidance for interpretating the scores. For example, in the SAPS, a total score of 0–10 indicates 'very dissatisfied' and 27 or 28 'very satisfied'. These types of scales are tested for validity and reliability during construction and later, in studies in a variety of settings. For the purpose of this chapter, we will make a distinction between the two terms.

SELECTING DATA COLLECTION METHODS FOR A STUDY

Questionnaires are most appropriate to collect quantitative descriptive and correlational data, in particular relating to prevalence and incidence of phenomena. They can provide a wealth of demographic data that can be used to explore and examine relationships between these (e.g. employment, age, etc.) with behaviours (e.g. use of services), perceptions (e.g. respondents' views on the quality of services) and attitudes, knowledge and beliefs (e.g. respondents' knowledge about attitudes to social distancing during the COVID-19 pandemic).

Researchers should provide a rationale to explain why a questionnaire is the most appropriate data collection method for their study. This may not be obvious to reviewers. For example, if the research question is 'How and when do people with common colds access medical services?', there are different methods that can assist in collecting these data. Researchers can examine and analyse patients' records. They can also ask patients themselves how they access services because these records are not available or reliable. Another reason for choosing questionnaires may be because this is the most common data collection tool for this type of study; this may provide opportunities for comparing findings with other studies. However, researchers should balance the need for originality and innovation with current best practice. Whatever the reasons for selecting a questionnaire to collect data for a study, these should be made clear in the proposal.

Having selected the questionnaire as the appropriate data collection tool, researchers have to decide whether they will construct (or have constructed) their own questionnaire or use an existing one. There are advantages and disadvantages for both approaches, and this is a decision that should be carefully thought out. Constructing and testing one's own questionnaire requires expertise and this process can be a study in itself. There are many texts and articles on how to construct questionnaires. Useful ones include:

- Tsang et al. (2017), 'Guidelines for developing, translating, and validating a questionnaire in perioperative and pain medicine'.
- Price et al. (2017), Chapter 7 in *Research Methods in Psychology*.

- Mathers et al. (2007), 'Surveys and questionnaires'.
- Yaddanapudi and Yaddanapudi (2019), 'How to design a questionnaire'.
- Robb and Shellenbarger (2020), 'Mastering survey design and questionnaire development'.

For an example of a description of the development of a questionnaire, see Proposal Example 8.1.

Researchers can also 'borrow' questions from other existing questionnaires to construct their own. Hyman et al. (2006) explained that researchers often do not consider using existing questions in their questionnaires, mainly because of 'pressures of being "original" in the academic and research worlds' or 'because of a general lack of awareness of the availability of ready-made questions used in UK social surveys' (p. 1). They point out the existence of 'question banks' such as the UK Data Service (https://ukdataservice.ac.uk/help/other-data-providers/question-banks/). Such 'banks' also exist in other countries such as Canada, the USA, Denmark and Sweden (for a list of these question banks and archives, see the UK Data Service above). The most obvious advantage of using existing questions is that 'pre-existing questions' have been 'extensively tested at the time of first use' (Hyman et al., 2006, p. 1). However, when borrowing questions from other questionnaires researchers must ensure that the 'borrowed' questions fit their questionnaires and that permission for use has been obtained.

Sometimes researchers can borrow a whole questionnaire for their study. However, local circumstances and the specific population that the questionnaire targets can make it difficult to find suitable questionnaires. Making changes to existing questionnaires can affect their reliability and validity so adapted questionnaires should also be tested for reliability and validity, prior to use.

PROPOSAL EXAMPLE 8.1
DESCRIBING THE DEVELOPMENT OF A QUESTIONNAIRE IN A PROPOSAL

Geidl et al. (2018), 'Exercise therapy in medical rehabilitation: study protocol of a national survey at facility and practitioner level with a mixed method design'.

In this study the authors decided to develop a questionnaire to survey 'concepts and processes of exercise therapy practice in medical rehabilitation Germany-wide' (p. 39).

COMMENTS

1. Geidl et al. (2018) described the questionnaire development in four steps. In step 1, a 'pool of comprehensive items' was compiled after a search and review of existing documents and instruments that record concepts and process features in rehabilitation and from expert knowledge. Step 2 'involved designing quality dimensions, quality-relevant action/content areas of exercise therapy and allocating items' (Geidl et al., 2018, p. 39).

2. In step 3, a preliminary version of the questionnaire was piloted with experts from an 'exercise therapy group' and 'selected executives in exercise therapy' to evaluate its 'completeness, answerability, acceptance and understandability' (p. 40). Based on this evaluation and the experts' suggestions for improvement, the final version was prepared. The questionnaire was included as an appendix in the proposal.

3. The detailed description of how the questionnaire was developed would help readers to assess the rigour of the process and the quality of the questionnaire.

Scales

Developing scales is also time-consuming and laborious. This is why researchers tend to use existing ones, where they can, to measure common concepts such as depression, quality of life or self-esteem. There are established and rigorous processes for developing scales. For an example of this, see Mavrinac et al. (2010), who explained in detail how they constructed and validated an Attitudes Toward Plagiarism Questionnaire in a Croatian population. This questionnaire was later adapted by Khairnar et al. (2019) in their 'survey on attitudes of dental professionals about plagiarism in Maharashtra, India'. They modified the scoring system of the Likert-type scale from 5 points to 3 points. They carried out an internal consistency reliability test by calculating the Cronbach's alpha coefficient. Khairnar et al. (2019) also assessed the test–retest reliability of the scale. Researchers aiming to adapt a scale should explain how they intend to change an existing scale and the tests they will carry out before using the modified version. Ideally, the modification and tests for reliability and validity should be carried out prior to developing the proposal.

For some concepts or constructs, there may be a number of scales or instruments to select from. For example, Bergman and Laviana (2014) identified 15 quality of life assessment tools for men with prostate cancer. Which one to choose depends on a number of factors, including how appropriate the tool is for the type of data to be collected. Each of these tools has core areas (domains) such as physical, social, emotional, etc. All these tools include some of the main domains, but some may focus more on some aspects than others (e.g. functional rather than social). The number of domains and items can vary so some of these tools are longer than others. The choice of tool depends on whether 'quality of life' is the primary outcome and requires a comprehensive tool or a secondary outcome that can be measured with a 'brief' scale, with fewer items. The known validity and reliability of the tools and how widely they have been used in other studies are other factors to be taken into account when selecting tools. The target population is another consideration in terms of how easy it is for participants to understand the questions and the time it takes to respond to them.

Showing an awareness of the main tools that are used to measure a concept or outcome and providing a rationale for the choice of instruments will add strength to the proposal. In their proposal for the 'economic evaluation of a complex intervention to improve the mental health of maltreated infants and children in foster care in the UK', Deidda et al. (2018) provide this rationale for selecting the Paediatric Quality of Life Inventory (PedsQL):

The PedsQL questionnaire is used to measure HRQoL in children aged 2–18. The PedsQL is a validated measure of child quality of life which has recently been mapped to utility values for use in health economic evaluations. The PedsQL has demonstrated responsiveness, construct validity and predictive validity in paediatric patients. The PedsQL scores can be mapped to generic EQ-5D utilities, facilitating calculation of QALYs [quality-adjusted life years], thus meeting most recent NICE guidance for public health interventions.

(p. 5)

Deidda et al. (2018) also supported some of the statements made above by citing the relevant literature. More information on how this tool fits into the overall objectives of the study is also provided by the authors.

It is good practice to report the known reliability of the tool, as Schofield et al. (2021) did in their proposal for 'a randomised controlled trial of an online treatment decision aid for men with low-risk prostate cancer and their partners':

> *Prostate cancer-specific quality of life is assessed at baseline and every follow-up with the 26-item Expanded Prostate Cancer Index Composite short-form (EPIC-26). The EPIC-26 comprises four subscales: urinary, bowel, sexual and hormonal. The hormonal subscale is not relevant in this context, so will not be administered. Subscales have shown acceptable internal consistency (all Cronbach's α > 0.70), test-retest reliability (all r > 0.69) and responsiveness when used independently.*

(p. 8)

Quemada-González et al. (2022) went further and provided a table listing all the scales, their 'domains' and their 'concurrent validity', 'interrater reliability' and 'internal consistency' in their proposal for a 'a randomised, controlled trial of a nurse navigator program for the management of hepatitis C virus in patients with severe mental disorder'.

Translation of Questionnaires or Scales

If the proposed study aims to translate a questionnaire or a scale for use with participants speaking a different language, the process of translation should be briefly described in the proposal. This process is itself laborious and time-consuming, and requires expertise. Translating a questionnaire can be a study in itself. If the protocol is about a study that involves the translation of one or more instruments, full consideration to the resource implications should be given. Although 'it is potentially less resource intensive to adapt an existing instrument with reliability and validity evidence than to develop an entirely new one' (Toma et al., 2017, p. 1), the cost of translation, back-translation and psychometric testing can also be significant.

For an example of the translation of an instrument in a protocol, see Winnige et al.'s (2020) study on 'cardiac rehabilitation in the Czech Republic'. They explained the rigorous process they followed for the translation of an English version of a 'cardiac rehabilitation barriers scale' into Czech. Their aim was to ensure that translation 'was accurate, high quality, and culturally-relevant' (p. 2). The translation process also included a psychometric validation of the translated instrument.

Mode of Delivery

In proposals, consideration should be given to the best mode for administering questionnaires. Traditional methods of collecting data include posting questionnaires, administering them via phones and 'face-to-face' interviews. The advantages and disadvantages of these modes of delivery are well documented in the literature. With the increasing use of digital technology, conducting research via the internet has become an established practice, alongside more traditional methods. According to Russell et al. (2018), 'intensifying interest in the potential of new, portable technology tools such as mobile phones and wearables to transform the conduct of clinical trials is a natural outgrowth of the broader societal trend towards digitisation' (p. 127). Russell et al. (2018), who carried out a pilot study to assess the feasibility of collecting and transmitting clinical trial data with mobile technologies, concluded that a wireless data transmission and processing platform was dependable and reliable.

Whatever the mode of delivery (traditional or online), they all have implications. These include compatibility with the population in terms of how to reach them, level of comprehension, vulnerability, fatigue, burden, potential distress, cost, expertise, recruitment, potential response rates, impact on participants, ethical issues, and data storage and management. Useful references for online questionnaires include:

- Ball (2019), 'Conducting online surveys'.
- Ford et al. (2021), 'Toward an ethical framework for the text mining of social media for health research: a systematic review'.
- Levi et al. (2022), 'Survey fraud and the integrity of web-based survey research'.
- Singh and Sagar (2022), 'Safety and ethical concerns associated with conducting online survey studies among children and adolescents'.

PHYSIOLOGICAL MEASURES AND OTHER SOURCES OF DATA

In health and social care research it is quite common to measure physiological outcomes. These can include, for example, heart rate, blood pressure, oxygen saturation or glycaemic control. In their proposal for a trial of an 'intervention for diabetes with education, advancement and support (IDEAS)', Lee et al. (2016) aimed to measure changes, following the intervention, in HbA1c (glycated haemoglobin, which reflects blood glucose levels). This is how they described measuring some of the outcomes in their study:

Participants' blood pressure will be calculated using the mean of two measurements performed with participants seated after at least 10 min rest, with the cuff on the predominant arm at the level of the heart (A&D, UA-767, USA). Body height and weight will be measured in light indoor clothing and without shoes using a stadiometer and a scale (A&D, UC-321 PBT-C, USA), respectively. Blood oxygen saturation and pulse rate will be measured using an oximeter (Nonin Oximeter II, Model 9560, USA).

(p. 7)

The provision of accurate and detailed information on physiological, physical (body weight, height, arm circumference, etc.) and other measurements is crucial for referees (clinical experts) to assess the appropriateness, feasibility and rigour of the proposed strategies to measure the selected outcomes. It is equally important to explain who will collect these data (researchers trained in the technique or clinicians as part of their routine work). If the proposal relies on data from patients' records, the validity and reliability of these records should be commented on in the proposal. For examples of the measurement of physiological and physical outcomes in research proposals, see:

- Farquharson et al. (2013), 'Nursing stress and patient care: real-time investigation of the effect of nursing tasks and demands on psychological stress, physiological stress, and job performance: study protocol'.
- Schäfer et al. (2018), 'Effects of heart rate variability biofeedback during exposure to fear-provoking stimuli within spider-fearful individuals: study protocol for a randomized controlled trial'.

Questionnaires, scales and physiological measurement tools are not the only sources of data in quantitative research. Clinical notes and public records, for example, provide important data for researchers. For instance, in their proposal on the 'epidemiology of avoidable significant harm in primary care', Bell et al. (2017) aimed 'to conduct electronic searches of general practice (GP) clinical computer systems to identify patients with avoidable significant harm' (p. 1). Sometimes questionnaires can be used alongside other sources of data. In a proposal for a study on 'ethnicity and COVID-19 outcomes in healthcare workers', Woolf et al. (2021), aimed to link data from a baseline questionnaire to health records with 25-year follow-up.

DATA ANALYSIS

Proposals should also include plans for how the collected data will be analysed and managed. There are established and common tests for analysing quantitative data and these should be described in enough detail for reviewers to assess the appropriateness of these tests. The data analysis section will also give reviewers an opportunity to assess whether the proposed sample size is justified (see Chapter 9 for sample size calculation and power analysis). For lesser used or novel analysis methods or techniques, a brief explanation of the choice and information on what the analysis involves should be given as reviewers may not be familiar with them.

The data analysis section of a proposal requires input from statisticians. It is preferable that this section is written by someone with expertise in statistical analysis, in a form and language that other statisticians understand. Some funders refer proposals to statisticians for comments before assessing the proposals as a whole. Analysis is not an 'afterthought' – it is very much at the centre of the research process. Therefore, having a team member with statistical expertise who is involved at every step of the development of the research proposal is an asset. In the resources section, there is an opportunity to identify who has this experience on the team.

Specifying the data analysis software and the version that will be used is part of this section. SPSS, Stata and SAS are some of the well-known software packages. In a review of statistical software applications used in health services research, Dembe et al. (2011) reported that, of the 1139 articles published in US journals, 'Stata and SAS were overwhelmingly the most commonly used' (p. 1). Of particular concern was the finding that 'only 61% of these papers identified the particular type of statistical software application used for data analysis' (p. 1). One should bear in mind that new software is constantly being developed. It is also important to specify who will carry out the analysis as this may affect 'blinding', particularly in trials. The strategies to avoid bias and enhance rigour in data analysis should also be described. For a

---

PROPOSAL EXAMPLE 8.2
DESCRIBING DATA ANALYSIS IN A PROPOSAL

Quemada-González et al. (2022), 'Study protocol: a randomised, controlled trial of a nurse navigator program for the management of hepatitis C virus in patients with severe mental disorder'.

The aim of this study is 'to evaluate the impact of a nurse navigation program on treatment adherence and resolution of hepatitis C infection in patients with severe mental disorder' (p. 1).

COMMENTS

1. Apart from 'the cure rate' and 'adherence to treatment', some of the variables to be measured include: 'change in quality of life', 'changes in daily functioning' and 'negative symptoms'. All of these will be measured with validated tools. This is how the authors describe their data analysis:

   First, an exploratory data analysis will be performed to determine the distributions of the different variables and evaluate their normality using the Kolmogorov–Smirnov test, kurtosis analysis and skewness. Measures of central tendency and dispersion will be calculated, as well as percentage distributions. Subsequently, a bivariate analysis will be performed using the chi-square test for comparison of qualitative variables, and Student's t-test for independent groups for quantitative variables.

   (p. 7)

2. The authors go on to say that the Mann–Whitney *U*-test will be carried out in case there is non-parametric distribution. They also plan to construct a multivariate regression model using Cox regression to 'evaluate the primary endpoints (cure and adherence), with follow-up periods as time adjusted for the variables found to have a significant association on bivariate analysis' (p. 7).

3. Finally, they mention that all the analyses will be performed by intention to treat and will be done with estimation of 95% confidence intervals.

---

detailed plan of data analysis in a proposal, see Katowa-Mukwato et al. (2021), 'Study protocol on stroke management: role of nurses and physiotherapists at the Adult University Teaching Hospital, Lusaka Zambia'.

Proposal Example 8.2 shows how data analysis was reported in a proposal.

DATA HANDLING AND MANAGEMENT

As well as a plan for how the data will be analysed, researchers should show clearly their plan for managing and handling the data. In particular, they should identify who will have overall responsibility for ensuring data security and protection and for ensuring that ethical principles are followed. Where responsibilities are shared, this should be made clear as well. For large, funded projects, researchers may be required to provide a supplementary document to detail the data management plan.

Baysan et al. (2020) described their data handling plan in their proposal for a study 'evaluating effect of red blood cell transfusion on oxygenation and mitochondrial oxygen tension in critically ill patients with anaemia'. They explained that all patients will be assigned a 'random patient identification code' (p. 7) generated electronically and recorded in a code book, which will be stored digitally, with restricted access, and encrypted with a password. They went on to explain that:

> All handling of personal data complies with the EU General Data Protection Regulation and the Dutch Act on Implementation of the General Data Protection Regulation. Extracted study data will be coded and entered in the electronic case report form Castor and stored for further publication. To ensure data quality, a data dictionary was made before start of the study and implemented digitally in the electronic case report, including range checks. Only the coordinating investigator, the principal investigators, the study monitor and Health and Youth Care Inspectorate will have access to the final dataset. Multiple times a year, the study will be monitored, and source data verification will be applied as depicted in the monitor plan in the study protocol, via the independent monitor pool of Leiden University Medical Center. No data safety monitoring board was set up, as it was deemed unnecessary by an independent expert.

(p. 7)

STRUCTURED INTERVIEWS

In quantitative studies, sometimes researchers have to administer questionnaires to participants in person (land-based face-to-face, by telephone or online). The main reason for this strategy is to provide an opportunity for researchers to clarify 'terms' or 'questions' for which participants need clarification. Although questionnaires should be developed to reflect the reading age of the target population, some participants may need help to complete questionnaires. Another reason for administering questionnaires personally is to increase the response rate, as the latter tends to be higher than for self-administered questionnaires.

In structured interviews (also known as standardised interviews), researchers ask all participants the same questions listed in the questionnaire. Researchers do not vary nor add or remove any questions. The aim is for them to be as neutral as possible and only to provide clarification and record the answers. Often even the recording of responses is also systematic. For example, Chetty Mhlanga et al. (2018) aimed to use standardised interviews in their 'prospective cohort study of school-going children investigating reproductive and neuro-behavioural health effects due to environmental pesticide exposure, in Western Cape, South Africa'. They explained that all personal interviews using a structured questionnaire would be installed on mobile devices. They added that to 'ensure quality of data collection, standard operating procedures (SOPs) are developed and all field workers are trained over a week prior to data collection' (p. 8).

Training of researchers to undertake standardised interviews is crucial to ensure that all researchers provide the same clarifications and record the data in the same way. Issues relating to the management and analysis of data are the same for standardised interviews as for questionnaires, as the data collection tool in these interviews is 'the questionnaire'. In research proposals of studies using standardised interviews, researchers should provide the same information as for studies using questionnaires. Additionally, they should provide justifications for why it is necessary for data collectors to administer the questionnaire personally. The steps taken to ensure standardisation in the method of administering questionnaires, such as training and piloting, should also be described.

CLINICAL INTERVIEWS

Clinical interviews share many of the features of structured interviews in terms of the structure and standardisation of the process. Nursing, health and social care researchers often have to assess or measure clinical symptoms or psychological states (e.g. depression, anxiety, etc.) in order to answer their research questions. Clinical interviews for research purposes differ from clinical assessments carried out by health or social care professionals as part of their clinical practice. The main difference is that, in research clinical interviews, data are collected to answer research questions. In clinical interviews, the aim is to diagnose or assess the progress of illnesses or other conditions; such interviews have a therapeutic purpose: to help people get better.

Research clinical interviews interviews use structured and standardised tools to measure outcomes. For example, in a proposal for a study by Swart et al. (2017), five structured clinical interviews will be used to chart the 'clinical course of trauma–related disorders and personality disorders' over a 2-year period. 'Personality disorder' will be measured by the Structured Interview for DSM Personality Disorders (SIDP-IV). Swart et al. (2017) also explained that all the tools/scales they were using 'have good to excellent psychometric properties, including test-retest reliability' (p. 5). Clinical interviews, for research purposes, should also be carried out by people trained to do so. Sometimes health professionals are enlisted to carry out these interviews. In Swart et al.'s (2017) study, well-trained psychologists with clinical expertise conducted these interviews.

Structured and clinical interviews also provide opportunities for researchers to collect qualitative data by undertaking qualitative interviews alongside structured ones. However, researchers have to be mindful of the burden that this may put on participants, especially those whose energy levels and concentration time span are low. In research proposals using clinical interviews, information should be provided on the outcomes or variables to be measured, the justification for the choice of measurement tools, the validity and reliability of the tools, the extent of their use in other studies, the background of the interviewers, the training provided, inter-rater reliability, whether different data collectors are involved and the practical and ethical implications of clinical interviews.

For an example of a proposal using both structured interviews and clinical interviews see Proposal Example 8.3.

REPORTING DATA COLLECTION AND ANALYSIS IN RESEARCH PROPOSALS

The information required in a research proposal can be summarised by asking the following questions:

What methods of data collection and analysis are selected for this study? In this section, the actual method of data collection should be stated (e.g. questionnaire, scale or other measuring tool).

Why has this method been selected? A rationale for choice should be provided (e.g. that it is the best method to answer the research question; it is an acceptable tool with established validity and reliability; it is commonly used to measure the concepts/outcomes in similar studies). As part of the rationale, researchers should quote or reference information demonstrating the validity and reliability of the method. If the questionnaire or scale is translated from another

PROPOSAL EXAMPLE 8.3
STRUCTURED INTERVIEWS AND CLINICAL INTERVIEWS IN A PROPOSAL

Woods et al (2009), 'Reminiscence groups for people with dementia and their family carers: pragmatic eight-centre randomised trial of joint reminiscence and maintenance versus usual treatment: a protocol'.
    The aim of this study is to carry out a randomised trial to assess the effectiveness and cost-effectiveness of joint reminiscence groups for people with dementia and their family caregivers.

COMMENTS
1. This study uses a battery of structured tools/instruments to collect data on primary and secondary outcomes, including Quality of Life in Alzheimer's Disease, General Health Questionnaire and Quality of the Carer-Patient Relationships.
2. Some of the structured tools used in this study (e.g. General Health Questionnaire) are completed by the carers themselves. Persons with dementia will also complete them, 'wherever possible'. Woods et al. (2009) explain that they will carry out structured interviews using the Rating Anxiety in Dementia scale, to rate anxiety in people with dementia.
3. The information required in proposals for studies using structured interviews and clinical interviews are the same as for questionnaires. In this proposal, the authors provided clear information on the aims of the study, the outcomes to be measured, the scales or instruments to be used and how data would be managed and analysed.

language or adapted for use in a particular population, the process of translation/adaptation should be briefly described and the implications of this should be highlighted. The rationale for the method of data analysis and the tests to be carried out should be provided.

How will it be administered? The mode of delivery (e.g. face-to-face, online, by phone, etc.) of the questionnaire should be described and the strengths and limitations of this choice should be highlighted.

When will it be administered? The information required here refers to the timing of the administration (e.g. the different time points if it is a longitudinal study). The approximate time it will take for participants to complete the questionnaire should also be mentioned.

Where will be it administered? This is related to the mode of delivery. If it is an online questionnaire, information on how participants can access, complete and submit it should be given. If the participants are patients in a hospital, the process of accessing them should also be described.

Who will the participants be? While this information is normally provided in the 'sample' section, readers and reviewers need to know how appropriate the method of data collection is for the participants in the study. The information will help reviewers to assess appropriateness in relation to 'participant burden' (e.g. whether the questionnaire is too long or there are too many scales) or 'cognitive level' (e.g. whether the questionnaire is appropriate for the participants' reading level).

Proposal Example 8.4 shows how quantitative data collection and analysis were reported in a proposal.

PROPOSAL EXAMPLE 8.4
REPORTING QUANTITATIVE DATA COLLECTION AND ANALYSIS IN PROPOSALS

Shimizu et al. (2020), 'Study protocol for a nationwide questionnaire survey of physical activity among breast cancer survivors in Japan'.

This study aims 'to identify the levels of physical activity among breast cancer survivors, to examine factors-related physical activity among breast cancer survivors, and to identify breast cancer survivors' preferences for and interest in exercise programmes' (p. 1).

COMMENTS

1. The authors propose to use questionnaires and scales (e.g. the Exercise-related Social Support Scale) to answer quantitative descriptive questions and correlational questions. These methods (questionnaires and scales) are appropriate for answering these types of question.

2. In the proposal, the authors explain how they developed their 'self-reported' questionnaire. This includes a review of previous studies, team discussion, focus groups and in-depth personal interviews with 'medical personnel' and breast cancer survivors. They also 'conducted cognitive checks with 5 breast cancer survivors to evaluate whether the questions were measuring the construct' they intended (p. 4).

3. In the proposal, Shimizu et al. (2020) link each scale to the outcomes they were expected to measure. For example, this is how they describe how they will measure quality of life with the EuroQol 5 Dimension (EQ-5D):

   [This] is a comprehensive evaluation scale developed by the EQ group established in 1987 to measure HRQOL [health-related quality of life]. We will use the 5-level EQ-5D version, which has improved the instrument's sensitivity and reduced ceiling effects. The reliability and validity of the Japanese version have also been confirmed. The scale consists of five items, and complete health can be converted to 1 and death to 0 as standardized utility values based on the results.

   (p. 4)

   The authors also provide references to support some of the statements made above.

4. In the data analysis section, the researchers outline the tests and calculations (e.g. logistic regression, univariate logistic analysis, *F*-test) they would carry out and explained what each test would achieve. Shimizu et al. (2020) also maintain that 'the analysis will be carried out using the SAS V.9.4 (SAS Institute)' (p. 7). The data analysis section should be written by proposal team members who have statistical experience and who can use the appropriate statistical language that reviewers will recognise so they are able to make their assessment of whether these tests are appropriate and feasible.

5. The limitations listed in the proposal include the possibility that participants interested in physical activity 'may participate and complete questionnaires more readily than those who are not'. The authors also acknowledge that 'a self-reported measure of physical activity may overestimate or underestimate participants' physical activity' (p. 8). It is important to list some of the potential and actual limitations of the study in a proposal as this shows that the researchers have given some thoughts to some of the difficulties/drawbacks that they may face.

Checklist for the quantitative data collection and analysis sections of a research proposal:

1. Are the data collection methods clearly described? How are they aligned/matched to each of the research questions and objectives?
2. Are the methods of data collection appropriate for answering the research questions? Are they suitable for the target population?
3. Is a justification for the choice of data collection methods given?
4. Are existing questionnaires and scales to be used in the proposed study? If so, how widely are they used in previous studies? Are they valid and reliable? If a number of tools exist for the same outcome, is a justification given for the one(s) selected?
5. If modifications or adaptions are to be made to existing tools, how will the reliability and validity of the modified tool be tested?
6. Will the existing tool require translation into another language? Is this process briefly described? How will the reliability and validity of the translated tool be tested?
7. If new tools are to be developed for the study, is a rationale/justification given for this decision?
8. How are the tools to be developed (process)? How will their reliability and validity be tested?
9. Will the development of a new questionnaire or tool be carried out before the proposal is submitted (as part of pre-proposal preparation)?
10. How will the tools be administered (e.g. face to face, online or via the telephone)? Is a justification given for the choice of delivery mode?
11. For clinical outcomes, are the measurement tools and techniques the most appropriate, reliable and valid? Who will carry out the measurements or recordings (clinical staff, researchers specially trained for this task, etc.)?
12. What is the process for the recording and analysis of the data?
13. Who will analyse the data and how will rigour be ensured?
14. What statistical calculations will be carried out? Are they appropriate and justified?
15. What data analysis/management software will be used? Is the choice appropriate and justified?
16. How will the data be managed and by whom? How will the security and protection of data be ensured? In the case of clinical samples, where will these be stored? And for how long? Who will have access to them?

SUMMARY AND CONCLUSIONS

In this chapter, we have listed the main data collection methods (questionnaires and scales) and data sources that quantitative researchers have at their disposal when designing a study. We have explained the type of information that researchers should highlight in the data collection, data analysis and data handling sections of proposal. Examples from real research proposals and a checklist of items to include in proposals have been provided.

REFERENCES

Ball, H. L. (2019). Conducting Online Surveys. *Journal of Human Lactation, 35*(3), 413–417.

Baysan, M., Arbous, M. S., Mik, E. G., Juffermans, N. P., & van der Bom, J. G. (2020). Study protocol and pilot results of an observational cohort study evaluating effect of red blood cell transfusion on oxygenation and mitochondrial oxygen tension in critically ill patients with anaemia: The INsufficient Oxygenation in the Intensive Care Unit (INOX ICU-2) study. *BMJ Open*, *10*(5), e036351. https://doi.org/10.1136/bmjopen-2019-036351

Bell, B. G., Campbell, S., Carson-Stevens, A., Evans, H. P., Cooper, A., Sheehan, C., Rodgers, S., Johnson, C., Edwards, A., Armstrong, S., Mehta, R., Chuter, A., Donnelly, A., Ashcroft, D. M., Lymn, J., Smith, P., Sheikh, A., Boyd, M., & Avery, A. J. (2017). Understanding the epidemiology of avoidable significant harm in primary care: Protocol for a retrospective cross-sectional study. *BMJ Open*, *7*(2), e013786. https://doi.org/10.1136/bmjopen-2016-013786

Bergman, J., & Laviana, A. (2014). Quality-of-life assessment tools for men with prostate cancer. *Nature Reviews Urology*, *11*(6), 352–359.

Chetty-Mhlanga, S., Basera, W., Fuhrimann, S., Probst-Hensch, N., Delport, S., Mugari, M., Van Wyk, J., Röösli, M., & Dalvie, M. A. (2018). A prospective cohort study of school-going children investigating reproductive and neurobehavioral health effects due to environmental pesticide exposure in the Western Cape, South Africa: Study protocol. *BMC Public Health*, *18*(1), 857. https://doi.org/10.1186/s12889-018-5783-0

Deidda, M., Boyd, K. A., Minnis, H., Donaldson, J., Brown, K., Boyer, N., McIntosh, E., & BeST Study Team. (2018). Protocol for the economic evaluation of a complex intervention to improve the mental health of maltreated infants and children in foster care in the UK (The BeST? services trial). *BMJ Open*, *8*(3), e020066. https://doi.org/10.1136/bmjopen-2017-020066

Dembe, A. E., Partridge, J. S., & Geist, L. C. (2011). Statistical software applications used in health services research: Analysis of published studies in the U.S. *BMC Health Services Research*, *11*, 252. https://doi.org/10.1186/1472-6963-11-252

Farquharson, B., Bell, C., Johnston, D., Jones, M., Schofield, P., Allan, J., Ricketts, I., Morrison, K., & Johnston, M. (2013). Nursing stress and patient care: Real-time investigation of the effect of nursing tasks and demands on psychological stress, physiological stress, and job performance: Study protocol. *Journal of Advanced Nursing*, *69*(10), 2327–2335. https://doi.org/10.1111/jan.12090

Ford, E., Shepherd, S., Jones, K., & Hassan, L. (2021). Toward an ethical framework for the text mining of social media for health research: A systematic review. *Frontiers in Digital Health*, *2*, 592237. https://doi.org/10.3389/fdgth.2020.592237

Geidl, W., Deprins, J., Streber, R., Rohrbach, N., Sudeck, G., & Pfeifer, K. (2018). Exercise therapy in medical rehabilitation: Study protocol of a national survey at facility and practitioner level with a mixed method design. *Contemporary Clinical Trials Communications*, *11*, 37–45.

Hawthorne, G., Sansoni, J., Hayes, L. M., Marosszeky, N., & Sansoni, E. (2006). Measuring patient satisfaction with incontinence treatment (final report). Centre for Health Service Development, University of Wollongong and the Department of Psychiatry, University of Melbourne.

Hyman, L., Lamb, J., Bulmer, M. (2006). *The use of pre-existing survey questions: Implications for data quality*. Proceedings of Q2006 European Conference on Quality in Survey Statistics. https://ec.europa.eu/eurostat/documents/64157/4374310/22-Use-of-pre-existing-survey-questions-implications-for-data-quality-2006.pdf/e953a39e-50be-40b3-910f-6c0d83f55ed4

Katowa-Mukwato, P., Banda, M., Kanyanta, M., Musenge, E., Phiri, P., Mwiinga-Kalusopa, V., Chapima, F., Simpamba, M., Kapenda, C., & Shula, H. (2021). Study protocol on stroke management: Role of nurses and physiotherapists at the adult university teaching hospital, Lusaka Zambia. *Journal of Biosciences and Medicines*, *9*, 25–37.

Khairnar, M. R., Wadgave, U., Shah, S. J., Shah, S., Jain, V. M., & Kumbhar, S. (2019). Survey on attitude of dental professionals about plagiarism in Maharashtra, India. *Perspectives in Clinical Research*, *10*(1), 9–14.

Lee, J. Y., Chan, C. K., Chua, S. S., Ng, C. J., Paraidathathu, T., Lee, K. K., & Lee, S. W. (2016). Intervention for Diabetes with Education, Advancement and Support (IDEAS) study: Protocol for a cluster randomised controlled trial. *BMC Health Services Research*, *16*(1), 524. https://doi.org/10.1186/s12913-016-1782-y

Levi, R., Ridberg, R., Akers, M., & Seligman, H. (2022). Survey Fraud and the Integrity of Web-Based Survey Research. *American Journal of Health Promotion: AJHP*, *36*(1), 18–20.

Mathers, N., Fox, N., & Hunn, A. (2007). *Surveys and questionnaires*. The NIHR RDS for the East Midlands/ Yorkshire & the Humber. https://www.rds-yh.nihr.ac.uk/wp-content/uploads/2013/05/12_Surveys_and_ Questionnaires_Revision_2009.pdf

Mavrinac, M., Brumini, G., Bilić-Zulle, L., & Petrovecki, M. (2010). Construction and validation of attitudes toward plagiarism questionnaire. *Croatian Medical Journal*, *51*(3), 195–201.

Nishi, D., Imamura, K., Watanabe, K., Obikane, E., Sasaki, N., Yasuma, N., Sekiya, Y., Matsuyama, Y., & Kawakami, N. (2020). Internet-based cognitive-behavioural therapy for prevention of depression during pregnancy and in the post partum (iPDP): A protocol for a large-scale randomised controlled trial. *BMJ Open*, *10*(5), e036482. https://doi.org/10.1136/bmjopen-2019-036482

Price, C., Jhangiani, R. S., Chiang, I. A., Dana, C. Leighton D C Cuttler C (2017) Research methods in psychology (3rd American Edition). Washington University: Washington. https://opentext.wsu.edu/carriecuttler/part/ chapter-9-survey-research/

Quemada-González, C., Morales-Asencio, J. M., Hurtado, M. M., & Martí-García, C. (2022). Study protocol: A randomised, controlled trial of a nurse navigator program for the management of hepatitis C virus in patients with severe mental disorder. *BMC Nursing*, *21*(1), 92. https://doi.org/10.1186/s12912-022-00870-w

Robb, M., & Shellenbarger, T. (2020). Mastering survey design and questionnaire development. *Journal of Continuing Education in Nursing*, *51*(6), 248–249.

Russell, C., Ammour, N., Wells, T., Bonnet, N., Kruse, M., Tardat, A., Erales, C., Shook, T., Kirkesseli, S., Hovsepian, L., & Pretorius, S. (2018). A pilot study to assess the feasibility of collecting and transmitting clinical trial data with mobile technologies. *Digital Biomarkers*, *2*(3), 126–138.

Schäfer, S. K., Ihmig, F. R., Lara, H. K. A., Neurohr, F., Kiefer, S., Staginnus, M., Lass-Hennemann, J., & Michael, T. (2018). Effects of heart rate variability biofeedback during exposure to fear-provoking stimuli within spider-fearful individuals: Study protocol for a randomized controlled trial. *Trials*, *19*(1), 184. https://doi.org/10.1186/ s13063-018-2554-2

Schofield, P., Gough, K., Hyatt, A., White, A., Frydenberg, M., Chambers, S., Gordon, L. G., Gardiner, R., Murphy, D. G., Cavedon, L., Richards, N., Murphy, B., Quinn, S., & Juraskova, I. (2021). Navigate: A study protocol for a randomised controlled trial of an online treatment decision aid for men with low-risk prostate cancer and their partners. *Trials*, *22*(1), 49. https://doi.org/10.1186/s13063-020-04986-9

Shimizu, Y., Tsuji, K., Ochi, E., Arai, H., Okubo, R., Kuchiba, A., Shimazu, T., Sakurai, N., Narisawa, T., Ueno, T., Iwata, H., & Matsuoka, Y. (2020). Study protocol for a nationwide questionnaire survey of physical activity among breast cancer survivors in Japan. *BMJ Open*, *10*(1), e032871. https://doi.org/10.1136/bmjopen-2019-032871

Singh, S., & Sagar, R. (2022). Safety and ethical concerns associated with conducting online survey studies among children and adolescents. *Indian Journal of Psychological Medicine*, *44*(2), 199–200.

Spasojevic, N., Hrabac, B., & Huseinagic, S. (2015). Patient's satisfaction with health care: A questionnaire study of different aspects of care. *Materia Socio-medica*, *27*(4), 220–224.

Swart, S., Wildschut, M., Draijer, N., Langeland, W., & Smit, J. H. (2017). The clinical course of trauma-related disorders and personality disorders: Study protocol of two-year follow-up based on structured interviews. *BMC Psychiatry*, *17*(1), 173. https://doi.org/10.1186/s12888-017-1339-6

Toma, G., Guetterman, T. C., Yaqub, T., Talaat, N., & Fetters, M. D. (2017). A systematic approach for accurate translation of instruments: EXPERIENCE with translating the Connor–Davidson Resilience Scale into Arabic. *Methodological Innovations*, *10*(3), 1–10. https://doi.org/2059799117741406

Tsang, S., Royse, C. F., & Terkawi, A. S. (2017). Guidelines for developing, translating, and validating a questionnaire in perioperative and pain medicine. *Saudi Journal of Anaesthesia*, *11*(suppl 1), S80–S89.

Winnige, P., Batalik, L., Filakova, K., Hnatiak, J., Dosbaba, F., & Grace, S. L. (2020). Translation and validation of the cardiac rehabilitation barriers scale in the Czech Republic (CRBS-CZE): Protocol to determine the key barriers in East-Central Europe. *Medicine*, *99*(11), e19546. https://doi.org/10.1097/MD.0000000000019546

Woods, R. T., Bruce, E., Edwards, R. T., Hounsome, B., Keady, J., Moniz-Cook, E. D., Orrell, M., & Russell, I. T. (2009). Reminiscence groups for people with dementia and their family carers: Pragmatic eight-centre randomised trial of joint reminiscence and maintenance versus usual treatment: A protocol. *Trials*, *10*, 64. https://doi.org/10.1186/1745-6215-10-64

Woolf, K., Melbourne, C., Bryant, L., Guyatt, A. L., McManus, I. C., Gupta, A., Free, R. C., Nellums, L., Carr, S., John, C., Martin, C. A., Wain, L. V., Gray, L. J., Garwood, C., Modhwadia, V., Abrams, K. R., Tobin, M. D., Khunti, K., Pareek, M., & UK-REACH Study Collaborative Group+. (2021). The United Kingdom research study into ethnicity and COVID-19 outcomes in healthcare workers (UK-REACH): Protocol for a prospective longitudinal cohort study of healthcare and ancillary workers in UK healthcare settings. *BMJ Open*, *11*(9), e050647. https://doi.org/10.1136/bmjopen-2021-050647

Yaddanapudi, S., Yaddanapudi, L. N. (2019). How to design a questionnaire. *Indian Journal of Anaesthesia*, *63*(5), 335–337.

9 QUALITATIVE DATA COLLECTION AND ANALYSIS

INTRODUCTION

In this chapter, we will explore the range of qualitative research methods that researchers can choose from when designing a study. In particular, we will emphasise the need to consider carefully the appropriateness of the selected methods and the challenges and implications that they present. The main qualitative methods discussed here are face-to-face interviews and focus groups. Observations (quantitative and qualitative) will be explored in Chapter 10.

The information provided in research proposals relating to quantitative data collection methods, described in the last chapter, are more or less the same as for qualitative methods. Qualitative research proposals (and mixed methods ones) require the same amount of detail as do quantitative proposals. This will allow reviewers and others to assess the appropriateness and feasibility of the proposed data collection methods for answering the research question(s).

QUALITATIVE FACE-TO-FACE INTERVIEWS

There are different types of qualitative, one-to-one interview: face-to-face in person, via the telephone and online. In-person, face-to-face interviews are perhaps the most widely used in qualitative studies, although there is a growing trend towards online interviews, and the COVID-19 pandemic has increased the use of online communication platforms for research purposes. In research proposals, researchers should demonstrate an awareness of the strengths, implications and challenges of the type of interview they have selected for their study.

The choice of interview format depends mainly on the type of information to be collected (aligned to research questions or objectives), the topic or focus of the study and the type of participant. Face-to-face interviews are appropriate (and are the method of choice) for exploring personal experience and issues, in particular those that are sensitive. For example, investigating participants' experience of losing a close family member through disease or accident requires a sensitive approach in the interview. If there are others present (as in focus groups), it is unlikely that participants will reveal their experiences to any great depth. It is also more unlikely that researchers will be able to meaningfully probe these experiences in a group situation. To appreciate (and show empathy for) a participant sharing their experiences, researchers have to give their full attention to this individual. Face-to-face interviews may also be appropriate for some participants who, due to their age or ability (or disability), may require one-to-one communication with the researchers. Some participants may feel overwhelmed and only feel able to communicate with one person.

Providing a rationale in a proposal for the choice of interview format is evidence that the researchers have given some thought to this issue. One-to-one interviews are more appropriate for qualitative approaches such as phenomenology (Parahoo, 2014) that focus on how individuals experience phenomena in their consciousness. In these interviews, researchers aim to facilitate participants in 'revealing' these experiences and to probe as appropriate. There is less 'discussion' than in focus groups. In the proposal for a study on 'how Australian women cope with pelvic girdle pain during pregnancy', Ceprnja et al. (2018) explained that 'face-to-face, individual semistructured interviews' will 'provide a rich description of the lived experiences of women living with pregnancy-related pelvic girdle pain' (p. 2). Such experiences are intimate and personal, and therefore not appropriate to talk about in the presence of other participants. In Ceprnja et al.'s (2018) study, they intended to carry out focus groups as well to discuss and further explore issues raised during the individual interviews.

Another issue to consider when selecting face-to-face interviews is how feasible it is to carry out the proposed interviews. Feasibility depends on recruiting suitable participants in sufficient numbers (this is discussed in Chapter 12). Equally important are the time, resources (in particular, funding) and expertise required to undertake these interviews. It is helpful to point out the qualitative interviewing expertise in the team or the training to be provided to those who will undertake the interviews.

Some interview scripts will need to be translated if they are to be analysed and reported in a different language from that in which the interviews were conducted. This will have to be explained in the proposal. This is how Rousham et al. (2019) described the issue of translation in their proposal for a study on 'pathways of antibiotic use in Bangladesh'. After explaining that their team comprised English speakers, Bangla (a native language in Bangladesh) speakers and some bilingual researchers, they had to take a decision on how much and at what point to translate, given the constraints of cost and time:

> *Our chosen solution is to translate one-third of transcripts in full into English, by native Bangla researchers. The translated transcripts will reflect the variety of our samples and will be used as the basis for the framework for analysis. The remaining Bangla transcripts will be coded in Bangla, and then the text in the framework will be translated into English. This method will allow the whole team (including non-Bangla speakers) to contribute to the development of the analysis structure and first draft analysis, while allowing the early analyses to be conducted in Bangla.*

(p. 5)

Data collection and analysis often occur simultaneously in qualitative studies. Measures to ensure rigour in these processes should also be clearly identified. The data analysis software and analysis framework to be used should be carefully selected and adequately described in a proposal. Below is an example from Edib et al. (2020) from their proposal for a study 'exploring the facilitators and barriers to using an online infertility risk production tool (FORECAST) for young women with breast cancer'. They explained that the 'processes of data collection and analysis' would be ongoing and that they would use a data analysis software (QRS NVivo V.12—QRS International, Doncaster, Victoria, Australia) and the Miles and Huberman (1994) data analysis framework. This is how they aimed to ensure rigour in the analysis process:

> To ensure the integrity and consistency of the codes and reduce bias, codes will be reviewed by the qualitative research specialist. The research team will discuss the coding tree and reach consensus. Subsequently, content analysis will also be performed for each code, to support results from thematic analyses by identifying essential aspects of the content and highlighting the recurrence of themes, to present results clearly and effectively. A final list of themes and subthemes will be determined through patterns as soon as further data that will emerge from the study add little to the emerging theory. Theoretical saturation is reached once no new themes emerge.
>
> *(p. 4)*

As with quantitative studies, the issue of data management is equally important. In their study of the 'experiences of peer support for newly qualified nurses in a dedicated online group', Webster et al. (2019) explained how data would be managed and protected:

> All data will be stored on password protected computers and only accessible by the research team. Paper data and all identifiable personal information will be destroyed at the end of the study. No one outside the study team will have access to the anonymized data unless they are from a research governance authority. The data will be archived and stored for 10-years.
>
> *(p. 1589)*

Proposal Example 9.1 describes face-to-face qualitative interviews in a proposal.

Qualitative Telephone Interviews

Novick (2008) believed that 'telephone interviews are largely neglected in the qualitative research literature and, when discussed, they are often depicted as a less attractive alternative to face-to-face interviewing' (p. 391). She explained that this might be because the lack of visual cues may 'compromise rapport, probing, and interpretation of responses' (p. 1). Yet, according to Novick (2008), 'telephones may allow respondents to feel relaxed and able to disclose sensitive information'. Williams et al. (2020), in their proposal for a qualitative exploration of the experiences and support requirements of men living with multiple miscarriages, pointed out that there is 'evidence to suggest that telephone communication may facilitate a sense of anonymity, privacy and freedom, and thereby confer more relational power to interviewees' as well as 'reduce any personal safety risks' (p. 4).

PROPOSAL EXAMPLE 9.1
FACE-TO-FACE QUALITATIVE INTERVIEWS

Sihre et al. (2019), 'Understanding the lived experiences of severe postnatal psychiatric illnesses in English speaking South Asian women, living in the UK: a qualitative study protocol'.

As the authors explained, the aim of this study was to 'explore South Asian women's narrative of living with a severe postnatal psychiatric illness and experiences of Perinatal Mental Health Services, care and support' (p. 1).

COMMENTS

1. In this study, an interpretive phenomenological analysis (IPA) approach was used to collect and analyse data. Sihre et al. (2019) pointed out that 'IPA is a methodological framework in qualitative research that focuses on exploring in-depth how individuals make sense of their lived experiences, including how they experience living through events and what meaning they attribute to a given phenomenon' (p. 3). These 'events' and 'experiences' are unique and personal; the topic itself (postnatal psychiatric illness) is sensitive. Researchers (interviewers) have to build a rapport and trust with individual participants and pay attention to their body language and other 'non-verbal' signals in order to show empathy and get the most out of the interviews. This is not feasible in focus groups as they involve a number of participants. Therefore, face-to-face, semistructured interviews are appropriate for this study.

2. The second objective, focusing on the participants' experience of their use of services, can be explored via either face-to-face or focus group interviews, because using services involves social interactions. 'Lived experience', on the other hand, is unique to the individual and each narrative is different.

3. In this proposal, the authors gave details of how the semistructured questions were developed, how many participants would be approached, how the interviews would be conducted, how long each interview might take, where they would be held and how data would be recorded.

4. Finally, Sihre et al. (2019) provided a rationale for the use of IPA in this study and how the IPA framework would be used to analyse data.

On the other hand, it may be argued the telephone interviews may be limited in connecting the participant with the researcher. In their qualitative study of the 'experiences of health care providers during the COVID-19 crisis in China', Liu et al. (2020) pointed out that a limitation of interviewing participants by telephone, in their study, was the difficulty of building a rapport with participants over the phone, and 'non-verbal cues could not be obtained' (p. 9). As Wuhan (where the study was carried out) was in lockdown and the authors could not go to hospitals (Liu et al., 2020), the choice of telephone interviews was justified.

Most of the issues identified for face-to-face, 'in-person' interviews apply equally to telephone interviews. The rationale for the choice of this type of interview should be provided. The process of telephone interviewing should also be considered at the design stage and described in proposals to give an idea of how the interviews will be conducted. This includes how the questions for the interview are developed, who will conduct the interview, how long the interviews are expected to last, informed consent and how data are to be recorded. In their proposal for a study on 'patient-centred and family-centred care [PFCC] of critically ill patients who are potential organ donors', Zheng et al. (2020) explained that they would employ a semi-structured interview guide which would be created 'by an interdisciplinary team of investigators with expertise in critical cares, palliative, organ donor, medical, education and sociological and qualitative research methods' (p. 3). They went on to explain that the content of the interview guide included:

> *a series of open-ended questions; participants will be guided to discuss their experience starting when they first learnt that their loved one was critically ill, through their in-hospital experience and finally, their posthospital bereavement. Interviews will explore the communication about the critical illness and donation, as well as the care and support provided during that time. Family members will be specifically asked their perspectives on the provision of PFCC and the ways in which care could have been enhanced and improved.*

(p. 3)

Zheng et al. (2020) also estimated that the interviews would last 45–60 minutes and that they would be carried out by several highly trained and qualified researchers. The process of translation and back-translation (English and French) is also described in the proposal.

As with face-to-face, in-person interviews, the process of data analysis as well as data management requires description in research proposals. Williams et al. (2020) described, in their proposal, how they would use a data analysis framework (Ritchie and Lewis, 2003) and NVivo software to analyse their data. An example of data handling, including protection of data, comes from Williams et al.'s (2020) study.

They explained that they would follow data protection regulations by keeping 'consent forms, demographic questionnaires, audio recording transcriptions and field notes securely in the custody of the chief investigator for 10-years after first publication of the project findings' in order 'to prevent inadvertent loss or disclosure of personally identifiable and other information' (p. 6)

An example of qualitative telephone interviews in a study, is given in Proposal Example 9.2.

Online Face-to-face Interviews

One growth area in qualitative research (and likely to develop even more) is the use of modern online technology for collecting, analysing and managing data. There are different purposes and ways of collecting data via the internet. In this section, we will briefly explore some of the issues that researchers should consider when proposing to conduct face-to-face, in-depth online interviews. For more information on qualitative research online, in particular online qualitative interviews, see Salmons (2016).

The first thing to bear in mind is that the principles involved in online interviews are the same as those for in person, face-to-face qualitative interviews, but with technology as an important

---

PROPOSAL EXAMPLE 9.2
QUALITATIVE TELEPHONE INTERVIEWS IN A PROPOSAL

Ibrahim et al. (2020), 'Recreational cannabis usage among young adults living with diabetes: protocol for a mixed methods study'.

This is a two-phase, mixed methods study. Phase 1 involves quantitative data and phase 2 is qualitative.

COMMENTS

1. The authors explained that 'Phase 2 will involve the collection of qualitative data through telephone, semi-structured one-on-one interviews to attain a more comprehensive understanding of the motivations for cannabis use and the management of diabetes among young adults living with diabetes' (p. 1409).

2. Ibrahim et al. (2020) justified the choice of telephone, face-to-face interviews on the basis that:

   it reduces the cost associated with traveling, mitigates the physical distance between participants and the researcher, reduces the power and response bias (i.e. social desirability) between the researcher and participants, and maintains anonymity and privacy, particularly given the sensitivity of the research topic.

   (p. 1424)

3. The process of data collection by phone is well described in the proposal, including how participants were to be contacted and informed about the project. They gave details of the broad content of the interviews as well as their duration. The topic of this study (recreational cannabis usage) is a sensitive topic and, as such, may lend itself more to telephone than face-to-face interviews. The authors also pointed out that participants would be afforded the opportunity to not answer questions they were not comfortable with or interested in discussing.

4. Ibrahim et al. (2020) explained that the interviews would be audio-taped but that the name of participants and of the healthcare institution 'will be removed from the transcripts to ensure the audio-recordings cannot be traced and/or associated to any of the participants' (p. 1412). The data analysis process is also well described.

---

dimension (Salmons, 2016). According to the author, we need to reflect on the effects that the use of technology has on 'the research design, conduct, and ultimately on the study's conclusions and on generalizations the researcher offers' (p. 178). The implications and processes of conducting online interviews are becoming clearer as more and more researchers conduct their studies online and reflect upon their experiences and challenges. For examples of these reflections, see:

- Carter et al. (2021), 'Conducting qualitative research online: challenges and solutions'.
- Topping et al. (2021), 'General considerations for conducting online qualitative research and practice implications for interviewing people with acquired brain injury'.
- Roberts et al. (2021), 'It's more complicated than it seems: virtual qualitative research in the COVID-19 era'.

There are a number of online technologies such as email, instant messaging, chat rooms, podcasting, blogs, etc. There are also a number of video conferencing platforms, such as Zoom, Skype and Microsoft Teams. While researchers are likely to choose the technologies or platforms that they are comfortable with, it is advisable to review the growing literature on their advantages and disadvantages and learn from the experiences of those who have used them. For example, Gray et al. (2020), in their paper on expanding qualitative research interviewing strategies, offer researchers some practical recommendations for using Zoom, including 'test Zoom ahead of interview', 'provide technical information', 'have a backup plan' and 'plan for distraction' (p. 1296).

Lo Iacono et al. (2016) highlighted the 'advantages of using Skype to conduct qualitative interviews' and 'weigh these advantages against any limitations and issues' that may arise when using this tool (p. 1). They based their reflections on two qualitative studies that they conducted. This paper (Lo Iacono et al., 2016) also offered some comparisons between Skype and email interviews. Hawkins (2018) examined the 'practical utility and suitability of email interviews in qualitative research' and discussed the potential advantages and disadvantages of email interviews and their 'relative appropriateness' in qualitative research. They concluded that:

Deciding on the best interview technique for each study should be based on an assessment of several factors. The research aims, confidence of credible findings, potential advantages and disadvantages of the data collection method such as time required to conduct interviews, costs and accessibility, researcher familiarity with the technology, and relative comfort level of the subject population with the technology are important factors when considering the email interview for conducting research.

(p. 493)

While these online technologies and facilities may be convenient and effective, they are not without implications, complications and costs. There are also issues relating to security, privacy, confidentiality, consent and human rights. Recording, handling and managing online collected data can have serious ethical and legal issues (see Chapter 13 for more discussion). For more information on some of these issues, see:

■ Saarijärvi and Bratt (2021), 'When face-to-face interviews are not possible: tips and tricks for video, telephone, online chat, and email interviews in qualitative research'.

Proposal Example 9.3 describes face-to-face online interviews in a proposal.

FOCUS GROUPS

As with other methods of data collection, the rationale for selecting the focus group for a study should be clearly thought out and stated in the proposal. Normally, the focus group is the method of choice when responses from one or more participants can trigger reactions from others by supporting or rejecting what is said and/or offering alternative perspectives on a topic. It is not enough in focus groups to obtain a range of perspectives; it is equally important

PROPOSAL EXAMPLE 9.3
FACE-TO-FACE ONLINE QUALITATIVE INTERVIEWS IN A PROPOSAL

White and Palmieri (2022), 'Women caring for husbands living with Parkinson's Disease: a phenomenological study protocol'.

The aim of this study is to 'understand the lived experience of women caregivers of husbands living with Parkinson's Disease' (p. 1).

COMMENTS

1. The authors chose face-to-face interviews 'to encourage the women to express themselves freely as they describe their caregiving experiences and identify their perceptions about caring for their husbands' (p. 8). Since the experiences are personal and the topic is sensitive, face-to-face interviews are appropriate. However, in-person, face-to-face interviews were not possible in this study because of COVID-19 restrictions. Therefore, the interviews were to be conducted face-to-face, via Zoom.

2. White and Palmieri (2022) recognised the limitations of conducting the interviews over Zoom. One potential limitation is that participants who lack the technological ability to use email or Zoom may not enrol in the study. The authors pointed out that potential participants may be able to 'request assistance from the Colorado Parkinson Foundation for assistance with the Zoom© interview' (p. 13). The choice of Zoom as a platform for the interviews is also justified in the proposal.

3. Both the interview and data analysis processes are explained in detail. Data management is also well described. For example, this is how the researchers described 'digital data management' in the proposal:

    All paper documents, including field notes, will be uploaded into the primary investigator's password-protected computer, and the paper document will be stored in secured file cabinet for 5 years. For the coding process, the audio recordings will be sent through a secure portal to the transcription service. The completed transcript will then be downloaded to the primary investigator's computer for upload into Atlas.ti (version 11). Only deidentified data will be shared between the researchers assisting in data analysis.

    (pp. 12–13)

to facilitate discussion on the views and experiences of the participants. While the findings of focus groups are not normally generalisable (due mainly to the small sample size and the recruitment procedures), one can seek consensus on some of the issues that are discussed in the focus groups.

While time and cost may be less of an issue for focus groups than for one-to-one interviews, they should not be the only or main reasons why focus groups are selected. In their study exploring the 'content and feature preferences for a physical activity app for adults with physical disabilities', Olsen et al. (2019) explain that they used focus groups to 'encourage interaction and generation of ideas related to the proposed fitness tracking app' (p. 3). They justified their selection based on the potential for focus groups to offer opportunities for 'discussion, debate and idea sharing' (p. 3). In this study (Olsen et al., 2019) the authors reported that focus group participants discussed and ranked a wide variety of features and content for the app. Consensus was also achieved 'for features that would make this app unique to people with physical disabilities' (Olsen et al., 2019, p. 16).

Another feature of focus groups to include in proposals is the suitability of this method of data collection for the specific population based on their vulnerability or condition. According to McParland and Flowers (2012), 'patient groups have specific requirements and the conduct of focus groups should be driven by these needs to maximise inclusion and quality contributions in the group' (p. 492). They offered nine lessons based on their experience of conducting focus groups with people with chronic pain:

> *The lessons relate to (1) translating study interest into group attendance, (2) ensuring the environment maximizes the opportunity to learn from participants, (3) understanding participant motivations for attendance as well as (4) what participants take from the group, (5) ensuring adequate question specificity, accommodating the needs of particular groups in (6) moderation style and (7) discussion time scales, (8) considering the function of conflict in the group and (9) paying due attention to simultaneous dialogue.*

> *McParland and Flowers (2012, p. 492)*

Llewellyn (2009) chose focus groups for her study on the advocacy role of learning disability nurses based on the 'convenience of interviewing more than one person with intellectual disabilities at the same time' and that 'participants tend to feel empowered and supported by the group dynamic and are more likely to share their opinions in the presence of others who they perceive to be like them in some way' (p. 846). However, she pointed out that some of 'the pitfalls associated with the method', in particular, that some 'people with learning disabilities are likely to require support from people who work with them when participating in focus groups' (p. 846). This can cause difficulties such as 'censoring' and 'conformity'. Llewellyn (2009) concluded that the 'attitudes of the supporters to their clients with intellectual disabilities affected both the interactions of the participants and the resultant information' and that 'this can cause a dilemma for researchers, who must be aware of these effects and attempt to counteract them' (p. 855).

These two examples of focus group research with specific populations are presented here to alert researchers designing a study that they need to think carefully about the population they seek to collect data from and the difficulties and challenges that they may face in their proposed study. Other groups include children, adolescents as well as older people with cognitive impairment.

Online Focus Groups

As online data collection becomes more popular, the need to discuss its benefits and challenges and for researchers to learn from one another has also increased. While most of the principles of, and expertise in, using 'land-based' data collection methods are applicable and useful for conducting online research, the online setting has its own practical, methodological, logistical, ethical and legal implications for focus groups. According to Wilkerson et al. (2014) 'researchers should reflect on administrative, population, and data collection considerations when deciding between online and offline data collection' (p. 561). The following recommendations by Wilkerson et al. (2014) should be helpful to researchers, in particular those designing a study and developing research proposals:

> *Decisions must be made regarding whether to conduct interviews or focus groups, to collect data using asynchronous or synchronous methods, and to use only text or to incorporate visual media. Researchers should also reflect on human subjects, recruitment, research instrumentation, additional data collection, and public relations considerations when writing protocols to guide the research team's response to various situations.*

> *(p. 561)*

Online focus group interviews can be synchronous or asynchronous (see, for example, Daniels et al., 2019). In synchronous focus groups, all participants engage in discussion at the same time, as is the case in traditional focus groups. This discussion led by a moderator, can be text based (e.g. via email, chat, instant messaging, discussion boards, etc.) or via an audio/video virtual conferencing platform such as Zoom or Teams. Kite and Phongsavan (2017) conducted real-time synchronous online focus groups via a web conference service, Blackboard Collaborate, to evaluate a 'postgraduate subject in public health' at a university. In this study, the authors carried out both face-to-face 'traditional' focus groups as well as online ones. All the groups were moderated in the same style and by the same person.

Asynchronous focus groups involve the collection of text-based data over a period of time during which participants can, in their own time, post messages via email and other social media. The moderator usually posts daily questions for the participants to discuss. Ripat and Colatruglio (2016) explored 'winter community participation among wheelchair users'. The online focus group took place over a period of seven consecutive days. The process was described by the authors as follows:

> *A moderator posted a new set of questions daily for the participants to discuss, and encouraged additional thoughts and reflections. Participants were asked to respond to the daily questions, to one another, and/or to previous days' questions throughout the entire week. On the final day, participants were asked to reflect on their own answers and the answers of others, and to post any additional comments that may not have been addressed by the topic questions.*

> *(p. 97)*

In research proposals, the choice of format of online focus groups (synchronous or asynchronous) should be justified. Ripat and Colatruglio (2016) explained that an asynchronous online focus group was selected because it had 'several advantages over a traditional focus group', including 'time for more in-depth and reflective responses from participants', 'greater participant anonymity', 'increased convenience in terms of participating from any location at any time' and 'automatic capture of discussion data' (p. 97).

An increasing number of publications offer reflections and recommendations for researchers contemplating online qualitative studies in general, and online focus groups in particular. The following papers are a good place to start:

- Jowett et al. (2011), 'Online interviewing in psychology: reflections on the process'.
- Wilkerson et al. (2014), 'Recommendations for internet-based qualitative health research with hard-to-reach populations'.
- Tuttas (2015), 'Lessons learned using Web conference technology for online focus group interviews'.
- Keen et al. (2022), 'From challenge to opportunity: virtual qualitative research during COVID-19 and beyond'.

There are benefits and challenges with any online focus group formats. The main benefits are well documented in the literature. These include reaching out to participants across large geographical areas and those who are unable to travel due to time, disability, the potential to remain anonymous and costs. Another benefit is that the degree of control of the discussion by participants is likely to be higher in synchronous online focus groups where they converse or discuss among themselves, with minimum 'control' by the moderator. Wirtz et al. (2019) conducted online focus groups in a feasibility study for qualitative HIV research among transgender women living in six cities in the eastern and southern USA. They observed that these focus groups:

were found to facilitate geographic diversity; allow participants to control anonymity and privacy (e.g., use of pseudonyms and option to use video); ease scheduling by eliminating challenges related to travel to a data collection site; and offer flexibility to join via a variety of devices.

(p. 1)

As with one-to-one online interviews, one of the main challenges is the need for participants to have good internet access and technological competence. After conducting a study that involved collecting data through online and face-to-face focus groups, Kite and Phongsavan (2017) concluded that the level of discussion and the quality of the data was similar in both groups. However, they noted that 'some issues remain such as managing technical issues experienced by participants and ensuring adequate recording quality to facilitate transcription and analysis' (p. 1).

Anticipating the challenges of computer mediated communication, the researchers in the study by Wirtz et al. (2019) informally assessed technological literacy during initial screening telephone calls. This enabled these researchers to address individuals' needs and preferences for communicating. Participants 'who appeared to have lower levels of technological literacy or lower levels of comfort with technology' were advised to call 'into the focus group discussion, rather than use a computer or tablet' (Wirtz et al., 2019, p. 3). It is clear that online focus groups can offer a fair degree of flexibility compared with traditional focus groups.

Researchers conducting online research, especially beginners, also need training and support. In addition, data security and the risk of data being intercepted by a third party (Jowett et al., 2011) should be of concern to researchers. There are many ways in which researchers have addressed some of these challenges. This is why it is important for those planning to conduct online focus groups to familiarise themselves with the literature on the topic. Recording and analysing potentially large amounts of data, sound quality and ensuring that all participants can fully participate in the discussion are some of the other issues that may present difficulties to researchers. Kite and Phongsavan (2017) used Blackboard Collaborate, which had an in-built facility to record; however, not all video conferencing platforms have this facility. There are also cost implications for acquiring or hiring these communication platforms. This, as well as technicians' input (prior to, during and after the focus groups), should be costed in proposals, as appropriate. Kite and Phongsavan (2017) also recommended that several conferencing platforms are explored when designing studies involving online focus groups. They also suggested the use of headsets with a microphone to ensure good quality sound.

The analysis of online focus group data is the same as for traditional focus groups. Some of the non-verbal 'messages' of participants may, however, be missed. There may be a need to conduct some individual interviews to clarify some of the participants' responses. On the other hand, taped videos of the focus groups can allow researchers opportunities to review the recordings as many times as they need. The same ethical and safety principles in handling and managing data of other qualitative online designs apply to data from online focus groups. Additional attention should be paid to how data recorded by such platforms as Zoom or Blackboard Collaborate can be removed from them and safely kept, according to research governance requirements. An example of data analysis for online focus groups comes from Wirtz et al. (2019), who explained that the discussions were recorded via the Zoom software platform and transcribed by a professional transcription company. These were read in conjunction with the 'detailed notes and debriefing meetings with study staff following the discussions' (p. 3). The analysis of data involved the use of NVivo qualitative analysis software by trained qualitative analysts who met 'to discuss agreement and resolve discrepancies in coding' (Wirtz et al., 2019, p. 3).

Data analysis for online focus groups is not without its own challenges. In their proposal for a study to explore membership of healthcare professionals in an intensive care virtual community, Rolls et al. (2016) anticipated the potential challenge relating to a high volume of data that may make data analysis more difficult. Pointing out the challenges of the design in a protocol is crucial in order to show that the researchers have carefully considered the strengths and limitations of what they are proposing. This type of observation adds credibility to the proposal.

Tuttas (2015) offered valuable lessons learned using web conference technology for online focus group interviews. These lessons included 'testing and retesting the technology', 'establishing effective lines of communication', 'assessing the technological capacity of participants', 'establishing rapport', 'connectivity: access to the virtual meeting space' and 'sound quality management'. These lessons are useful to researchers designing and conducting studies involving online focus groups.

An example of an online focus group is given in Proposal Example 9.4.

PROPOSAL EXAMPLE 9.4
DESCRIBING ONLINE FOCUS GROUPS IN A PROPOSAL

Brady et al. (2022), 'Physiotherapist beliefs and perspectives on virtual reality–supported rehabilitation for the assessment and management of musculoskeletal shoulder pain: a focus group study protocol'.

COMMENTS

1. The authors selected a qualitative research approach because it 'is appropriate for this research question as it provides preliminary insight into a novel clinical intervention' (p. 4). According to them, qualitative description is an 'excellent choice for the healthcare environments designer, practitioner or health sciences researcher because it provides rich descriptive content from the subject's perspective' (p. 5).

2. Brady et al. (2022) chose online focus groups to collect data because they wanted to encourage discussion between participants, and between researchers and participants. According to them, 'focus groups allow for the emergence of important themes that may be overlooked in individual interviews with a more structured question schedule' (p. 5). Another reason given for choosing them is that 'focus groups have also been identified as an appropriate method for informing product or intervention development' (p. 5).

3. The authors explained, below, in detail how they intended to undertake the online focus groups:

Interviews will be conducted via Microsoft Teams and will be video recorded using Microsoft Team's native recording function. Permission for video recording will occur at two time-points; via completion of the consent form with attached information sheet which outlines the interview and recording process, and at the start of the focus group interview, before commencing the recording function. On completion of the focus group interview, the built-in recording function in Microsoft Teams stores the video recording directly to UCC One Drive which is secure and private. The recordings will then be transcribed into text by the [principal investigator] and the transcription will be saved in Microsoft Teams in Microsoft word format. The original video recording will then be deleted.

(p. 7)

4. Brady et al. (2022) mentioned that data collection and analysis would be carried out concurrently. They also gave details of their 'six-phase process of thematic analysis'.

Checklist for the qualitative data collection and analysis sections of research proposals:

1. Are the data collection methods stated and explained? (e.g. If 'in-depth interview' is the choice, what type of interview is it – land based or online?)

2. Is the choice of method justified to achieve the aim(s) of this study? (e.g. What makes the 'interview' or 'focus group' [or both], the method[s] of choice?)

3. Does the data collection method suit the topic of the study and/or the population being studied? Are relevant references provided to support the choice of methods?

4. Is the process of data collection clearly explained? (e.g. How will interviews or focus groups be conducted?)

5. Are details about the method(s) provided (e.g. number, duration, timing, setting of interviews/focus groups, etc.)?

6. Is the interviewer or focus group moderator trained or experienced? Or will training be provided?
7. If the interview or focus group is online, has the relevant information been provided (e.g. type of online focus group [synchronous or asynchronous]; choice and justification of platform; data recording facility and process; technical support prior to, during and after the focus group; assessment of the level of technical support that participants may need, etc.)?
8. What is the process for the recording and analysis of the data?
9. Who will analyse the data and how will rigour be ensured?
10. Is a particular analysis framework to be used (e.g. grounded theory, IPA, framework analysis etc.) ? Are they appropriate and justified?
11. What data analysis/management software will be used? Is the choice appropriate and justified?
12. How will the data be managed and by whom? (e.g. How will the security and protection of the data be ensured? How long will the data be stored? Who will have access to them?)

SUMMARY AND CONCLUSIONS

The main types of qualitative interview (one-to-one and focus groups) have been explored. The implications of using each when designing a study have been explained. The benefits and challenges of each method have also been highlighted. Examples from real research proposals have been provided.

This chapter has shown that choosing appropriate qualitative data collection and analysis methods for a study is a laborious but crucial process for the study to be completed successfully. Providing relevant and adequate information in the proposal about why and how these methods will be used in the study also requires careful thought. The checklist provided can help to remind researchers of the key items that they should include in their research proposals.

REFERENCES

Brady, N., Lewis, J., McCreesh, K., Dejaco, B., & McVeigh, J. G. (2022). Physiotherapist beliefs and perspectives on virtual reality–supported rehabilitation for the assessment and management of musculoskeletal shoulder pain: A focus group study protocol. *HRB Open Research*, 4, 40. https://doi.org/10.12688/hrbopenrcs.13239.2

Carter, M., Shih, P., Williams, J., Degeling, C., & Mooney-Somers, J. (2021). Conducting qualitative research online: Challenges and solutions. *Patient*, 14, 711–718.

Ceprnja, D., Chipchase, L., Liamputtong, P., & Gupta, A. (2018). How do Australian women cope with pelvic girdle pain during pregnancy? A qualitative study protocol. *BMJ Open*, 8(7), e022332. https://doi.org/10.1136/bmjopen-2018-022332

Daniels, N., Gillen, P., Wilson, I., & Casson, K. (2019). STEER: Factors to consider when designing online focus groups using audio-visual technology in health research. *International Journal of Qualitative Methods*, 18, 1. https://doi.org/10.1177/1609406919885786

Edib, Z., Jayasinghe, Y., Hickey, M., Stafford, L., Anderson, R. A., Su, H. I., Stern, K., Saunders, C., Anazodo, A., Macheras-Magias, M., Chang, S., Pang, P., Agresta, F., Chin-Lenn, L., Cui, W., Pratt, S., Gorelik, A., & Peate, M. (2020). Exploring the facilitators and barriers to using an online infertility risk prediction tool (FoRECAsT) for young women with breast cancer: A qualitative study protocol. *BMJ Open*, 10(2), e033669. https://doi.org/10.1136/bmjopen-2019-033669

Gray, L. M., Wong-Wylie, G., Rempel, G. R., & Cook, K. (2020). Expanding qualitative research interviewing strategies: Zoom video communications. *The Qualitative Report*, *25*(5), 1292–1301.

Hawkins, J. E. (2018). The practical utility and suitability of email interviews in qualitative research. *The Qualitative Report*, *23*(2), 493–501.

Ibrahim, S., Sidani, S., Lok, J., Mukerji, G., & Sherifali, D. (2020). Recreational cannabis usage among young adults living with diabetes: Protocol for a mixed methods study. *Diabetes Therapy*, *11*(6), 1407–1417. https://doi.org/10.1007/s13300-020-00818-w

Jowett, A., Peel, E., & Shaw, R. (2011). Online interviewing in psychology: Reflections on the process. *Qualitative Research in Psychology*, *8*(4), 354–369.

Keen, S., Lomeli-Rodriguez, M., & Joffe, H. (2022). From challenge to opportunity: Virtual qualitative research during COVID-19 and beyond. *International Journal of Qualitative Methods*, *21*, 16094069221105075. https://doi.org/10.1177/16094069221105075

Kite, J., & Phongsavan, P. (2017). Insights for conducting real-time focus groups online using a web conferencing service. *F1000Research*, *6*, 122. https://doi.org/10.12688/f1000research.10427.1

Liu, Q., Luo, D., Haase, J. E., Guo, Q., Wang, X. Q., Liu, S., Xia, L., Liu, Z., Yang, J., & Yang, B. X. (2020). The experiences of health-care providers during the COVID-19 crisis in China: A qualitative study. *Lancet Global Health*, *8*(6), e790–e798. https://doi.org/10.1016/S2214-109X(20)30204-7

Llewellyn, P. (2009). Supporting people with intellectual disabilities to take part in focus groups: Reflections on a research project. *Disability & Society*, *24*(7), 845–856. https://doi.org/10.1080/09687590903283431

Lo Iacono, V., Symonds, P., & Brown, D. H. (2016). Skype as a Tool for Qualitative Research Interviews. *Sociological Research Online*, *21*, 103–117.

McParland, J. L., & Flowers, P. (2012). Nine lessons and recommendations from the conduct of focus group research in chronic pain samples. *British Journal of Health Psychology*, *17*(3), 492–504.

Miles, M. B., & Huberman, A. M. (1994). *Qualitative data analysis: An expanded sourcebook*. California: Sage.

Novick, G. (2008). Is there a bias against telephone interviews in qualitative research? *Research in Nursing & Health*, *31*(4), 391–398.

Olsen, S. H., Saperstein, S. L., & Gold, R. S. (2019). Content and feature preferences for a physical activity app for adults with physical disabilities: Focus Group Study. *JMIR Mhealth and Uhealth*, *7*(10), e15019. https://doi.org/10.2196/15019

Parahoo, K. (2014). *Nursing research: Principles, process and issues* (3rd ed.). London: Palgrave Macmillan.

Ripat, J., & Colatruglio, A. (2016). Exploring winter community participation among wheelchair users: An Online Focus Group. *Occupational Therapy in Health Care*, *30*(1), 95–106.

Ritchie, J., & Lewis, J. (2003). *Qualitative research practice: A guide for social science students and researchers*. London: Sage.

Roberts, J., Pavlakis, A., & Richards, M. (2021). It's more complicated than it seems: Virtual qualitative research in the COVID-19 era. *International Journal of Qualitative Methods*, *20*, 160940692110029. https://doi.org/10.1177/16094069211002959

Rolls, K., Hansen, M., Jackson, D., & Elliott, D. (2016). Why we belong – Exploring membership of healthcare professionals in an intensive care virtual community via online focus groups: Rationale and protocol. *JMIR Research Protocols*, *5*(2), e99. https://doi.org/10.2196/resprot.5323

Rousham, E. K., Islam, M. A., Nahar, P., Lucas, P. J., Naher, N., Ahmed, S. M., Nizame, F. A., & Unicomb, L. (2019). Pathways of antibiotic use in Bangladesh: Qualitative protocol for the PAUSE study. *BMJ Open*, *9*(1), e028215. https://doi.org/10.1136/bmjopen-2018-028215

Saarijärvi, M., & Bratt, E. L. (2021). When face-to-face interviews are not possible: Tips and tricks for video, telephone, online chat, and email interviews in qualitative research. *European Journal of Cardiovascular Nursing*, *20*(4), 392–396.

Salmons, J. (2016). *Doing qualitative research online.* Los Angeles: Sage.

Sihre, H. K., Gill, P., Lindenmeyer, A., McGuiness, M., Berrisford, G., Jankovic, J., Patel, M., Lewin, J., & Fazil, Q. (2019). Understanding the lived experiences of severe postnatal psychiatric illnesses in English speaking South Asian women, living in the UK: A qualitative study protocol. *BMJ Open*, *9*(8), e025928. https://doi.org/10.1136/bmjopen-2018-025928

Topping, M., Douglas, J., & Winkler, D. (2021). General considerations for conducting online qualitative research and practice implications for interviewing people with acquired brain injury. *International Journal of Qualitative Methods*, *20*, 160940692110196. https://doi.org/10.1177/16094069211019615

Tuttas, C. A. (2015). Lessons learned using Web conference technology for online focus group interviews. *Qualitative Health Research*, *25*(1), 122–133.

Webster, N., Jenkins, C., Oyebode, J., Bentham, P., & Smythe, A. (2019). Experiences of peer support for newly qualified nurses in a dedicated online group: Study protocol. *Journal of Advanced Nursing*, *75*(7), 1585–1591.

White, D. R., & Palmieri, P. A. (2022). Women caring for husbands living with Parkinson's Disease: A phenomenological study protocol. *Journal of Personalized Medicine*, *12*(5), 659. https://doi.org/10.3390/jpm12050659

Wilkerson, J. M., Iantaffi, A., Grey, J. A., Bockting, W. O., & Rosser, B. R. (2014). Recommendations for internet-based qualitative health research with hard-to-reach populations. *Qualitative Health Research*, *24*(4), 561–574.

Williams, H. M., Jones, L. L., Coomarasamy, A., & Topping, A. E. (2020). Men living through multiple miscarriages: Protocol for a qualitative exploration of experiences and support requirements. *BMJ Open*, *10*(5), e035967. https://doi.org/10.1136/bmjopen-2019-035967

Wirtz, A. L., Cooney, E. E., Chaudhry, A., Reisner, S. L., & American Cohort to Study HIV Acquisition Among Transgender Women. (2019). Computer-mediated communication to facilitate synchronous online focus group discussions: Feasibility study for qualitative HIV research among transgender women across the United States. *Journal of Medical Internet Research*, *21*(3), e12569. https://doi.org/10.2196/12569

Zheng, K., Sutherland, S., Cardinal, P., Meade, M., Landriault, A., Vanderspank-Wright, B., Valiani, S., Shemie, S., Appleby, A., Keenan, S., Weiss, M., Werestiuk, K., Kramer, A. H., Kawchuk, J., Beed, S., Dhanani, S., Pagliarello, G., Chasse, M., Lotherington, K., Gatien, M., ... Sarti, A. J. (2020). Patient-centred and family-centred care of critically ill patients who are potential organ donors: A qualitative study protocol of family member perspectives. *BMJ Open*, *10*(6), e037527. https://doi.org/10.1136/bmjopen-2020-037527

10 QUANTITATIVE AND QUALITATIVE OBSERVATION IN PROPOSALS

INTRODUCTION

Observation plays an important part in nursing, health and social care research because it allows the exploration of actual behaviour and events. It is a useful method to collect data to answer research questions in quantitative, qualitative and mixed methods studies. It can be used on its own or in conjunction with other methods such as interviews. The aim of this chapter is to give examples of what observations can be used for and what to take into account when designing a study using observation as a data collection method. The main types of observation used in quantitative and qualitative research will be briefly discussed. A checklist to remind researchers what to include in proposals of studies using observation will also be provided.

In some disciplines, an observational study is a broad term that refers to studies other than randomised controlled trials. For example, Song and Chung (2010) identified two primary types of observational study: cohort and case studies. These types of study may or may not involve observation as a data collection method. The term 'observational study' will be used here to denote studies with observation as the main method of data collection.

COMMON TYPES OF OBSERVATION IN RESEARCH STUDIES

There are three main types of observation: structured, unstructured and semistructured. Semistructured and unstructured observation are mostly used in qualitative studies (see the section on qualitative observation, later in the chapter). Structured observations are appropriate for quantitative studies where the aim is to measure phenomena. Catchpole et al. (2017) pointed out that 'non-participant direct observation of health care processes offers a rich method for understanding safety and performance improvement' (p. 1015). Structured observations have been used to study 'the types, frequency and severity of adverse events that occur in different domains, including drug administration, emergency departments, operating theatres, anaesthesia, obstetrics and intensive care units' (Carthey, 2003, p. ii13). Gathara et al. (2018) developed a proposal for a study aimed at quantifying nursing delivered in Kenyan newborn units, using direct, structured observation to collect data. Johnson et al. (2023) carried out an observational study of physiotherapists' use of motor learning principles in stroke rehabilitation.

Ferguson (2016) believed that 'observing encounters between social workers and service users as they naturally occur' is necessary for 'producing knowledge of what actually goes on when social workers and children and families are face to face' (p. 154).

Structured observation can be defined as the systematic collection of data by direct observation using predetermined categories. Researchers decide, in advance of data collection, what components and sub-components of the behaviour or event will be observed and recorded using a checklist or observation schedule. For example, in their proposal for a study 'to measure and map community pharmacists' time and workspace as a means of informing the feasibility of implementing extended pharmacy services' (p. 443), Karia et al. (2020) carried out a workflow analysis using the Work Observation Method By Activity Timing (WOMBAT) tool. They explained that 'data will be collected across four dimensions', as follows:

1. *What (the task being observed);*
2. *Where (the location where the observed task is being undertaken);*
3. *With (the person/people with the pharmacist at the time the observed task is being undertaken);*
4. *How (how is the task being completed, for example, using a phone?).*

(p. 444)

It is beyond the scope of this chapter to give a fuller discussion of observation as a data collection method. For more information on structured observation, see:

- Carthey (2003), 'The role of structured observational research in healthcare'.
- Fix et al. (2022), 'Direct observation methods: a practical guide for health researchers'.
- Parkinson et al. (2017), 'Observation in health and social care: applications for learning, research and practice with children and adults'.
- Catchpole et al. (2017), 'Framework for direct observation of performance and safety in healthcare'.
- Mansell (2011), 'Structured observational research in services for people with learning disabilities'.

ISSUES TO CONSIDER WHEN USING STRUCTURED OBSERVATION

There are a number of issues or aspects of observation to think about when designing a study using this method. These are: what is to be observed, how the observations will be carried out, when and where data will be collected and who will undertake the observations. Other issues to consider are recruitment, sampling of participants (or events), access to potential observation sites and ethical implications (these will be discussed in Chapters 11, 12 and 13).

What Is to Be Observed

The target of observation is mainly the behaviour of people (patients, clients, health professionals) during selected events. This can vary between simply observing and counting, for example, the number of times a health professional 'interrupts' when a client is talking during a counselling session, to a detailed observation of the non-verbal communication between them. What is to be observed can be stated in the research question(s) or aims. For example, Duxbury et al. (2010) carried out observations to answer the following questions:

1. *What occurs during a medication round?*
2. *What interaction takes place between nursing staff and service users?*
3. *How is consent established and addressed?*
4. *To what extent is information shared?*

(p. 2483)

After stating what is to be observed, key concepts such as 'medication round' should be operationally defined. In this case the term 'round' referred to 'set daily periods during which time prescribed medications are administered routinely' (Duxbury et al. 2010, p. 2583). 'Factors influencing interaction' itself is a broad concept that also needs to be defined. In this study it comprised 'several subsections including practical issues, understanding administration, inter-action, information exchange, assessing the patient's ability to take medication, collaboration, "prn" and "the end of the round" ' (p. 2583).

Sometimes the definition of concepts or behaviours to be observed can be taken from well-established and recommended sources. For example, direct observation of 'hand hygiene com-pliance' has been based on the World Health Organization (2012) five moments when health care workers should perform hand hygiene:

1. *before touching a patient*
2. *before clean/aseptic procedure*
3. *after body fluid exposure risk*
4. *after touching a patient*
5. *after touching a patient's surroundings.*

This definition was used in a proposal for the study of hand hygiene compliance in nursing homes by Teesing et al. (2020).

How the Observations Will Be Carried Out

This phase of the design includes selecting the instrument or observation schedule/checklist to be used to record the observations, how the recordings will be made and how the data will be stored and analysed.

Nurses and health and social care professionals are familiar with the assessment tools they use in their practice with patients or students. For example, Westlake et al. (2020) developed an evidence-informed practice tool to assess social work communication through direct observa-tion. In physiotherapy, the Assessment of Physiotherapy Practice instrument can be used to measure 'professional competence' (Dalton et al., 2012). For research purposes, an observation tool has to be valid (i.e. the items should adequately represent the concept being observed, e.g. 'professional competence') and reliable (the tool has to be consistent in measuring professional competence and able to differentiate between a poor, mediocre or high level of competence). Researchers have to develop and test their own observation tools or use existing ones. For an example of an observation tool, see Appendix 1 in Duxbury et al. (2010).

For proposals competing for funding, it is advisable to use existing, validated tools or construct and test the observation tool in advance of the proposal's submission. The section on how observations will be carried out should include how the concept to be observed is defined and broken into components and subcomponents, and how the tool will be tested for feasibility (i.e. whether it is actually possible to observe what is in the checklist) and reliability (including inter-rater reliability). In their proposal for a study of 'community pharmacist workflow', Karia et al. (2020) explain how this will be done in their study:

> *During the training, observers will jointly practice observing and categorising tasks undertaken by a pharmacist participant. Discrepancies between observers will be discussed and corrected. Consistency will then be tested with both the trainer and the trainee research assistant independently recording observations of the same pharmacist, at the same time until there are reasonable uniformity and good inter-rater reliability scores between all observers. Repeated training sessions and assessments will be scheduled to clarify observations, rectify discrepancies and achieve consistency before any further data collection occurs. Task list and definitions will also be amended during observer trainings if clarification is required.*

> *(p. 444)*

The need for describing how the observation tool will be tested for validity, reliability and feasibility should not be underestimated. This type of information in a proposal can instil confidence in reviewers that the data collection tool will be rigorously developed and tested.

Where and When Data Will Be Collected

The observation of phenomena depends on when and where they manifest themselves. Some events, such as team meetings or assessment of clients, happen regularly. Others, such as medical errors or aggressive behaviour, are less predictable. Deciding on when, where, for how long and how frequently to observe an event or behaviour depends on how often and in what circumstances they reveal themselves. In the pharmacist workflow study (Karia et al., 2020), the phenomenon to be observed is the work of pharmacists; this is ongoing between set hours. Therefore, researchers can choose the number and size of pharmacies, the number of observations to be carried out and the duration and timing of each observation session.

In the study by Duxbury et al. (2010) of interactions during 'medical rounds', they explained that a sample of rounds on each ward was observed to ensure that the 24-hour period was covered and that these took place at 8:30 a.m., 12:30 p.m., 5:30 p.m. and 10 p.m. A total of 20 rounds were observed and the observations ranged between 20 minutes and 1 hour (Duxbury et al., 2010). The process of sampling is known as 'event' sampling; the event (or phenomenon) to be observed in this case is the 'round'. The choice of times at which the observations took place is called 'time sampling'. In this study the sample of times at which observations happened was 8:30 a.m., 12:30 p.m., etc. Justification for both event and time sampling should be given in research proposals.

Observers

Researchers have to decide, in advance, who will carry out the observations, and any training they may require prior to undertaking the task of observing and recording data. Observing minute behavioural detail (e.g. non-verbal communication) and multiple, simultaneous behaviours and recording them as accurately as possible are difficult tasks. Sometimes experienced professionals are recruited to carry out the observations because they have an understanding of the behaviours and interactions taking place. In Duxbury et al.'s (2010) study of medication rounds, there were three observers (two mental health nurses and one psychologist). However, familiarity with what is being observed can also lead observers to take things for granted. This can be avoided by training observers, giving clear instructions and pilot testing of the observation tool.

An important issue to be considered when designing structured observation studies is the effect that the presence of observers has on the behaviour of those being observed. This is known as the Hawthorne effect (see Paradis and Sutkin, 2017, for a discussion of this concept). For example, in a study by Ram et al. (2010), there was some evidence that hand washing behaviour was significantly increased when observed by researchers. Halder et al. (2013) recommended a 'prolonged duration of structured observation', and the development of innovative models to 'reduce reactivity to observation and improve the measurement of hand washing behaviour' (p. 1). In their proposal, Karia et al. (2020) explained how they intended to address any potential reactivity effect of observation:

It is acknowledged that the direct, open observational method adopted here may influence pharmacists' work patterns where the participant (and other staff or consumers) may feel anxious and possibly present an enhancement in performance in the presence of an external observer. However, these may be reduced with the pharmacist being observed for extended periods, on multiple occasions and for up to two hours per session, and by the observer being positioned out of the way of usual practices but close enough to observe the participant.

(p. 445)

The plans for data management, handling and analysis are also issues that should be planned in advance and explained in the proposal. This process should be no different from that explained in the previous chapter in relation to questionnaires. In Karia et al.'s (2020) study, collected data were to be stored 'primarily in digital format' on 'password protected computers'; data on paper (such as consent forms) would be stored in locked cabinets for 'at least seven years following results publication and destroyed in line with current local guidelines' (p. 443).

In proposals, the choice of structured observation in a study should be justified. In the proposal by Karia et al. (2020), the study's objectives were to quantify the proportion of time spent on different work tasks, the frequency of each task and of consumer contact, the time spent on multitasking and the rate of interruptions, and to 'relate these observations to metrics analysis of existing spacial capacity and pharmacy layouts' (p. 443). Questionnaires and interviews rely on self-reports and are not appropriate to meet these objectives. Semistructured and unstructured observations will not be systematic enough to collect the quantifiable data required.

For an example of a proposal using structured observation, see Proposal Example 10.1.

PROPOSAL EXAMPLE 10.1
A PROPOSAL FOR A STRUCTURED OBSERVATION STUDY

Gathara et al. (2018), 'Quantifying nursing care delivered in Kenyan newborn units: protocol for a cross-sectional direct observational study'.

The aim of this study was to describe 'essential neonatal nursing care given or missed within newborn units' (p. 1) in six hospitals in Nairobi, Kenya, by means of structured observation.

COMMENTS

1. The authors 'adopted the definition of missed care reported in the wider literature' (p. 6). A list of 'routine and critical tasks' to be observed were identified by the nursing advisory group of the project. The authors explained that 'where necessary, tasks are broken down into manageable observable task components to facilitate observation' (p. 5). These tasks constituted the 'observation checklist'.

2. To ensure that it was feasible to undertake observations, the authors stated that the 'observation checklist will be extensively piloted over a period of 6 weeks' (p. 5). According to them, this would 'determine the quantity and quality of data that can be reasonably gathered and will be adapted as needed' (p. 5). The pilot phase also helped to explore whether it would be possible, feasible and practical to observe everything that the authors were setting out to observe. Pilot testing the observation tool in real-life settings is crucial prior to undertaking the main study. In proposals, it is crucial to describe the aim, process and expected outcome of the piloting phase.

3. In this study, six observers were to be trained for 2 weeks. Although the term 'inter-rater reliability' is not mentioned, the authors aimed to compare observations made by the observers during the 2 weeks' training, discuss any differences and adjust the checklist and observation instructions, as necessary.

4. Gathara et al. (2018) acknowledged that 'nurses might change the way they provide care when they are being observed (the Hawthorne effect)' (p. 6). To reduce this effect, the observer would spend at least 1 week in the observation setting 'to familiarise themselves with the environment, to explain the study to staff and parents and for the staff within the newborn unit to get used to them' (p. 6). Formal observation would start after the 1-week familiarisation.

5. The authors also explained that they had considered collecting data by means of video recording, but for ethical, medical and legal reasons they could not do so.

6. In this study the recording of observation will be paper-based. Data will then be transferred to an electronic file thereafter. For the accurate transfer of data, measures should be put in place to ensure the reliability of the transfer.

Checklist for quantitative structured observation in a proposal:
1. Does the research question reflect clearly what is to be observed?
2. Is the structured observation data collection method appropriate for answering this question?
3. What is the rationale/justification for the choice of structured observation?
4. What is the event or behaviour that will be observed?
5. Has the event or behaviour been defined? Who has defined it (i.e. researchers in the team or an existing definition)? Is there likely to be a consensus among professionals/academics for this definition?
6. How will the event or behaviour be observed? Will an instrument be constructed or will an existing one be used?
7. If the instrument is to be constructed, has the process been explained (who will construct it, how the content of the instrument will be determined and how it will be tested)?
8. If an existing tool is used, has it been tested for validity and reliability? Has it been used in other studies? Will the tool be adapted? Why? How will the tool be tested?
9. Who will carry out the observation? Will they be trained? Has this process been explained?
10. Will inter-rater reliability be tested? How?
11. How will the event or behaviour be selected (event sampling)? What is the justification for this selection?
12. What is the timing, duration and frequency of the observations? Will this provide a valid representation of the event or behaviour?
13. Where will the observation take place? How many sites are involved and how (and why) are these selected? Has some preliminary contact been made with stakeholders or 'gatekeepers' to assess the feasibility of observation?
14. When will the observation be carried out? How long will it take to complete all the observations?
15. What other potential issues (e.g. the Hawthorne effect) and implications or complications may arise? How will these be addressed?
17. How will the data be recorded, handled and analysed? Who will analyse the data?
18. If non-participant observation is being used, in what circumstances would the observer intervene?

QUALITATIVE OBSERVATIONS

The purpose of qualitative research is to explore how people think about phenomena and behave the way they do (and why), from their own perspectives and, as far as possible, in their natural environment. Unstructured and semistructured observations are best suited to this type of exploration. In unstructured observations, researchers focus on a broad topic and then allow their attention to be drawn on aspects that they find revealing and worth exploring. This type of observation is normally carried out in anthropological studies where researchers live for prolonged periods among communities, participate in their activities and learn about people's lives as an insider. It involves total or full participation, and is rarely used in nursing, health and social research.

Gold (1958) identified four observational roles in sociological research: 'complete observer', 'observer-as-participant', 'participant-as-observer' and 'complete participant'. The complete observer role is one in which the observer does not take part in the social setting at all, for example when watching people's behaviour from behind a two-way mirror (Gold 1958). This role is the one that quantitative researchers aim to achieve in structured observations, described earlier. The 'observer-as-participant' role is one in which the main role of researchers is to observe but they may be drawn into the 'action', for example when a health professional looking after a patient needs the researcher to fetch a glass of water for a patient or help in an emergency, such as a patient falling. In the 'participant-as-observer' role, the researcher is involved as a health or social care professional and makes observations during the course of their work. The 'complete participant' is the anthropological one described above, where the researcher is fully involved in the life of the community and (tries to) behave as they do.

A brief scan of the literature on health studies involving qualitative observations shows that researchers describe their methods as participant or non-participant observation. They then describe the type and extent of participation. For example, in a study of the 'relationship between community-based physical activity and wellbeing in people with dementia', Wright (2018) conducted 'participant observation'. Participation was described as engaging 'in physical activity alongside participants in each of the seven locations' and occasionally accompanying people with dementia and their carers 'as they walked around their neighbourhood' (p. 526).

In their proposal for a study evaluating the feasibility of a randomised controlled trial of an intervention to support stroke survivors and their carers in the longer term, Hardicre et al. (2018) explained that during 'non-participant' observation of the study site, 'researchers will not seek to become involved in conversations, meetings or interactions, so as not to influence local processes, but may seek clarification about what has been observed through conversation at an appropriate later time' (p. 8).

Participant and non-participant observations can be unstructured or semistructured. The literature shows that the degree or extent of structure varies from study to study. Unstructured observations may be too unspecific, free-flowing and flexible to fit proposals that require every detail of what will happen. Researchers can, however, give as much information as possible on what the focus of the study is and how observations will be carried out. For example, Hunter et al. (2016) explained the focus and process of the unstructured observations that they conducted in their study of psychosocial intervention use in long-stay dementia care:

Unstructured observation explored the manner in which psychosocial interventions were used within the long-stay setting by viewing staff–resident with dementia interactions. The amount of time spent in each site varied between 4 and 12 hours. The researcher placed himself in resident sitting rooms, dining rooms, staff offices, and reception areas. As the researcher became more familiar with how psychosocial interventions were used by participants in the long-stay settings and the emergent theory, the observation and resultant memoing became more focused on the emergent codes and categories.

(p. 2027)

With semistructured observations, as the term suggests, researchers select some areas to focus upon. While they are open to other findings that are not related to the aspects of the topic they have pre-selected, they use the subcomponents of the topic to guide their observations (and their subsequent data analysis). In their study of 'daytime drinking spaces in the London

Borough of Islington', Thompson et al. (2018) developed a semistructured observation guide 'which allowed for open-ended observations and impressions' of 'the establishment in terms of its clientele, atmosphere, design, and place in the wider alcohol environment' (p. 3). The four 'observation criteria', which provided some structure to the observations, were: 'general observations' (e.g. external appearance, location, opening times, etc.); 'sensory impressions' (e.g. internal design, sound, music, etc.); 'impressions about clientele' (e.g. observations of other customers, their alcohol consumption, age, gender, etc.); and 'alcohol specific observation' (e.g. alcohol on display, deals and promotions, etc.). These items were 'open-ended' as opposed to the 'closed-ended' items in tools used in quantitative structured observations described at the beginning of this chapter.

Other terms that have been used in conjunction with qualitative observations include 'ethnography' and 'focused ethnography'. Wright (2018), in his study of physical activity and wellbeing in people with dementia, described his approach as 'broadly ethnographic'. von Gaudecker et al. (2019) described the method used in their study of 'women's experiences with epilepsy treatment in Southern India' as 'focused ethnography'. They explained that the characteristics of 'focused ethnography' include small samples of participants, 'short-term but intensive field work, participant observation that can occur episodically, and structured interview topics' (p. 1036).

One common feature in studies using qualitative observations is the use of interviews alongside, or following, observations. This makes sense since behaviour can best be explained when we know the thoughts and feelings of the participants. von Gaudecker et al. (2019) used interviews to 'validate observations and to collect information on phenomena that cannot be observed' (p. 1037). Wright (2018) found that 'the process of observation helped to identify potential interviewees and inform interview questions' (p. 527). Interviews in participant observational studies can be formal and informal. The latter normally takes the form of a conversation during which clarifications or justifications of actions and behaviours are sought.

As well as interviews, other data collection methods can also be used in observation studies. Saberi Zafarghandi et al. (2019), in their proposal for a study of 'drug-related community issues' in Tehran, Iran, list three methods – interviews, field observation and focus groups – to answer their research questions. It is also common for researchers to collect demographic and contextual information about participants. In research proposals, each of the data collection methods and sources of information should be fully described, even when they are complementary or subordinate to the main method.

As with quantitative observations, proposals of qualitative observations should include information on what is to be observed, the rationale for the choice of observation type, the process of how, when, where and by whom observations will be undertaken, plans for handling and analysing data and strategies to ensure rigour. Each of these aspects of the proposal will be discussed below. Sampling and ethical issues will be dealt with in Chapters 11, 12 and 13.

Focus of Observation

The focus of qualitative observations should be clearly stated in the research question(s) or aim(s). There are numerous examples of how this can be done in published research proposals and studies. For example, Lillehagen et al. (2013) developed a proposal for a qualitative study of knowledge translation in a participatory research project. Their 'area of study', or focus is the FYSIOPRIM, a programme designed to 'meet some of the challenges for physiotherapy research in primary healthcare' (p. 2). The objective of the study was 'to investigate how KTs (knowledge translations) take place in the interaction between participants in a participatory research project' (p. 2). Lillehagen et al. (2013) gave more information on the particular aspects of interactions that they would focus on. Below are some examples of questions that they sought answers for:

What sort of topics and dilemmas do the participants take a common interest in? Who are responding to what sort of questions in various situations, in what way and with what effect? What sort of arguments are raised as the participants reflect, discuss and try to define a particular problem? What problem-solving approaches are suggested with what effect?

(p. 3)

The focus of qualitative observation can also be broad, with little or no preconceived ideas of the aspects of the topic that will be focused upon. In Hunter et al.'s (2016) study, the objective was 'to develop a substantive grounded theory of staff psychosocial intervention use with residents with dementia in long-stay care' (p. 2024). They carried out unstructured observations of the interactions between staff and residents with dementia, to explore the manner in which psychosocial interventions were used. In accordance with the principles of grounded theory (Glaser and Strauss, 1967), they allowed the codes and categories to begin to emerge from the data to form the emergent theory. Subsequent observations focused on the emerging categories and theory.

Rationale for Qualitative Observation

In a proposal there should be a justification of why qualitative observation is selected for the study. While it makes sense that behaviours and activities are well suited to observation, it is not necessarily the case that observation is always the most appropriate data collection method for all behaviours. Selecting an appropriate method depends on several factors, including what is to be observed, the participants involved in the study, the actual mode of observation, stakeholders' and gatekeepers' approval for access to sites and ethical approval. What is ideal, however, is not always practical or feasible. The choice of data collection method should be carefully considered. Sometimes the obstacles and challenges are so great that collecting data that are valid and reliable may be compromised. In these cases, it may be better to rely on interviews and self-reports, despite their limitations.

The reason why participant observation is selected instead of non-participant (or vice versa) should also be given. There are two types of justification: 'generic' and 'specific'. The generic rationale makes the case that observation of behaviour can reveal what actually happens rather than rely on self-reports (from interviews and questionnaires). This rationale can apply to most studies using observation. A specific rationale makes the case for why participant observation, for example, is best suited to a particular study. Zhao and Ji (2014) chose participant observation and semi-structured interviews in their study of 'Chinese-born immigrant women' in

North Carolina, USA. The specific rationale they offered was that participant observation 'can help researchers to gain an understanding about the sociocultural context where the study informants' daily activities occur' (p. 1) and that this type of observation is particularly appropriate for any community health research.

Depending on the aim of the study, non-participant observation may be a better choice than participant observation. For example, participant observation in a study of interactions at meetings may change the dynamics of the group and influence the interactions. On the other hand, participant observation may reduce the discomfort that participants may feel in the presence of observers. In their participant observations of interactions between adults with severe intellectual disability and their communication partners, Johnson et al. (2011) concluded that:

> *discomfort for all involved can be reduced by the researcher embracing the role of participant-as-observer to allow for family members to include the researcher more fully in the interactions, along with discussing beforehand the purpose of the visits and how the research goals might best be achieved.*
>
> *(p. 276)*

Johnson et al. (2011) went on to state that 'perhaps in situations in which the researcher requires engagement with the person with a severe intellectual disability, a participant-as-observer role may allow for more opportunities to develop trust and interaction than the role of observer' (p. 275).

The use of a particular qualitative approach in observational studies should also be justified. Saletti-Cuesta et al. (2017) in their proposal for a study of 'patient and relative/carer experience of hip fracture in acute care', explained that their choice of hermeneutical phenomenology to underpin their study was because it 'allows exploration of how participants come to know and understand the world through their embodied experience within a wider historical and social context' (p. 37). They also stated that they would use semistructured interviews and participant observation because 'interviews are normally the method of choice in phenomenology as language is a key way of expressing experience' (p. 38).

There are no set rules for choosing one method over another. As explained earlier, there are many factors to take into account and many issues to be considered. The papers by Zhao and Ji (2014) and Johnson et al. (2011) are particularly useful in discussing the difficulties and challenges in observational research.

The Observation Process

Researchers should justify the selected type of observation and explain how it will be carried out in the study. As outlined earlier, not all participant observations are the same. They vary according to the extent of participation and structure. Therefore, how they will be operationalised needs to be clarified in the proposal. Saletti-Cuesta et al. (2017), in their proposal, explained that 'participant observation will take the form of sitting alongside participants and experiencing the daily activities of ward life with them at various times of the day as appropriate' (p. 38).

In their proposal for a study to develop 'an intervention to support the reproductive health of Cambodian women who seek medical abortion', Oreglia et al. (2020) gave details of how the participant observations were to take place, including how 'researchers will live in a guesthouse in the area to experience the environment and familiarize themselves with life in the neighborhood' (p. 4). They will also spend the first week '*hanging out* at both the factory and outside, befriending different potential participants, having meals with them, and, if they agree, joining them for activities outside the factory or to visit their living quarters' (p. 4, original emphasis). In addition, they intended to conduct participant observation at local pharmacies and a clinic.

The number, duration and frequency of observations, as well as who will carry them out and whether, in the case of participant-as-observer, they will be employed as health workers, should be included in a proposal. For example, in their proposal to investigate how knowledge transfer takes place, Lillehagen et al. (2013) stated that they planned to observe 15 coordination meetings. They also identified the three observers (from the authors of proposal) who would conduct the observations. Non-participant observations requires the same amount of detail as well as information on aspects of the behaviour or activities that will be focused upon. There should also be some explanation of where non-participant observers will position themselves, so as not to be conspicuous.

Data Recording, Management and Analysis

How data will be recorded during or after observations should be well planned and adequately described in proposals. Normally, researchers aim to be as inconspicuous as possible when writing notes, as this may cause some discomfort or even concern among participants. In the study of physical activity and wellbeing of people with dementia, Wright (2018) reported that 'brief contemporaneous notes were discretely made during the sessions with more detailed descriptions written up immediately afterwards and discussed with colleagues' (p. 526). Manias et al. (2019) explained that, in their study of 'communicating with patients, families and health professionals about managing medications in intensive care', 'audio-recordings were undertaken of communication interactions using an audio digital recorder with a lapel microphone' (p. 17). The use of audio or video recording should be described and justified in research proposals.

The strategies for recording, storing and analysing data are normally the same as for qualitative interviews, in particular if approaches such as phenomenology or grounded theory are used in the study. For example, Fernández-Sola et al. (2018), in their proposal on the 'characterization, conservation and loss of dignity at the end-of-life in the emergency department', aimed to use a qualitative data management software package to analyse their data. They also explained that they would use four steps to analyse their data, based on a Gadamerian framework.

ADDITIONAL NOTES ON OBSERVATION IN PROPOSALS

Observation is nearly always accompanied or supplemented by data from other sources such as documents, records and other artefacts (Parahoo, 2014). The collection of data from these sources should also be described in detail in the proposal. As many qualitative observational studies tend to include interviews, both methods (or indeed other methods such as focus groups or questionnaires) should be treated equally in terms of how they are described in a proposal, no matter which method is the main or primary one.

Observation as a data collection method has a number of practical implications and challenges that have been highlighted in this chapter. Unlike interviews, which focus on participants' self-reports, observation focus on people, their interactions and their activities in their natural settings, mostly their work sites such as clinics, hospitals, offices and people's homes. In the process of developing proposals, it is crucially important to make preliminary enquiries to explore the feasibility of access to, and observation of, the targeted sites or events. This should then be reported in the proposal.

A checklist for qualitative observations in proposals is given below. Examples of proposals involving participation and non-participation observations are given in Proposal Example 10.2 and 10.3, respectively.

PROPOSAL EXAMPLE 10.2
A PROPOSAL OF A STUDY USING PARTICIPANT OBSERVATION

Dunger et al. (2017), Nurses' decision-making in ethically relevant clinical situations using the example of breathlessness. study protocol of a reflexive grounded theory integrating Goffman's framework analysis'.

The aim of the study in this proposal was to explore which factors influence nurses' decision making to use nursing interventions in situations where patients suffer from severe breathlessness.

COMMENTS

1. Decision making can be studied by several methods including questionnaires, focus groups, interviews and observations. In this study, a combination of methods – qualitative interviews and participant observation – is proposed. The rationale for this choice is that the two methods provide an opportunity for triangulation of the data. Participant observations, qualitative interviews and the observer's self-reflection will help to answer the core question in the study (factors that influence nurses' decision making). The study will be underpinned by the work of Goffman (1974), whose framework analysis integrates participants' observable behaviours and their accounts within their social context. Some components of grounded theory will also be used in this study.

2. The authors recognised, in their proposal, the many challenges they might face in accessing sites, patients and nurses.

3. Participant observations will be carried out by a trained nurse who will 'cover one shift including overtime'; this is 'comparable to an internship or job shadowing' (p. 4). It seems that no predetermined questions will be used to structure the observation other than 'open questions' guided by the 'researcher's perception (Who? What? How? Where? With whom? Why? When?)'.

4. The data analysis process was described in detail in the proposal. Data will be analysed using 'F4 to transcribe the audiotaped interviews' and 'MAXQDA to analyse the observation' data and interview transcripts (p. 4). The authors provided a graphic representation of the process of data collection and analysis as well as the integration of reflexive grounded theory and Goffmann's framework analysis. This is a good example of the effective use of graphics in a proposal.

5. The authors also showed, in the proposal, their awareness of potential challenges that may arise during participant observations, including 'conflicting interests', the sensitivity involved in observing 'intimate interactions', etc. This showed that they had carefully thought out the implications of using participant observation in the study.

PROPOSAL EXAMPLE 10.3
A PROPOSAL OF A STUDY INVOLVING NON-PARTICIPANT QUALITATIVE OBSERVATION

Anagnostou et al. (2017), 'Development of an intervention to support patients and clinicians with advanced lung cancer when considering systemic anticancer therapy: protocol for the PACT study'.

This proposal is about a study that aimed to 'identify the information and decision support needs of patients, leading to the development of an intervention to support patients with advanced lung cancer when considering treatment options' (p. 1).

COMMENTS

1. This study, described by the authors as 'multi-method', will use a combination of data collection methods, including non-participant qualitative observation and interviews. The aim was further detailed in five objectives, representing the five stages of the study. There will be non-participant qualitative observation of four lung multidisciplinary team meetings in each of the four health boards. Non-participant observers 'will be seated away from observed communications and will keep field notes and manage the digital recorder' (p. 4).
2. Aspects of the meetings to be observed (qualitatively) will be broad, and 'in-depth, descriptive and reflective notes recording the researcher's observations will be completed as soon as possible after each observed consultation' (p. 4). These 'aspects' constituted what could be termed 'semistructured qualitative observations', since they will be pre-selected but not measured.
3. The 'description and reflective notes' of the observer will be analysed using the thematic analysis framework of Braun and Clarke (2006).
4. This study also will include the use of a 'structured observation tool' to measure patient consultation in stage 2 of the study. The Observing Patient Involvement in Shared Decision-Making instrument will be used collect quantitative observation data. Therefore, this study uses both qualitative and quantitative observation to collect data.

Checklist for qualitative observations in a proposal:
1. Is the overall research question clearly stated? If there are a number of questions or objectives, is the link between them and the data collection methods clearly shown?
2. If a particular qualitative approach (e.g. grounded theory, phenomenology, etc.). is used, is this explained and justified? What would it add to the design, analysis and findings?
3. What is the type of qualitative observation (participant or non-participant) to be used? If participant, what is the extent to which the observer will participate in the participants' activities? Will the researcher be a paid employee? Is there a potential for conflict between the clinical or professional role and the observer's role?
4. If a non-participant observation format is used, is this justified? Does the proposal provide a semistructured list of areas on which the observer will focus?
5. Where will observations take place? How many sites are there? Who are the participants? Has preliminary conversation with stakeholders/gatekeepers (if appropriate) taken place?
6. How many observations will be conducted? Is information on the timing, duration and frequency of observation provided?
7. How will the event or case to be observed be selected?
8. Who will carry out the observations? Are they trained professionals? Do they have experience as observers? Will training be provided?

Continued

9. Will there be a period of familiarisation or immersion before the actual observations take place?
10. When will the observations commence and what is the projected overall period when all the observations will be completed?
11. How will the observations be recorded? If audio/visual or other equipment is to be used, is its use justified? How will recordings take place?
12. How will data be managed, handled and analysed? What data analysis framework and software, if any, will be used?
13. How will rigour be ensured in the analysis and interpretation of the data?
14. If multiple methods are used (e.g. observation, interviews, etc.) how will they be integrated?

SUMMARY AND CONCLUSIONS

In this chapter, the key issues to consider at the design stage and the information required in proposals for studies involving quantitative and qualitative observation have been highlighted. Questions to address in detail in proposals of studies using observations are: Why is observation selected? What is to be observed? Why? How? Where? When? By whom? Examples of how others have described observations in the proposals have been given. The checklists should also be helpful to those developing proposals for the first time. Chapters 11–13 will go on to discuss sampling, recruitment and ethical issues to consider when designing studies and writing proposals.

REFERENCES

Anagnostou, D., Sivell, S., Noble, S., Lester, J., Byrne, A., Sampson, C., Longo, M., & Nelson, A. (2017). Development of an intervention to support patients and clinicians with advanced lung cancer when considering systematic anticancer therapy: Protocol for the PACT study. *BMJ Open*, 7(7), e015277.

Braun, V., & Clarke, V. (2006). Using thematic analysis in psychology. *Qualitative Research in Psychology*, 3, 77–101. https://doi.org/10.1191/1478088706qp063oa

Carthey, J. (2003). The role of structured observational research in health care. *Quality and Safety in Health Care*, 12(Suppl 2):ii13–ii16. https://doi.org/10.1136/qhc.12.suppl_2.ii13

Catchpole, K., Neyens, D. M., Abernathy, J., Allison, D., Joseph, A., & Reeves, S. T. (2017). Framework for direct observation of performance and safety in healthcare. *BMJ Quality & Safety*, 26, 1015–1021.

Dalton, M., Davidson, M., & Keating, J. L. (2012). The Assessment of Physiotherapy Practice (APP) is a reliable measure of professional competence of physiotherapy students: A reliability study. *Journal of Physiotherapy*, 58(1), 49–56.

Dunger, C., Schnell, M. W., & Bausewein, C. (2017). Nurses' decision-making in ethically relevant clinical situations using the example of breathlessness: Study protocol of a reflexive grounded theory integrating Goffman's framework analysis. *BMJ Open*, 7, e012975. https://doi.org/10.1136/bmjopen-2016-012975

Duxbury, J. A., Wright, K. M., Hart, A., Bradley, D., Roach, P., Harris, N., & Carter, B. (2010). A structured observation of the interaction between nurses and patients during the administration of medication in an acute mental health unit. *Journal of Clinical Nursing*, 19, 2481–2492.

Ferguson, H. (2016). Researching social work practice close up: using ethnographic and mobile methods to understand encounters between social workers, children and families. *British Journal of Social Work*, 46(1), 153–168.

Fernández-Sola, C., Granero-Molina, J., Díaz-Cortés, M. D. M., Jiménez-López, F. R., Roman-López, P., Saez-Molina, E., Aranda-Torres, C. J., Muñoz-Terrón, J. M., García-Caro, M. P., & Hernández-Padilla, J. M. (2018). Characterization, conservation and loss of dignity at the end-of- life in the emergency department. A qualitative protocol. *Journal of Advanced Nursing, 74*, 1392–1401.

Fix, G. M., Kim, B., Ruben, M. A., & McCullough, M. B. (2022). Direct observation methods: A practical guide for health researchers. *PEC Innovation, 1*, 100036. https://doi.org/10.1016/j.pecinn.2022.100036

Gathara, D., Serem, G., Murphy, G. A. V., Abuya, N., Kuria, R., Tallam, E., & English, M. (2018). Quantifying nursing care delivered in Kenyan newborn units: Protocol for a cross-sectional direct observational study. *BMJ Open, 8*, e022020. https://doi.org/10.1136/bmjopen-2018-022020

Glaser, B. G. & Strauss, A. L. (1967). *The discovery of grounded theory. Strategies for qualitative research.* Chicago: Aldine.

Goffman, E. (1974). *Frame analysis: An essay on the organization of experience.* New York: Harper & Row.

Gold, R. L. (1958). Roles in sociological field observation. *Social Forces, 36*, 217–223.

Halder, A. K., Molyneaux, J. W., Luby, S. P., & Ram, P. K. (2013). Impact of duration of structured observations on measurement of handwashing behavior at critical times. *BMC Public Health, 13*, 705. https://doi.org/10.10.1186/1471-2458-13-705

Hardicre, N. K., Crocker, T. F., Wright, A., Burton, L. J., Ozer, S., Atkinson, R., House, A., Hewison, J., McKevitt, C., Forster, A., & Farrin, A. J. (2018). LoTS2Care Programme Management Group. An intervention to support stroke survivors and their carers in the longer term (LoTS2Care): Study protocol for the process evaluation of a cluster randomised controlled feasibility trial. *Trials, 19*(1), 368. https://doi.org/10.1186/s13063-018-2683-7

Hunter, A., Keady, J., Casey, D., Grealish, A., & Murphy, K. (2016). Psychosocial intervention use in long-stay dementia care: A classic grounded theory. *Qualitative Health Research, 26*(14), 2024–2034.

Johnson, L., Burridge, J., Ewings, S., Westcott, E., Gayton, M., & Demain, S. (2023). Principles into practice: An observational study of physiotherapists use of motor learning principles in stroke rehabilitation. *Physiotherapy, 118*, 20–30.

Johnson, H., Douglas, J., Bigby, C., & Iacono, T. (2011). The challenges and benefits of using participant observation to understand the social interaction of adults with intellectual disabilities. *Augmentative and Alternative Communication (Baltimore, Md.: 1985), 27*(4), 267–278. https://doi.org/10.3109/07434618.2011.587831

Karia, A. M., Balane, C., Norman, R., Robinson, S., Lehnbom, E., Durakovic, I., Laba, T. L., Joshi, R., & Webster, R. (2020). Community pharmacist workflow: Space for Pharmacy-based Interventions and Consultation TimE study protocol. *International Journal of Pharmacy Practice, 28*(5), 441–448.

Lillehagen, I., Vøllestad, N., Heggen, K., & Engebretsen, E. (2013). Protocol for a qualitative study of knowledge translation in a participatory research project. *BMJ Open, 3*, e003328. https://doi.org/10.1136/bmjopen-2013-003328

Manias, E., Braaf, S., Rixon, S., Williams, A., Liew, D., & Blackburn, A. (2019). Communicating with patients, families and health professionals about managing medications in intensive care: A qualitative observational study. *Intensive and Critical Care Nursing, 54*, 15–22.

Mansell, J. (2011). *Structured observational research in services for people with learning disabilities.* SSCR methods review, 10. London, UK: NIHR School for Social Care Research. https://www.sscr.nihr.ac.uk/wp-content/uploads/SSCR-methods-review_MR010.pdf

Oreglia, E., Ly, S., Tijamo, C., Ou, A., Free, C., & Smith, C. (2020). Development of an intervention to support the reproductive health of Cambodian women who seek medical abortion: Research protocol. *JMIR Research Protocols, 9*(7), e17779. https://doi.org/10.2196/17779

Paradis, E., & Sutkin, G. (2017). Beyond a good story: from Hawthorne Effect to reactivity in health professions education research. *Medical Education, 51*, 31–39.

Parahoo, K. (2014). *Nursing research: Principles, process and issues* (3rd ed.). Basingstoke: Palgrave Macmillan.

Parkinson, C., Hingley-Jones, H., & Allain, L. (2017). *Observation in health and social care: Applications for learning, research and practice with children and adults.* London: Jessica Kingsley Publishers.

Ram, P. K., Halder, A. K., Granger, S. P., Jones, T., Hall, P., Hitchcock, D. R., Wright, R., Nygren, B. L., Islam, M. D., Molyneaux, J. W., & Luby, S. P. (2010). Is structured observation a valid technique to measure handwashing behavior? Use of acceleration sensors embedded in soap to assess reactivity to structured observation. *American Journal of Tropical Medicine and Hygiene, 83*(5), 1070–1076.

Saberi Zafarghandi, M. B., Eshrati, S., Vameghi, M., Ranjbar, H., Arezoomandan, R., Clausen, T., & Waal, H. (2019). Drug-related community issues and the required interventions in open drug scenes in Tehran, Iran: A qualitative study protocol. *BMJ Open, 9,* e030488. https://doi.org/10.1136/bmjopen-2019-030488

Saletti-Cuesta, L., Tutton, E., langstaff, D., & Willett, K. (2017). Understanding patient and relative/carer experience of hip fracture in acute care: A qualitative study protocol. *International Journal of Orthopaedic and Trauma Nursing, 25,* 36–41.

Song, J. W., & Chung, K. C. (2010). Observational studies: Cohort and case-control studies. *Plastic and Reconstructive Surgery, 6,* 2234–2242.

Teesing, G. R., Erasmus, V., Petrignani, M., Koopmans, M. P. G., de Graaf, M., Vos, M. C., Klaassen, C. H. W., Verduijn-Leenman, A., Schols, J. M. G. A., Richardus, J. H., & Voeten, H. A. C. M. (2020). Improving hand hygiene compliance in nursing homes: Protocol for a cluster randomized controlled trial (HANDSOME study). *JMIR Research Protocols, 9*(5), e17419. https://doi.org/10.2196/17419

Thompson, C., Milton, S., Egan, M., & Lock, K. (2018). Down the local: A qualitative case study of daytime drinking spaces in the London Borough of Islington. *International Journal of Drug Policy, 52,* 1–8.

von Gaudecker, J., Taylor, A. G., Buelow, J., Benjamin, S., & Draucker, C. (2019). Women's experiences with epilepsy treatment in Southern India: A focused ethnography. *Qualitative Report, 24*(5), 1034–1051.

Westlake, D., Stabler, L., & McDonnell, J. (2020). Direct observation in practice: Co-developing an evidence-informed practice tool to assess social work communicatio'. *Journal of Children's Services, 15*(3), 123–140.

WHO. (2012). *Hand hygiene in outpatient and home-based care and long-term care facilities: A guide to the application of the WHO multimodal hand hygiene improvement strategy and the 'My Five Moments for Hand Hygiene' approach.* Geneva: World Health. https://apps.who.int/iris/bitstream/handle/10665/78060/9789241503372_eng.pdf;jsessionid=5323786B5125752D161D8CA92B23D413?sequence=1

Wright, A. (2018). Exploring the relationship between community-based physical activity and wellbeing in people with dementia: A qualitative study. *Ageing & Society, 38,* 522–542.

Zhao, M., & Ji, Y. (2014). Challenges of introducing participant observation to community health research. *ISRN Nursing, 2014,* 802490. https://doi.org/10.1155/2014/802490

SAMPLES AND SAMPLING IN QUANTITATIVE STUDIES AND PROPOSALS

INTRODUCTION

In nursing, health and social care research, the main source of data are people. We seek their responses (through interviews and questionnaires), observe their behaviour and the events they participate in (e.g. how clients/patients interact with health professionals), collect samples (e.g. blood, urine or saliva) and take physical, physiological and psychological measurements from them (e.g. weight, temperature or self-esteem). We also obtain information from documents (e.g. registers, patients' records, etc.). Therefore, it is important that researchers pay particular attention to who they recruit for their study, how this is done and what the implications of these decisions are. In this chapter, we will discuss the issues that researchers designing a study and writing research proposals should consider in relation to samples and sampling in quantitative studies. In Chapter 12, we will explore samples and sampling in qualitative studies.

SAMPLES AND SAMPLING

The term 'sample' refers to a smaller number of people to represent those from the larger group they are drawn from (a subset of the population). Sampling refers to the technique, method or procedure to make the selection (e.g. select every fifth name from a list or use computer-generated numbers to do so).

Individuals who are recruited to a study are referred to as 'participants' or 'subjects'. The latter is often not used as it can signify an unequal power relation between researchers and those who take part in studies – historically the term 'subject' meant somebody who is subordinate to a 'master' or 'king'. However, different health disciplines use different terms. The target population describes the population being studied and to whom the findings could be generalised (e.g. first-time mothers or newly qualified social workers). A sample frame is simply a list or record of the target population from which a sample can be drawn. For example, the Australian Physiotherapy Association keeps a record of its members. This list was used as a sample frame for recruitment in a proposal for a study of the 'views and perceptions of Australian physiotherapists and physiotherapy students about the potential implementation of physiotherapist prescribing in Australia' (Noblet et al., 2018).

Sometimes the target population is the same as the sample frame. For example, if the study is about the first-year students on a particular occupational therapy degree programme, the target population or the sample frame consists of all students undertaking the course in that year. More often, the target population and the sample frame can be too large for a study, so researchers 'draw' or recruit a proportion of this population. They may want to draw a sample (rather than use the entire population, where possible) for a number of reasons. Some of these may be ethical (recruiting a greater number of people than required) or related to budgetary limitations, logistics, time restrictions or an unknown target population size (Martínez-Mesa et al., 2016). Selecting participants for a study has ethical implications, which will be discussed in Chapter 13).

The decision of who to include in a study depends on the research question(s) or hypothesis (e.g. who is being studied), the methodological approach (qualitative or quantitative), the research design (e.g. randomised controlled trial [RCT] or survey) and the methods of data collection (e.g. questionnaires or interviews). Each of these aspects influences the choice, size and composition of the sample. The sample or population section of a proposal should demonstrate that the right population or event (to be observed) is selected, the size of the sample is adequate and the method of selection is clearly described. The decisions underpinning sample selection should also be justified. This section should demonstrate evidence that the author(s) of the proposal are aware of the size of the target population (or a realistic estimation of it), and how a sample frame (if available) would be accessed or constructed. This means providing figures and statistical data on the targeted population and information on how to access this population.

Gatekeepers (e.g. doctors or social workers, who have a degree of control over access to participants for study purposes) should be consulted prior to making any decision about the selection of participants in clinical or health and social care settings. Information regarding whether gatekeepers have been consulted will give others the confidence that you have done preparatory work and that you know what you are writing about. One of the common mistakes that new researchers make is to assume they will be able to access their population and obtain the required sample size, only to find out later on that this is a challenge. The successful completion of a study depends largely on whether the target population is accessible, in sufficient numbers and willing or able to participate.

Consulting the literature on studies on the same topic as in the proposal will help the authors of proposals to be aware of the pitfalls and challenges they may face. For example, some topics or populations may be associated with low response rates, high participant refusal to take part in the research studies and high attrition (loss of participants to a study when they drop out or die). When such challenges are anticipated, the strategies that will be used to increase participation should be mentioned and justified (e.g. by quoting recent, relevant literature). For proposals seeking significant funding, feasibility or pilot studies prior to the main study would give proposal authors and funding panels the confidence that the proposed sampling plan is appropriate and realistic.

Sometimes the presentation of complex information on samples and sampling in proposals can be enhanced graphically, through the use of tables and figures. Flow charts are particularly useful when the study sample consists of different groups of people. In their protocol for 'a prospective, longitudinal cohort study of the medical and psychosocial outcomes of the UK combat casualties from the Afghanistan war', Bennett et al. (2020) provided a flow chart to give details of the various groups to be selected (e.g. 'battle casualties with amputations', 'non-amputee battle casualties', etc.).

To design a study and write a proposal one needs to have a basic knowledge of samples and sampling. This can be obtained from any research textbook. For an overview of how to select sampling in a study and sampling issues, see Martínez-Mesa et al. (2016). Their article provides basic information on types of sampling and when to use them. For information on sampling in randomized controlled trials, see White et al. (2014).

The rest of this chapter will expand on the some of the issues mentioned above. It will also highlight the essential information that should be provided in the sampling or population section of proposals for studies using the following research designs: quantitative descriptive and correlational (e.g. survey, cohort, case-control), experimental (RCT) and quasi-experimental. Many of the sampling issues (e.g. sample definition, setting criteria for inclusion/exclusion) are the same regardless of the research design but some of the issues are only applicable to particular designs (e.g. allocation of participants to control or experimental groups in RCTs compared with selecting a sample for a survey).

There are two types of sampling: probability and non-probability. Probability sampling is mainly used in quantitative studies as their findings are expected to be generalised to the target population. For this to happen, everyone in the target population should be given an equal chance of being selected. This is why researchers use one or more random selection methods in their studies. There are four main types of probability sampling: simple random (everyone has an equal chance of being selected), systematic (participants are selected at a regular interval from a list, for example choosing every fifth name until the required sample size is reached), stratified (participants are divided into groups before the required number from each group are selected (by means of a simple or systematic random method) and cluster (groups of people such as those in schools, factories or hospitals, rather than individuals, are selected by means of simple or systematic random sampling). Each random selection method has its uses and limitations. For more information on types of sampling, see a basic research methods text.

With non-probability sampling, the chances of being selected is not known. This approach is used mainly in qualitative studies (see Chapter 12). The aim in these studies is not to generalise or make inferences about the population from whom the sample is drawn. Qualitative studies explore phenomena (such as the meaning of depression or the experience of receiving good news) rather than how they are distributed in a population (e.g. the percentage of the population who has depression according to the various age groups).

SAMPLING IN PROPOSALS FOR SURVEYS AND CORRELATIONAL STUDIES

Surveys, cohort and case-control studies are quantitative in nature and are therefore expected to use probability sampling methods as they seek to make inferences or generalisations to the population under study. In this section, the key information to be included in the sampling section of a proposal will be highlighted. This includes detail regarding the target population, sample frame, definition of the population, units or cases, inclusion and exclusion criteria, sample size, and recruitment and retention strategies.

In a proposal for 'a case-control study of the determinants of suicide attempts in young people in India' (Balaji et al., 2020), the study population was people 15–29 years of age in India. Because it would be impossible to include everyone in India in this age group, these researchers focused on three hospitals, including a 750-bed hospital that served an urban population of about a million people (Balaji et al., 2020). The records of suicide attempts, kept at the hospital, were used as a sample frame.

Defining the study population clearly is the first step in the sampling procedure. The research question or aim of the study contains the terms or concepts that need to be defined. In Rang et al.'s (2020) case-control study, the aim was 'to examine the association between maternal secondhand smoking during pregnancy and preterm birth' (p. 1). 'Secondhand exposure' was defined as exposure to 'husband or family members who smoked on a daily basis of more than 5 cigarettes a day at home' (p .2) while 'preterm birth' was defined as babies born before the 37th gestational week (Rang et al., 2020). In defining the cases or population, one must be cautious in using terms or descriptors that may also require further definition. For example, in a proposal for a 'survey of physical activity among breast cancer survivors in Japan', Shimizu et al. (2020) use this National Cancer Institute (USA) definition:

> *A cancer survivor is 'a person who lives after being diagnosed with cancer'. Family members, friends and loved ones are also included as 'survivors', as they too are affected.*
>
> *(p. 3)*

This definition of cancer survivor is broad as it includes 'family members' and 'loved ones'. However, it was not clear, in the proposal, whether these 'family members' would also be included in Shimizu et al.'s (2020) study. The term 'loved ones' also needs to be defined.

Setting Inclusion and Exclusion Criteria

One of the many ways to be as precise as possible regarding the study participants is to list the inclusion and exclusion criteria. There are some factors to take into account when deciding who, among the target population, to include in a study. The inclusion criteria are those factors or features that the target population must have in order to be included in a study. For example, in a study examining the relationship between 'exercise' and 'wellbeing' among residents in a care home, researchers may set inclusion criteria such as all residents should 'be aged over 65', 'have been in the home for over 1 year' and 'be able to walk short distances'. However, among those who meet these criteria there may be other factors that would restrict residents from participating, such as a severe cardiac condition (e.g. arising from chronic obstructive pulmonary disease [COPD]), or the fact that they are already taking part in another exercise programme. These factors (COPD and taking part in another exercise) would then constitute the 'exclusion' criteria.

Patino and Ferreira (2018) define exclusion criteria as 'features of the potential study participants who meet the inclusion criteria but present with additional characteristics that could interfere with the success of the study or increase their risk for an unfavorable outcome' (p. 1).

Exclusion criteria are sometimes stated as a mirror image of the inclusion criteria. For example, if the inclusion criterion is 'those over 18 years old', there is no need to state the exclusion criterion as those under 18 years. Rather, the exclusion criteria should refer to those over 18 who can potentially participate but have characteristics or features that would exclude them. In a proposal for an 'observational cohort study investigating cognitive outcomes, social networks and well-being in older adults', Siette et al. (2019) set the following criteria for selecting participants:

Inclusion criteria:

- *≥ 55 years of age*
- *Receiving home and community-based social support aged care services from an aged care provider.*

Exclusion criteria:

- *Advanced cognitive impairment or unable to follow simple commands (as determined by aged care staff or from client's medical records).*
- *Primary neurological injury (e.g., anoxic injury, stroke or traumatic brain injury).*
- *Not fluent in English.*
- *Requiring institution-based rehabilitation or nursing home placement.*
- *Terminally ill.*
- *No capacity to provide consent at any time point of the study.*

(p. 3)

All the inclusion and exclusion criteria must be justified as anyone reading the proposal, especially funding panel members, may question these criteria. Therefore, careful consideration should be given to deciding who or what to include or exclude. For example, in Balaji et al.'s (2020) study on suicide among young people in India, only those aged between 15 and 29 years were included. The reason given by the authors is that '40% of all suicides' (p. 1) occur in this age group. In a study of 'occupational burnout among active physiotherapists working in clinical hospitals during the COVID-19 pandemic in South-eastern Poland', Pniak et al. (2021) set an inclusion criterion for participants as those aged between 25 and 60. The reason they gave was that 'typically, in Poland those graduating from Master's degree courses in physiotherapy and acquiring a licence to work in the profession are 25 years old' (Pniak et al., 2021, p. 287). People are sometimes excluded from a study because it makes the study easier to undertake. For example, excluding those not 'fluent in English' or not having 'sufficient English' can, by default, exclude people from ethnic minority groups.

Screening those who are included or excluded also requires explanation. What does 'not fluent in English' or 'does not have sufficient English' mean and how are participants to be assessed? There are also implications for criteria that are too narrow or two broad. Findings from studies with narrow criteria tend to be applicable to fewer people, while broad criteria can lead to findings applicable to a broad population, thereby lacking specificity. Hornberger and

Rangu (2020) explain that a balance between 'broad' and 'narrow' criteria should be achieved in order that the study can successfully answer the research question(s) and be of benefit to a broader population. As they explain:

> *You can find the perfect balance of specificity through understanding the purpose of your criteria, reading key studies with similar goals to yours, and measuring the impact on study feasibility. It is important to consider potential problems that could arise and the reality of how many participants you will be able to screen. Remaining focused on the purpose of your study will allow you to create effective inclusion/exclusion criteria for collecting the most significant data.*

(p. 1)

Hornberger and Rangu (2020) also suggest the following steps in determining effective criteria: 'brainstorm as a team', 'carefully look through key studies from your literature review', 'refer to valid sources for medical conditions to include/exclude', 'look at past protocols' and 'justify the reasoning behind each criterion'. For examples of discussions on inclusion and exclusion criteria in research proposals (of survey, cohort and case-control studies), see Lee et al. (2020), Patino and Ferreira (2018), Hornberger and Rangu (2020) and Siette et al. (2019).

Sample Size and Sample Calculation

An adequate sample size is crucial to the successful completion of a quantitative study. If a study is underpowered (i.e. it does not have sufficient participants or cases to allow statistical calculations to produce reliable findings), it is a waste of resources and an abuse of participants' time, efforts and goodwill as the study is unlikely to be successful in fulfilling its aims. An overpowered study (i.e. one with a much larger a sample size than is required to answer the research question(s)) is also an abuse of participants' time and effort. The ethical implications of this are further discussed in Chapter 13.

There is a lack of information on sample size calculation in proposals (Flege and Thomsen, 2018). Clark et al. (2013), who conducted a review of 446 study protocols submitted to research ethics committees in the UK, concluded that 'most research protocols did not contain sufficient information to allow the sample size to be reproduced or the plausibility of the design assumptions to be assessed' (p. 1). In a more recent study in Denmark, Flege and Thomsen (2018) found that newer studies were more likely to include a sample size calculation in their protocol. They also found that intervention studies were more likely to report sample size calculations.

The reporting of the sample size and its calculation, implications and limitations is one of the key aspects that reviewers of proposals (in particular, potential funders) focus upon. Some research funding organisations have in-house statisticians who will undertake sample size calculations before sending the proposals to subject experts for their review. This is why it is important to include statisticians, health economists and other relevant experts at the design stage of a study and before a proposal is written.

Quantitative studies aim to measure variables and to establish relationships between them by using mathematical and statistical methods. For example, in a study by Al-Hanawi et al. (2020), the aim was 'to investigate the knowledge, attitudes and practices' of residents in the Kingdom of Saudi Arabia (KSA) 'towards COVID-19 during the pandemic spike' (p. 2). An adequate sample was required to make generalisations about the knowledge, attitude and practice related to COVID-19 in this population (residents of KSA) as otherwise the aim of this study would not have been achieved.

There are a number of factors that should be considered when calculating an adequate sample size and deciding on the sampling methods for a quantitative study. Only some of the key factors are listed below. It is beyond the scope of this chapter to deal adequately with sample size calculation, but most basic statistics textbooks will cover this topic. Some of these factors include the size of the target population (if this is small, there may not be a need to sample, although an adequate sample size is still needed). Underpowered sample sizes can lead to type 2 errors (accepting a null hypothesis when it is actually false). Comparative studies may require larger samples to adequately represent the different groups being compared. For an example of how sampling is carried out in comparative study, see the proposal by Anderson et al. (2020) of a study of 'multilevel influences on resilient healthcare in six countries'.

Other factors (for calculating sample size) include the confidence level that researchers set for the study. This is the probability that if the survey or test is repeated, the findings will match those of the original survey (if the level is set close to 100%) or will not (if the level is set close to 0%). The potential for attrition (when participants drop out of the study, if it is longitudinal), for low response rates as well as for the outcomes to be measured, is also an important consideration. Sample size calculation in RCTs will be discussed later in this chapter.

If a number of outcomes are to be measured, sample size calculations for each of them may be required. In a proposal by Chetty-Mhlanga et al. (2018) for 'a prospective cohort study of school-going children investigating reproductive and neurobehavioral health effects due to environmental pesticide exposure in the Western Cape, South Africa', a number of outcomes were to be measured. These included 'neurobehavioral health' and 'reproductive hormones'. This is how Chetty-Mhlanga et al. (2018) described the sample calculations for the neurobehavioural health outcomes in the proposal:

The sample size for neurobehavioral health outcomes is determined assuming a 0.2 standard deviation from the median neurobehavior score in the exposed group compared to the control group. This corresponds to observed differences found in studies investigating environmental exposure on neurobehavioral outcomes, using metabolites as the method to assess for pesticide exposure in the Western Cape of South Africa, in the United States and in Costa Rica. A sample size of 900 was judged to be adequate with a power of 80% and a 5% level of significance.

(p. 9)

Sample size calculations for each of the other outcomes were also described. It is worth noting that both the statistical analysis of the data and the outcomes to be measured are taken into account when sample sizes are calculated. Chetty-Mhlanga et al. (2018) also based their calculations of standard deviation [SD]) on previous studies. This, no doubt, adds credibility to their calculations. For another example, see the proposal by Siette et al. (2019).

Once the sample size has been calculated, the sampling strategy should be selected. In practice, researchers do not think in a linear fashion: they think of a number of issues at the same time in order to come to a final decision. Sampling strategies, here, refers to the actual process of selecting participants; some of these strategies were mentioned earlier in the chapter. It is important to explain the process of selection clearly. Sometimes a diagram can add clarity to the description. It is not enough to say a simple random selection will be carried out; the actual method of selection (e.g. using a random sampling selector) and the list (sample frame) from which the sample will be drawn should be described.

Determining the required sample size is only the beginning of the process of recruiting participants to a study. Researchers should familiarise themselves with the setting where the participants will be assessed. There may be gatekeepers such as nurses, doctors or social workers who need to be consulted before their clients or patients can be contacted. This is how Balaji et al. (2020) describe one of the settings in their proposal for a case-control study of the determinants of suicide attempts in young people in India:

> *Recruitment is ongoing at YCMH, in Pimpri-Chinchwad, Pune city, Maharashtra. This 750-bed hospital is owned and operated by the Pimpri-Chinchwad Municipal Corporation established under the Government of Maharashtra. It serves an urban population of about 2 million, nearly 10% of whom live in slum areas. The average literacy rate is 87%. Between 40 and 50 persons with suicide attempts present at the Emergency department of the hospital every month, and approximately 50% of them are treated as outpatients. About 15% come from neighbouring rural areas.*

(p. 3)

Such descriptions give readers of proposals an idea of the context in which the participants are being recruited and show that these researchers have attempted to find out some data on their target population in preparation for the study.

Recruitment and Retention

Sample recruitment brings its own challenges apart from access to the target population. Researchers use different strategies (depending on who they want to recruit) to enlist people into the studies. Usually, the more inaccessible or difficult it is to recruit, the more researchers have to explain in their proposals how they will proceed. Funding agencies will not want to invest money in studies that are unlikely to recruit the required sample size. An example of some of the recruitment strategies used by researchers is in the proposal by Westrupp et al. (2020) for a study on the 'adjustment of Australian parents of a child 0–18 years' (p. 1) to the COVID-19 pandemic. The authors explained that 'parents will be recruited via paid and unpaid social media advertisements' (in particular Facebook) and that a range of methods would be used, such as 'targeting via postcodes and demographic factors', tailoring the 'style and wording of advertisements', emphasising the affiliation to the university where the study was to be carried out, and writing all advertisements 'in engaging and yet plain language' (Westrupp et al., 2020, p. 3).

If incentives are to be offered to potential participants to take part in a study, this should be explained and justified. There are different forms of incentive, such as gift cards, goods/grocery vouchers and monetary compensation (e.g. for parking and travel costs). Whatever the justification for giving incentives, the ethical implications should be carefully considered (see Chapter 13). For a discussion of the arguments for and against incentives see 'Payments and incentives in research' (University of Oxford, 2020). Wong (2020) offers useful insights into incentives in longitudinal studies. The paper by Yu et al. (2017) discusses the effectiveness of monetary incentives in research. Booker et al. (2021) explore survey strategies to increase participants' response rates in primary care research studies.

SAMPLING IN TRIALS

Most of the issues and principles discussed in the previous sections are relevant and applicable when considering sampling in RCTs. However, issues such as allocation to groups in a trial is not the same as drawing a simple random sample. White et al. (2014) explain the difference between these two concepts:

Random assignment should not be confused with random sampling. Random sampling refers to how a sample is drawn from one or more populations. Random assignment refers to how individuals or groups are assigned to either a treatment group or a control group. RCTs typically use both random sampling (since they are usually aiming to make inferences about a larger population) and random assignment (an essential characteristic of an RCT).

(p. 3)

Random allocation or assignment to groups is carried out to prevent bias. Normally the person who carries out the allocation is unaware or 'blind' to which group is the experimental or the control group. Sometimes opaque envelopes containing either a letter A or B (signifying the experimental or control group) are used for the allocation. There are different types of randomisation used in RCTs, such as parallel, cluster and block (see Chapter 5). This is how Bird et al. (2019) report their randomisation process in their proposal for a trial on the 'efficacy of rhinothermy delivered by nasal high flow therapy in the treatment of the common cold':

Following the screening process, eligible participants who are enrolled in the study will be immediately randomised 1:1 to one of the following treatment arms:

- *rNHF (n=85 participants).*
- *'Sham' rhinothermy (n=85 participants).*

A permuted block randomisation method stratified by duration of illness, lesser versus greater than or equal to one day, will be used to allocate participants to either treatment arm. The computer-generated sequence will be supplied by the study statistician, independent of the investigators. The eCRF [electronic case report form] system will conceal the allocations and will release a participant's randomisation outcome at the time of randomisation. The randomisation schedule will only be accessed by the study statistician and the eCRF provider; study staff will not have access to the randomisation schedule.

(p. 3)

Whatever the randomisation method, researchers have to provide justification for their selection. In their proposal for a trial of 'exercise therapy for patients with depressive symptoms in healthcare services', Heissel et al. (2020) justified the choice of cluster randomisation on the basis that 'the study is aimed not only at patients but also at units within the health services that involve the restructuring of healthcare delivery' (p. 7). Other reasons given by Heissel et al. (2020) include the usefulness of cluster randomisation in determining 'the comparative effectiveness of two or more therapy options under conditions of actual use' and the 'considerable cost and time efficiency by simplifying the logistics of implementation' (p. 7). Heissel et al. (2020) also point out the limitations of cluster RCTs (CRCTs):

Compared with the individual-level RCT, a CRCT is more difficult to perform, which requires more participants to obtain the same statistical power and necessitates more complex statistical analysis (eg, adjustment for the ICC [intraclass correlation coefficient] coefficient of the cluster randomisation). Thus, in the present study, a relatively large sample of participants will be recruited to address these stipulations and a more rigorous data analysis strategy will be implemented.

(p .8)

The process of calculating sample sizes for surveys and RCTs is similar. Both have to take into account the outcomes to be measured. However, in RCTs researchers have to calculate the sample size based on what has been termed 'minimal clinically important differences' (MCIDs; Rai et al., 2015), not just statistical differences. As McGlothlin and Lewis (2014) explain:

When assessing the clinical utility of therapies intended to improve subjective outcomes, the amount of improvement that is important to patients must be determined. The smallest benefit of value to patients is called the minimal clinically important difference (MCID). The MCID is a patient-centered concept, capturing both the magnitude of the improvement and also the value patients place on the change.

(p. 1342)

For useful information on MCIDs and how to calculate sample size in trials, see:

- Salas Apaza et al. (2021), 'Minimal clinically important difference: the basics'.
- Mouelhi et al. (2020), 'How is the minimal clinically important difference established in health-related quality of life instruments? Review of anchors and methods'.
- Malec and Ketchum (2020), 'A standard method for determining the minimal clinically important difference for rehabilitation measures'.

Flow charts, in particular the CONSORT diagram (Schulz et al., 2010), are recommended when reporting the sampling process and the size of groups in RCTs. For an example of flow charts in a proposal, see Schitter et al. (2022).

Proposal Example 11.1 shows how sampling and recruitment issues were reported in a proposal for an RCT.

PROPOSAL EXAMPLE 11.1
SAMPLING AND RECRUITMENT ISSUES IN A PROPOSAL

García-Galant et al. (2020), 'Study protocol of a randomized controlled trial of home-based computerized executive function training for children with cerebral palsy'.

COMMENTS

1. This is a proposal for a single-blind RCT examining whether 'a computerized executive function (EF) training programme could provide superior benefits for executive functioning, participation, QOL [quality of life] and brain plasticity, as compared to usual care' (p. 1).

2. The authors set a number of inclusion criteria including age (8–12 years), ability to understand simple instructions, access to the internet at home, etc. The 'simple instructions' criteria were to be assessed by the Screening Test of Spanish Grammar. The exclusion criterion is: 'identified hearing or visual impairment that precludes neuropsychological assessment and cognitive training' (p. 3).

3. The authors explained that participants would be contacted by the medical staff of their reference health centre. The sample size calculation took into account the differences in the continuous primary outcomes after 12 weeks of the training programme. As they explained:

   to detect a large standardized difference (i.e. a difference of at least 0.8 SD) between the immediate intervention and waitlist groups, with 80% power and $\alpha = 0.05$, 26 children would be necessary in each group. Assuming 15% attrition, the required sample size was calculated as 60 participants.

   (p. 4)

4. Garcia-Galant et al. (2020) go on to explain how participants would be randomised to the two groups and provide a flow chart to show the design of the trial.

Checklist for the sample/sampling sections in proposals for surveys, cohort and case-control studies:

1. Has the target population been identified and defined? What are the inclusion and exclusion criteria? Are these criteria justified?

2. What size of sample is required and how is this calculated? Is there an existing sampling frame (e.g. list of patients/clients)? Has a sample size calculator been used? Is the calculation based on identified outcomes, statistical tests and confidence levels?

3. What type of sampling will be used (e.g. stratified or simple random)? Is the sampling strategy justified? How will the sampling strategy be implemented?

4. What strategies will be used to access and recruit participants and enhance response rates? If the study is longitudinal, how will attrition and retention be addressed? If incentives are to be used, what are they and are they justified and ethical?

Checklist for the randomisation section in proposals for trials:
1. Has the target population been identified and defined? Has an estimation of its size been made? What are the inclusion and exclusion criteria?
2. Has the sample size for each group (control, experimental, etc.) been calculated? Is the MCID taken into account in the calculation of effect size?
3. Have the sequence generation and concealment processes been described? Have sampling and randomisation processes been included in a CONSORT or CONSORT-type flow chart?
4. What type of sampling will be used (e.g. block or cluster randomisation) and has the rationale for this choice been given?
5. How will participants be accessed? Will gatekeepers be involved? Who are they and has initial contact with the gatekeepers been made? What records, if any, will be used? What setting(s) will be involved?
6. What strategies will be used to enhance recruitment, attrition and retention? If incentives are to be used, what are they and are they justified and ethical?

SUMMARY AND CONCLUSIONS

In this chapter, we have looked at the purpose of sampling, the different types of sampling and the issues and factors that researchers need to take into account when designing surveys and trials. They should be aware of the implications of their decisions and of the challenges that sampling and recruiting participants can bring. The need to identify the target population, draw an adequate sample size, set inclusion and exclusion criteria and select the strategies for accessing, recruiting and retaining participants has been emphasised.

The sampling section of a proposal should give readers a well thought out plan and ensure that all aspects of the sampling/randomisation processes and other issues such as recruitment and retention have been addressed. There should be evidence of preparatory work (e.g. pilot study, feasibility study, contact with gatekeepers, where appropriate). This will add to the credibility of the proposal.

Word limitations in proposals means that the description and justification for decisions should be clear, brief and succinct. Not all the decisions should be fully justified, particularly those that are based on a consensus among researchers and are self-explanatory. However, if what is proposed is different from the norm, an explanation is needed. Remember that 'a picture paints a thousand words'; therefore, flow charts, where appropriate, can save words.

REFERENCES

Al-Hanawi, M. K., Angawi, K., Alshareef, N., Qattan, A., Helmy, H. Z., Abudawood, Y., Alqurashi, M., Kattan, W. M., Kadasah, N. A., Chirwa, G. C., & Alharqi, O. (2020). Knowledge, attitude and practice toward COVID-19 among the public in the Kingdom of Saudi Arabia: A cross-sectional study. *Frontiers in Public Health*, *8*, 217. https://doi.org/10.3389/fpubh.2020.00217
Anderson, J. E., Aase, K., Bal, R. A., Bourrier, M., Braithwaite, J., Nakajima, K., Wiig, S., & Guise, V. (2020). Multi-level influences on resilient healthcare in six countries: An international comparative study protocol. *BMJ Open*, *10*, e039158. https://doi.org/10.1136/bmjopen-2020-039158

Balaji, M., Vijayakumar, L., Phillips, M., Panse, S., Santre, M., Pathare, S., & Patel, V. (2020). The Young Lives Matter study protocol: A case-control study of the determinants of suicide attempts in young people in India. *Wellcome Open Research*, 5, 262. https://doi.org/10.12688/wellcomeopenres.16364.1

Bennett, A. N., Dyball, D. M., Boos, C. J., Fear, N. T., Schofield, S., Bull, A. M. J., Cullinan, P., & ADVANCE Study. (2020). Study protocol for a prospective, longitudinal cohort study investigating the medical and psychosocial outcomes of UK combat casualties from the Afghanistan war: The ADVANCE Study. *BMJ Open*, 10(10), e037850. https://doi.org/10.1136/bmjopen-2020-037850

Bird, G., Braithwaite, I., Harper, J., McKinstry, S., Koorevaar, I., Fingleton, J., Semprini, A., Dilcher, M., Jennings, L., Weatherall, M., & Beasley, R. (2019). Protocol for a randomised, single-blind, two-arm, parallel-group controlled trial of the efficacy of rhinothermy delivered by nasal high flow therapy in the treatment of the common cold. *BMJ Open*, 9(6), e028098. https://doi.org/10.1136/bmjopen-2018-028098

Booker, Q. S., Austin, J. D., & Balasubramanian, B. A. (2021). Survey strategies to increase participant response rates in primary care research studies. *Family Practice*, 38(5), 699–702.

Chetty-Mhlanga, S., Basera, W., Fuhrimann, S., Probst-Hensch, N., Delport, S., Mugari, M., Van Wyk, J., Röösli, M., & Dalvie, M. A. (2018). A prospective cohort study of school-going children investigating reproductive and neurobehavioral health effects due to environmental pesticide exposure in the Western Cape, South Africa: Study protocol. *BMC Public Health*, 18(1), 857. https://doi.org/10.1186/s12889-018-5783-0

Clark, T., Berger, U., & Mansmann, U. (2013). Sample size determinations in original research protocols for randomised clinical trials submitted to UK research ethics committees: Review. *BMJ (Clinical Research Ed.)*, 346, f1135. https://doi.org/10.1136/bmj.f1135

Flege, M. M., & Thomsen, S. F. (2018). Sample size estimation practices in research protocols submitted to Danish scientific ethics committees. *Contemporary Clinical Trials Communications*, 11, 165–169.

García-Galant, M., Blasco, M., Reid, L., Pannek, K., Leiva, D., Laporta-Hoyos, O., Ballester-Plané, J., Miralbell, J., Caldú, X., Alonso, X., Toro-Tamargo, E., Meléndez-Plumed, M., Gimeno, F., Coronas, M., Soro-Camats, E., Boyd, R., & Pueyo, R. (2020). Study protocol of a randomized controlled trial of home-based computerized executive function training for children with cerebral palsy. *BMC Pediatrics*, 20(1), 9. https://doi.org/10.1186/s12887-019-1904-x

Heissel, A., Pietrek, A., Schwefel, M., Abula, K., Wilbertz, G., Heinzel, S., & Rapp, M. (2020). STEP.De study – a multicentre cluster-randomised effectiveness trial of exercise therapy for patients with depressive symptoms in healthcare services: Study protocol. *BMJ Open*, 10(4), e036287. https://doi.org/10.1136/bmjopen-2019-036287

Hornberger, B., Rangu, S. (2020). *Designing inclusion and exclusion criteria*. https://repository.upenn.edu/cgi/viewcontent.cgi?article=1000&context=crp

Lee, T. Y., Lee, J., Lee, H. J., Lee, Y., Rhee, S. J., Park, D. Y., Paek, M. J., Kim, E. Y., Kim, E., Roh, S., Jung, H. Y., Kim, M., Kim, S. H., Han, D., Ahn, Y. M., Ha, K., & Kwon, J. S. (2020). Study protocol for a prospective longitudinal cohort study to identify proteomic predictors of pluripotent risk for mental illness: the Seoul Pluripotent Risk for Mental Illness Study. *Frontiers in Psychiatry*, 11, 340. https://doi.org/10.3389/fpsyt.2020.00340

Malec, J. F., & Ketchum, J. M. (2020). A standard method for determining the minimal clinically important difference for rehabilitation measures. *Archives of Physical Medicine and Rehabilitation*, 101(6), 1090–1094.

Martínez-Mesa, J., González-Chica, D. A., Duquia, R. P., Bonamigo, R. R., & Bastos, J. L. (2016). Sampling: How to select participants in my research study? *Anais brasileiros de Dermatologia*, 91(3), 326–330.

McGlothlin, A. E., & Lewis, R. J. (2014). Minimal clinically important difference: Defining what really matters to patients. *JAMA*, 312(13), 1342–1343.

Mouelhi, Y., Jouve, E., Castelli, C., & Gentile, S. (2020). How is the minimal clinically important difference established in health-related quality of life instruments? Review of anchors and methods. *Health and Quality of Life Outcomes*, 18(1), 136. https://doi.org/10.1186/s12955-020-01344-w

Noblet, T., Marriot, J., Jones, T., Dean, C., & Rushton, A. (2018). Views and perceptions of Australian physiotherapists and physiotherapy students about the potential implementation of physiotherapist prescribing in

Australia: A survey protocol. *BMC Health Services Research*, *18*(1), 472. https://doi.org/10.1186/s12913-018-3300-x

Patino, C. M., & Ferreira, J. C. (2018). Inclusion and exclusion criteria in research studies: Definitions and why they matter. *Jornal brasileiro de pneumologia: publicacao oficial da Sociedade Brasileira de Pneumologia e Tisilogia*, *44*(2), 84. https://doi.org/10.1590/s1806-37562018000000088

Pniak, B., Leszczak, J., Adamczyk, M., Rusek, W., Matłosz, P., & Guzik, A. (2021). Occupational burnout among active physiotherapists working in clinical hospitals during the COVID-19 pandemic in south-eastern Poland. *Work (Reading, Mass.)*, *68*(2), 285–295.

Rang, N. N., Hien, T. Q., Chanh, T. Q., & Thuyen, T. K. (2020). Preterm birth and secondhand smoking during pregnancy: A case-control study from Vietnam. *PloS One*, *15*(10), e0240289. https://doi.org/10.1371/journal.pone.0240289

Salas Apaza, J. A., Franco, J., Meza, N., Madrid, E., Loézar, C., & Garegnani, L. (2021). Minimal clinically important difference: The basics. Diferencia mínima clínicamente importante: conceptos básicos. *Medwave*, *21*(3), e8149. https://doi.org/10.5867/medwave.2021.03.8149

Schitter, A. M., Frei, P., Elfering, A., Kurpiers, N., & Radlinger, L. (2022). Evaluation of short-term effects of three passive aquatic interventions on chronic non-specific low back pain: study protocol for a randomized crossover clinical trial. *Contemporary Clinical Trials Communications*, *26*, 100904. https://doi.org/10.1016/j.conctc.2022.100904

Schulz, K. F., Altman, D. G., Moher, D., for the CONSORT Group. (2010). CONSORT 2010 Statement: Updated guidelines for reporting parallel group randomised trials. *Annals of Internal Medicine*, *152*, 726–732.

Shimizu, Y., Tsuji, K., Ochi, E., Arai, H., Okubo, R., Kuchiba, A., Shimazu, T., Sakurai, N., Narisawa, T., Ueno, T., Iwata, H., & Matsuoka, Y. (2020). Study protocol for a nationwide questionnaire survey of physical activity among breast cancer survivors in Japan. *BMJ Open*, *10*(1), e032871. https://doi.org/10.1136/bmjopen-2019-032871

Siette, J., Georgiou, A., & Westbrook, J. (2019). Observational cohort study investigating cognitive outcomes, social networks and well-being in older adults: A study protocol. *BMJ Open*, *9*(6), e029495. https://doi.org/10.1136/bmjopen-2019-029495

University of Oxford. (2020). *Payments and incentives in research*. https://researchsupport.admin.ox.ac.uk/files/bpg05paymentsandincentivesinresearchv10pdf

Westrupp, E. M., Karantzas, G., Macdonald, J. A., Olive, L., Youssef, G., Greenwood, C. J., Sciberras, E., Fuller-Tyszkiewicz, M., Evans, S., Mikocka-Walus, A., Ling, M., Cummins, R., Hutchinson, D., Melvin, G., Fernando, J. W., Teague, S., Wood, A. G., Toumbourou, J. W., Berkowitz, T., Linardon, J., ... Olsson, C. A. (2020). Study protocol for the COVID-19 Pandemic Adjustment Survey (CPAS): A longitudinal study of Australian parents of a child 0-18 years. *Frontiers in Psychiatry*, *11*, 555750. https://doi.org/10.3389/fpsyt.2020.555750

White, H., Sabarwal S., & de Hoop, T. (2014). *Randomized Controlled Trials (RCTs), Methodological briefs: Impact evaluation 7*. Florence: UNICEF Office of Research.

Wong, E. (2020). *Incentives in longitudinal studies, CLS Working Paper 2020/1*. London: UCL Centre for Longitudinal Studies.

Yu, S., Alper, H. E., Nguyen, A. M., Brackbill, R. M., Turner, L., Walker, D. J., Maslow, C. B., & Zweig, K. C. (2017). The effectiveness of a monetary incentive offer on survey response rates and response completeness in a longitudinal study. *BMC Medical Research Methodology*, *17*(1), 77. https://doi.org/10.1186/s12874-017-0353-1

12 SAMPLES AND SAMPLING IN QUALITATIVE STUDIES AND PROPOSALS

INTRODUCTION

Deciding on the sample size and type of sampling at the design stage of a qualitative study and writing about them in research proposals are not as straightforward as for quantitative investigations. In qualitative studies, both the sample size and sample selection are fluid and evolving. This is mainly because data collection and data analysis in qualitative studies are iterative (i.e. they go back and forth) and often unpredictable. Researchers may need more or fewer participants than they expected at the start of the study. Some participants can be recruited well after the study has started through sampling methods such as a 'snowball' (initial participants referring others to the study). In the circumstances it is difficult to decide or calculate in advance the number of participants required for qualitative study. Quantitative terms such as 'probability' and sample size 'calculation', or even the term 'sampling', are contentious when applied to qualitative studies. For a useful discussion on whether sample size can be decided in advance, see Sim et al. (2018).

The difficulties that researchers experience in deciding the sample size and selection process in advance are matched by difficulties that reviewers experience when little information is provided for them to decide whether the study will be adequately resourced or whether the time frame is realistic. As Ayres (2007) explained, 'writers and reviewers of qualitative research proposals may struggle to define sample size' and 'reviewers insist on numbers' (p. 243). This problem is sometimes made worse by reviewers of proposals who apply quantitative research concepts or principles to qualitative studies. As early as 1969, Herbert Blumer pointed out how funding agencies were assessing qualitative research proposals by inappropriately using quantitative criteria (Blumer, 1969). Parahoo (2003), writing on this topic, compared the use of criteria for evaluating quantitative research to review qualitative proposals to 'forcing square pegs into round holes' (p. 156).

To address the complaint that qualitative proposals were not reviewed fairly when some funding agencies use quantitative criteria for the evaluation of qualitative proposals, Morse (2003) developed 'criteria to assess the relevance, rigor, and feasibility of qualitative research' (p. 833). Although much progress has been achieved in getting qualitative studies accepted on their own merits since then, there are still issues in reporting samples and sampling in qualitative studies and proposals. For example, Robinson (2014) reported that sampling in qualitative research has been poorly reported in journal articles. Gentles et al. (2015) reported that the 'literature regarding sampling in qualitative research is characterized by important inconsistencies and ambiguities' (p. 1772). Vasileiou et al. (2018), who carried out a systematic analysis of qualitative studies in the disciplines of psychology, sociology and medicine over a period of 15 years, concluded that 'the provision of sample size justifications in qualitative health research' (p. 1) was limited.

If some researchers find it difficult to report samples and sampling after their studies have been completed, it is no surprise that they may find it even more difficult to be clear and precise in their research proposals. In the rest of the chapter, we will examine the nature of samples and sampling in qualitative research and identify the key information to include in the relevant section of a proposal.

FACTORS DETERMINING SAMPLES AND SAMPLING IN QUALITATIVE RESEARCH

The difficulties researchers experience in deciding in advance sample size and sample selection in qualitative studies is mainly due to the nature of qualitative inquiry. Qualitative research comes in different forms, and well-known designs such as grounded theory or phenomenology are often adapted to suit the particular needs of the studies being undertaken. It is not rare to read that researchers have adapted the original version of grounded theory developed by Glaser and Strauss (1967) to suit their own studies. Even Strauss and Corbin went on to develop another version of grounded theory (see Strauss and Corbin, 1990).

As we have seen in Chapter 11, in quantitative studies an adequate sample size is important because, among other things, it allows conclusions to be drawn about how possible or not that the findings are due to chance. Random sampling methods are used to ensure that the findings are representative of the target population. Together the sample size and sampling methods determine that the findings are valid, reliable and generalisable to the target population. The focus in quantitative research is on 'population', in particular on how phenomena are distributed in a population. For example, in the survey of 'mental health of children in England in 2017' (Sadler et al., 2018), the focus was on, among other things, how mental illness was distributed among children (5–19 years old). The main aim of the survey was to estimate what proportion of children and young people in England were living with a mental disorder and the types of mental disorder they experienced. Sadler et al. (2018) explained that 'a stratified multistage random probability sample of children was drawn from the NHS [National Health Service] Patient Register in October 2016' (p. 31). Sadler et al. (2018) concluded that one in eight children and young people has at least one mental disorder (based on the 10th revision of the International Classification of Diseases). They also reported on trends; for example, they found that there was a slight increase in overall rates of mental disorder among those aged 5–15 years when compared with previous surveys.

Qualitative research, on the other hand, focuses on phenomena. The aim is to explore phenomena in order to increase our understanding of them. For example, Liberati et al. (2021) explored the experiences of UK NHS mental healthcare workers during the COVID-19 pandemic. One of the reasons a qualitative approach was used was because the difficulties mental healthcare workers experienced were 'less scrutinised and understood' and that there was a 'void in the literature' on this topic. The authors explained that their sampling strategy was 'not aiming to achieve statistical representation of the population but to identify a variety of experiences' (p. 2) related to their research questions (Liberati et al. 2021). It was important for them that their findings were representative of the phenomenon of the 'experience of working during the COVID-19 pandemic'.

Selecting samples for a qualitative study is almost like detectives deciding who to question when searching for witnesses and clues. Detectives will not know in advance how the investigation will develop and who (and how many) witnesses overall will be needed. Witnesses will be 'selected' for 'interview' because they are perceived to have some knowledge or information that may explain the crime.

In quantitative research, sampling methods or techniques are based on probability theory, hence the term 'probability sampling'. Not all quantitative studies use probability sampling (e.g. some use convenience sampling) but the aim is to do so as much as possible. On the other hand, sampling strategies in qualitative research have been described as 'non-probability'. The term 'non-probability' describes what it is not, but not what it is. One term that is commonly used to describe the sampling in qualitative studies is 'purposive' or 'purposeful'. The two terms have been used interchangeability to describe the selection of 'information-rich' cases that can provide both depth and breadth to the findings. Patton (2002) provided this rationale for the use of purposeful sampling:

> The logic and power of purposeful sampling lie in selecting information-rich cases for study in depth. Information-rich cases are those from which one can learn a great deal about issues of central importance to the purpose of the inquiry, thus the term purposeful sampling. Studying information-rich cases yields insights and in-depth understanding rather than empirical generalizations.
>
> *(p. 230)*

Patton (2015) went on to identify 40 types of purposeful sampling (including maximum variation, typical case, high-impact cases, etc.). While many researchers use the term 'purposeful' to describe their samples in qualitative studies, most rarely explain clearly how the participants were selected. Gentles et al. (2015) suggested that 'whenever researchers describe a sampling process as purposeful they should describe what this means in their specific context, rather than simply state that purposeful sampling was employed' (p. 1779). Anyone preparing purposeful sampling for a qualitative study would benefit from reading the typologies of Patton (2015).

As explained earlier, sample size and sample selection in qualitative studies depend on a number of factors, in particular the research approach or design and the data collection methods. To explain this further, we will look at three main approaches: grounded theory, phenomenology and ethnography. It must be acknowledged, however, that many qualitative studies do not specify the approach they used, if any.

SAMPLES AND SAMPLING IN GROUNDED THEORY STUDIES

In grounded theory (Glaser and Strauss, 1967; Strauss and Corbin, 1990; Charmaz, 2006), the aim is to develop theories from data. As Depoy and Gitlin (2016) explained, the research aim in grounded theory is to 'reveal theoretical principles about a phenomenon under study'(p. 319). To achieve this, grounded theory researchers seek participants who can offer different perspectives that can contribute to a full conceptual understanding of the phenomena they wish to investigate. A number of data collection methods, such as qualitative interviews and observations as well as quantitative methods such as surveys, can be used to achieve a conceptual or theoretical understanding.

Two main concepts determine sample selection and sample size in grounded theory studies: 'theoretical sampling' and 'saturation'. In simple terms, theoretical sampling means selecting participants and other data sources (such as diaries, notes and other documents) to enable a conceptual or theoretical development of phenomena. In grounded theory, data are analysed during and after data collection. As the theory develops researchers get an idea of where it is leading to and what gaps (in the emerging theory) need to be filled. More questions are asked and more participants are selected in order to find answers. In their seminal book on grounded theory, Glaser and Strauss (1967) explained that, in the process of data collection for generating theory, 'the analyst jointly collects, codes and analyses his data and decides what data to collect next and where to find them, in order to develop his theory as it emerges' (p. 45). Later, Strauss and Corbin (1998) expanded on this to explain that theoretical sampling helps to 'maximise opportunities to discover variations among concepts and to densify categories in terms of their properties and dimensions' (p. 201).

Typically, one would start a grounded theory study with a purposeful sample (i.e. people whom researchers know have experience of the phenomenon) and move to theoretical sampling as some components of the theory begin to emerge. How many participants to enlist at the beginning of the study may vary according to the topic and who is available. If the categories and dimensions of the concepts or theories emerge early, the researchers may have to move into the theoretical sample phase. Although it is possible to become theoretically-sensitive from the first few interviews or observations, one must be mindful of what Glaser (1978) calls 'premature closure' that 'can occur when the initial ideas or patterns that emerge out of the data are not sufficiently explored to enable the theory to fully describe the phenomenon under investigation' (Parahoo, 2014, p. 233). Premature closure may lead to fewer participants being selected than anticipated. For discussions on theoretical sampling in grounded theory studies, see Breckenridge and Jones (2009), Conlon et al. (2020) and Hood (2007). See Ligita et al. (2020) for an excellent practical example of how theoretical sampling was used in a grounded theory of 'the social processes of how people living with diabetes in Indonesia learn about their disease' (p. 117).

While theoretical sampling guides researchers toward selecting more participants (to add to data/insights already obtained), the concept of 'saturation' avoids the collection of more of the same data. Saturation happens when researchers find that new data no longer add to what has been revealed already. This is the point at which researchers have to decide whether or not to stop collecting data. The principle of 'diminishing returns' (when the amount of effort far outweighs the outcome) can be useful in making the decision that data collection has reached saturation point.

Saturation as a concept has been put into practice in studies other than grounded theory. The term 'informational redundancy' (Gentles et al., 2015) is sometimes used to describe 'saturation'. However, in their review of sampling in studies carried out in three research traditions – grounded theory, phenomenology and case study – Gentles et al. (2015) found that there was 'no mention of saturation outside grounded theory' (p. 1781). On the other hand, in the review of sampling practices in five approaches to qualitative research in education and health sciences, there was evidence of the use of saturation in some phenomenological studies (Guetterman, 2015). Vasileiou et al. (2018), in their systematic analysis of qualitative health research over a 15-year period, concluded that 'defence of sample size was most frequently supported across all three journals with reference to the principle of saturation and to pragmatic considerations' (p. 1).

Saturation is a complex concept and difficult to implement. It comes in different forms including 'theoretical', 'thematic', 'data' and 'meaning' (see, for example, Sebele-Mpofu 2020). For more discussion on saturation, see Saunders et al. (2018), Guest et al. (2006), Guest et al. (2020) and Hennink et al. (2017). In their proposal for a qualitative study on 'key stakeholders' perspectives and experiences with defining, identifying and displaying gaps in health research', Nyanchoka et al. (2020) explained in detail how saturation influenced their estimation of the required sample size for their study. After reviewing previous studies regarding when saturation was reached, Nyanchoka et al. (2020) stated that saturation in their proposed study would be guided by the seven parameters identified by Hennink et al. (2017), namely 'the study purpose, population, sampling strategy, data quality, type of codes, code book and saturation goal, and focus retrieved from the study' (p. 2).

Although theoretical sampling and saturation influence sample selection and sample size in grounded theory studies, they offer no indication of what a sample size should be prior to a study. Thomson (2010) carried out 'a content analysis of one hundred articles that utilised grounded theory and interviews as a data collection method' (p. 45). He reported that the average size was 25 participants. However, Thomson (2010) recommended that it was important 'to plan for thirty interviews to fully develop patterns, concepts, categories, properties, and dimensions of the given phenomena' (p. 45). These figures can only serve to indicate the parameters within which researchers may want to operate. Vasileiou et al. (2018) acknowledged that researchers might find that 'sample size community norms serve as useful rules of thumb' (p. 16). They recommended that 'methodological knowledge is used to critically consider how saturation and other parameters that affect sample size sufficiency pertain to the specifics of the particular project' (p. 16).

Proposal Example 12.1 shows how sample and sampling were reported in a grounded theory study proposal.

SAMPLES AND SAMPLING IN PHENOMENOLOGICAL STUDIES

In grounded theory, the concept of theory development determines sampling selection and sample size. Saturation is guided by theory development; to develop their theory, researchers ask questions and identify new avenues for exploration. In grounded theory, data collection

PROPOSAL EXAMPLE 12.1
SAMPLES AND SAMPLING IN A GROUNDED THEORY STUDY PROPOSAL

Low et al. (2017), 'A qualitative study protocol of ageing carers' caregiving experiences and their planning for continuation of care for their immediate family members with intellectual disability'.

In this proposal, the authors intended to use a 'constructivist grounded theory' approach to 'capture family caregiving experiences and the processes of carers in addressing caregiving needs, support received and plans to continue to provide care for themselves and their relatives with intellectual disability (ID) in their later life' (p. 1).

COMMENTS

1. The target population was 'carers who have an immediate family member with mild (ID 50–69) or moderate (25–49) grades of ID' (p. 4). The inclusion criteria were 'primary carer aged 50+ years', 'immediate family members (e.g., parents, siblings)', currently using services provided by sheltered workshops and living in Hong Kong.
2. The setting was described as three 'sheltered workshops'. In their proposal Low et al. (2017) also provided some description of the workshops, their target population, their activities and their overall aim.
3. According to the authors, the study would target 20 family carers in each of the three selected workshops, giving a total of 60 carers. They intended to start with the 'purposive sampling' of 'participants who are most likely to provide rich information about the experiences of the phenomena under study' (p. 4). Purposive sampling was to be followed by theoretical sampling in order to 'enrich and clarify the important data/information by sampling for people, circumstances, activities and incidents as guided by the codes and categories that are being developed by the emerging theory' (p. 4). The authors of this proposal have shown that their sampling strategies are in line with their chosen approach (grounded theory). They used concepts and terminologies from grounded theory to demonstrate this.

and analysis happen simultaneously and concurrently. This process helps researchers to know how theory development is progressing and where to take the data next. This does not happen in phenomenological studies, where the description of how phenomena are experienced is what researchers seek. There is little to guide researchers through the saturation process. However, phenomenological researchers may find that the data may lack both depth and richness (usually due to some participants not articulating their experience as fluently as the researchers expect). In these circumstances, phenomenological researchers may want to interview more participants than expected. Conversely, some researchers may begin to see that participants' descriptions are being 'repeated' in later interviews and may want to stop the data collection. Therefore, what determines sample selection and sample size in phenomenological studies is the quest for rich and meaningful descriptions.

The methodological literature shows that different terms are used in phenomenological studies to describe sample selections. These include 'purposive', 'convenient', 'criterion' and 'snowball' (although some studies use a combination of those terms). There is some ambiguity regarding the type of sampling suitable for phenomenological studies. van Manen (a prominent writer on phenomenology) believed that 'purposive' sampling may not be applicable when using this approach (van Manen, 2014). Yet purposive sampling is more commonly employed in phenomenological research because it 'allows selecting participants who have rich knowledge of the phenomenon (Frechette et al, 2020, p. 6). However, more than one sampling strategy can be used in the same study. In her doctoral study of the 'lived experience of parents of young children with autism receiving special education services', Barrow (2017) employed 'purposeful snowball sampling'.

It is more important to describe how participants are selected than to get tangled up in the choice of labels or terminology to describe sampling strategies. Groenewald (2003) gives a detailed account of a phenomenological study he carried out. He used the subheading 'locating the research participants/informants' to explain how and why he selected and accessed his participants. He chose purposive sampling based on 'his judgement and purpose on the research' and because the participants 'had experiences relating to the phenomenon to be researched' (p. 45). He went on to explain that he carried out internet searches and telephone enquiries to identify the people who were subsequently interviewed. Groenewald (2003) also used snowball sampling to trace additional participants. All his decisions were backed up by references to credible experts in the field.

Deciding the sample size in advance for proposals for phenomenological studies is a contentious issue. According to Frechette et al. (2020), 'the richness of the data collected takes precedence over the actual size of the sample' (p. 6). If the aim is to be descriptive, the sample size depends on how the initial participants are able to provide rich data. If these data are not forthcoming, researchers may have to seek more participants, hence the use of the snowball strategy. Small sample sizes are not unusual for phenomenological studies. In her doctoral study, Barrow (2017) reported that unstructured interviews and photo-elicitation (a methodology involving the use of family photographs as part of the interview process) with four parents 'generated 300 pages of transcripts from which the essential themes emerged' (p. 4). Barrow (2017) explained that these interviews 'generated extensive narrative data' and 'an in-depth and detailed picture of the participants' lived experiences' (p. 98).

Each of the different types of phenomenology (Husserlian, Heidegerian and interpretive phenomenological analysis) has its own approach to data collection and analysis. Generalising about an adequate sample size for all these approaches is not helpful. Different authors also make different recommendations on what an adequate sample size should be in these types of study. According to Noon (2018), there is no right answer to the question of sample size in interpretive phenomenological analysis . The sample size depends on how wide or narrow the aim of the study is and how homogeneous the sample is. Different disciplines may have different sample size norms. In his review of sample size and sampling practices, Guetterman (2015) reported that the mean average sample size of phenomenological studies in the field of education was 15 (range 8–31) and in health sciences was 25 (range 8–52). All these factors, mentioned above, complicate decisions of how many participants to sample in advance.

Researchers should also find out how easy or difficult it is for participants to be accessed and how likely it is that those selected will be able and willing to open up and articulate their lived experience. This depends on the phenomenon being investigated. In addition, researchers should consider the literature on the topic (in particular, previous studies) and the social and cultural normative practices and taboos that may influence how freely participants can talk about their experience. Researchers will, no doubt, be guided by the depth or richness (or lack of these) as they collect the data. For research proposals, researchers intending to carry out phenomenological studies should identify (through discussion with team members) the factors that may affect participant selection. They should also talk with stakeholders to find out about access and recruitment. An estimation of the upper end of the sample size should also be given, with an explanation of how this may change.

For an example of how samples and sampling occur for a phenomenological study see Proposal Example 12.2. The proposal by McKeaveney et al. (2020) is another example.

SAMPLES AND SAMPLING IN ETHNOGRAPHIC STUDIES

Compared with grounded theory and phenomenology, describing samples and sampling in research proposals for ethnographic studies can be even more challenging. This is because ethnographic studies involve a more fluid and evolving process. Ethnographers often have a topic they want to explore, and it is only when they are immersed in the setting that they can focus

---

PROPOSAL EXAMPLE 12.2
SAMPLES AND SAMPLING IN A PROPOSAL FOR A PHENOMENOLOGICAL STUDY

Fiori et al. (2019), 'Exploring patients' and healthcare professionals' experiences of patient-witnessed resuscitation: a qualitative study protocol'.

COMMENTS

1. This phenomenological study proposed recruiting two participant groups: hospital patients who witnessed cardiopulmonary resuscitation (CPR) on other patients and health care professionals involved in CPR on hospital wards. These participants would be taken from nine wards in a hospital. Under the heading 'Participants', the authors stated that they intended to use a 'criterion-based purposive sampling strategy' (based on the literature on phenomenological studies) to recruit 5–25 participants (patients) who met the criterion of having witnessed CPR undertaken on other patients. According to Fiori et al. (2019), this sample size was based on qualitative research guidelines. For the health professional group (nurses, doctors, healthcare assistants and other health care professionals), the authors make reference to the methodological literature to justify their estimation of sample size.

2. Fiori et al. (2019) also provided detailed plans of how they intended to recruit the participants. They described the setting where the study would take place and the procedures they would follow. They explained that recruitment would be 'through the co-operation between the resuscitation team, the clinical care team of the wards, the local research nurse and the research team' (p. 208). This process was presented in the form of a flow chart that would be helpful to all those involved in this study. It also would help readers (ethics panel members and others) to understand how and when recruitment would take place.

3. The authors indicated that the stakeholders had been consulted and that their views and advice had been taken into account when designing the study. This type of 'homework' can inspire confidence that this proposal has been carefully thought out.

on particular phenomena. Another difference (from grounded theory and phenomenology) is that ethnographers do not know in advance the specifics of who they will talk with or interview and what they will observe. What constitutes a 'sample' is also problematic and contentious. One does not necessarily 'select' who one talks with in the setting where the study takes place (as this often happens by chance or accident). Therefore, ethnography, in its traditional form (when ethnographers went to live among the people and in the culture they were studying) does not fit into the neat structure of a conventional research proposal. Contemporary or focused ethnography (e.g. observing interactions of health professionals in a work setting) is much more demarcated and lends itself to the provision of some of the required detail in a research proposal.

Focused ethnography (as opposed to traditional ethnography), 'applies to any small-scale research that is conducted in the everyday setting, explores shared practices and meanings from a cultural lens, and where the researcher may or may not have familiarity with the sub-culture under study' (Rashid et al., 2019, p. 2). With this type of ethnography, researchers can decide in advance who (and how many) participants to interview or observe, although this is likely to change during the course of the study. Chan et al. (2018) carried out a 'focused ethnographic' study of 'patients' perceptions of their experiences with nurse-patient communication in oncology settings'. After setting out the inclusion and exclusion criteria, they recruited 93 patients and 24 nurses on an oncology unit, using convenient, purposive and snowball sampling. Similarly, Harmon et al. (2019) used focused ethnography to study 'nurses' culturally mediated practices influencing pain care provision for older people in acute care'. They 'purposively sampled' nine nurses and 42 older persons in two hospital sites. Harmon (the first author) 'set aside two months to gain access and was immersed for six months in the field' (p. 23).

The more unstructured the ethnography, the less precise one can be in stipulating in advance the types and number of participants taking part in the study. During periods of observation in a particular setting, a number and types of people are likely to 'cross the researcher's path'. In true ethnographic style, researchers have to follow the data wherever they come from. Some participants can be formally interviewed (as is the case in qualitative studies using other approaches). However, there are situations when the interview is informal and happens 'in situ' (where the action takes place). In such circumstances, it is difficult, or even unproductive, to count the number of people with whom one talks. What constitutes an interview in the context of ethnographic studies should be described in a research proposal (e.g. formal, semistructured or even focus group).

The size of a sample in ethnographic studies tends to be large. In Guetterman's (2015) review of sampling practices in qualitative studies, the mean sample size for ethnographic studies was 128 (compared with 59 for grounded theory and 21 for phenomenology). This is probably due to ethnographers interacting with groups rather than individuals. During periods of observation, they also come into contact with many people, some of whom are then enlisted in the study.

Stipulating samples in proposals of ethnographic studies can be very problematic. Apart from estimating the number of participants who may be required for the study, ethnographic researchers have to give some detail regarding what they will observe, including how many times they will observe and the length of observations. Research proposals for ethnographic studies should also include information on who will be recruited and how. Key informants or facilitators should be contacted in advance of writing the proposal to gain some insight on access issues such the potential for participants to take part in the study and some of the difficulties or issues that may arise. The setting where the study will be carried out will need to be described. Finally, the person or people undertaking the data collection should be identified.

Proposal Example 12.3 shows how samples and sampling issues are dealt with in an ethnographic study proposal.

SAMPLES AND SAMPLING IN MIXED METHODS STUDIES

Most of the issues identified in this chapter and Chapter 11 with regards to samples and sampling apply to mixed methods studies as well (since they tend to combine quantitative and qualitative approaches in the same study). No matter how subordinate one method is to the other (in the same study), all the necessary information on how and why the data sources (including participants) are selected should be reported in enough detail in the proposal. To avoid confusion, it is better to deal with each method separately, using diagrams or flow charts, where appropriate, to present the required information. Mixed methods studies can be in a number of phases (see Chapter 7). Therefore, describing each phase clearly is important.

PROPOSAL EXAMPLE 12.3
SAMPLES AND SAMPLING IN A PROPOSAL FOR AN ETHNOGRAPHIC STUDY

Darbyshire et al. (2020), ' "Where have all the doctors gone?" A protocol for an ethnographic study of the retention problem in emergency medicine in the UK'.

COMMENTS

1. After giving the reasons why an ethnographic approach was appropriate for this study, Darbyshire et al. (2020) explained that the first author aimed 'to perform 4 days of observation each week by scheduling 48 days over the 12-week period' (p. 5), including days, evenings, nights and weekends at two sites.

2. They stated that the first author would conduct around 40 interviews. These interviews would be on both research sites, with doctors and individuals within key organisations relevant to retention in emergency medicine. Darbyshire et al. (2020) made a distinction between conversations as part of participant observation and formal interviews. They explained, that 'in addition to the participant-observation conversations' they would 'conduct interviews, reserving the term for the physically separate, planned, audio-recorded and transcribed encounters' (p. 5).

3. The estimated sample size was decided upon after discussion with the research team 'who have extensive experience with this methodology' and after 'consulting key texts' (p. 5). They also pointed out that the sample size was an estimation based on 'when theoretical saturation might be achieved' (p. 5). In this case, one can see that a grounded theory concept (theoretical saturation) was used to estimate sample size.

4. To select participants for interviews, they listed a number of inclusion criteria for eligibility, including the length of time the participants (doctors) had worked in emergency medicine. Participant observation sites were selected based on the 'presence of foundation, core and higher trainees', 'presence of staff and associate specialists' and 'type 1 ED [emergency department] (major ED, providing a consultant-led 24 hour service with full resuscitation facilities)' (p. 5).

If the same participants (or some of them) are to be used in the quantitative and qualitative phases of a study, this has to be explained in the proposal. In the proposal by Fitzpatrick et al. (2021) for a study on 'protecting older people living in care homes from COVID-19', the authors described each phase separately and provided sample and sampling-related information for each phase. For another example of how this was done in a proposal, see Proposal Example 12.4.

PROPOSAL EXAMPLE 12.4
SAMPLES AND SAMPLING IN A MIXED METHODS STUDY PROPOSAL

Climent-Sanz et al. (2020), 'A web-based therapeutic patient education intervention for pain and sleep for women with fibromyalgia: a sequential exploratory mixed-methods research protocol'.

COMMENTS

1. In this proposal, the authors aimed to conduct a study in three phases. Phase 1 comprised semistructured, qualitative interviews with adult women with fibromyalgia to develop the content of a web-based therapeutic patient education intervention (TPE). In phase 2, the TPE would be developed, based on the findings of the qualitative findings. In phase 3, the TPE would be tested in a parallel, double-blinded, randomised controlled trial.

2. The sample and sampling were reported separately for phases 1 and 3. In the qualitative phase, after setting the inclusion criteria, 'a theoretical sample will be recruited using the snowball technique' (p. 1429). Although no mention is made of sample size, the authors stated that 'saturation' would be used to guide the final size of the sample.

3. Similarly, the inclusion and exclusion criteria for the quantitative phase were stated. The list from which the participants for the trial would be recruited as well as the 'systematized and randomised sampling method and sample size calculation' (p. 1429) (based on clinically significant difference) were described in the proposal. Details about allocation concealment, blinding and the tests to calculate sample size are also provided.

Checklist for the sample/sampling section of proposals for qualitative studies:

1. Has the target population (or other sources of data) been identified and defined? What are the inclusion and exclusion criteria, if any? Are these criteria justified? Are they in line with the aim of the study?

2. Has an estimation of the sample size been provided? What is the justification for this? How many participants will initially be recruited? Will saturation and theoretical sampling (for grounded theory purposes) be used to guide the sampling requirements for the study?

3. What type of sampling (e.g. purposive, snowball, etc.), will be used in the study? Is the sampling strategy aligned with the qualitative approach selected (e.g. grounded theory or phenomenology)?

4. How will the participants or other data sources be accessed?

5. Is there a description of site(s) where the study will be conducted?

6. Are gatekeepers involved? Has preliminary contact been made with them? How will the participants be selected?

7. What strategies will be employed if more participants need to be recruited? Is there a statement regarding 'saturation', if appropriate?

SUMMARY AND CONCLUSIONS

This chapter has shown how samples and sampling in qualitative studies can be fluid and flexible. We have highlighted the various factors that affect the size of samples and the sampling strategies. Sampling-related issues in grounded theory, phenomenological and ethnographic studies have been examined.

The literature, in particular reviews of sampling practices in the different types of qualitative approach, shows that there is no consensus on what sample sizes should be in qualitative studies or how they can be calculated. There is a consensus that the sample size may increase or decrease when conducting a qualitative study. However, in research proposals of qualitative studies, especially those seeking funding, an estimation of the anticipated sample size and the initial number of participants should be given as far as possible. The estimated sample size is likely to consider the aim of the study, the type of participants, the potential for recruiting them, the research approach and previous studies on the topic.

REFERENCES

Ayres, L. (2007). Qualitative research proposals—part III: Sampling and data collection. *Journal of Wound, Ostomy, and Continence Nursing : official publication of The Wound, Ostomy and Continence Nurses Society, 34*(3), 242–244.

Barrow, D. M. (2017). A phenomenological study of the lived experiences of parents of young children with autism receiving special education services. Dissertations and Theses. Paper 4035. https://doi.org/10.15760/etd.5919

Blumer, H. (1969). *Symbolic interactionism. Perspective and method.* London: University of California Press.

Breckenridge, J., & Jones, D. (2009). Demystifying theoretical sampling in grounded theory research. *Grounded Theory Review, 8,* 113–126.

Chan, E. A., Wong, F., Cheung, M. Y., & Lam, W. (2018). Patients' perceptions of their experiences with nurse-patient communication in oncology settings: A focused ethnographic study. *PloS One, 13*(6), e0199183. https://doi.org/10.1371/journal.pone.0199183

Charmaz, K. (2006). *Constructing grounded theory: A practical guide through qualitative analysis.* Thousand Oaks, CA: Sage Publications.

Climent-Sanz, C., Gea-Sánchez, M., Moreno-Casbas, M. T., Blanco-Blanco, J., García-Martínez, E., & Valenzuela-Pascual, F. (2020). A web-based therapeutic patient education intervention for pain and sleep for women with fibromyalgia: A sequential exploratory mixed-methods research protocol. *Journal of Advanced Nursing, 76*(6), 1425–1435.

Conlon, C., Timonen, V., Elliott-O'Dare, C., O'Keeffe, S., & Foley, G. (2020). Confused about theoretical sampling? Engaging theoretical sampling in diverse grounded theory studies. *Qualitative Health Research, 30*(6), 947–959.

Darbyshire, D., Brewster, L., Isba, R., Body, R., & Goodwin, D. (2020). 'Where have all the doctors gone?' A protocol for an ethnographic study of the retention problem in emergency medicine in the UK. *BMJ Open, 10*(11), e038229. https://doi.org/10.1136/bmjopen-2020-038229

DePoy, E., & Gitlin, L. N. (2016). *Introduction to research: understanding and applying multiple strategies* (5th ed.). St Louis, Missouri: Elsevier.

Fiori, M., Endacott, R., & Latour, J. M. (2019). Exploring patients' and healthcare professionals' experiences of patient-witnessed resuscitation: A qualitative study protocol. *Journal of Advanced Nursing, 75*(1), 205–214.

Fitzpatrick, J. M., Rafferty, A. M., Hussein, S., Ezhova, I., Palmer, S., Adams, R., Rees, L., Brearley, S., Sims, S., & Harris, R. (2021). Protecting older people living in care homes from COVID-19: A protocol for a mixed-methods study to understand the challenges and solutions to implementing social distancing and isolation. *BMJ Open*, *11*(8), e050706. https://doi.org/10.1136/bmjopen-2021-050706

Frechette, J., Bitzas, V., Aubry, M., Kilpatrick, K., & Lavoie-Tremblay, M. (2020). Capturing lived experience: Methodological considerations for interpretive phenomenological inquiry. *International Journal of Qualitative Methods*, *19*. https://doi.org/10.1177/1609406920907254

Gentles, S. J., Charles, C., Ploeg, J., & McKibbon, K. A. (2015). Sampling in qualitative research: Insights from an overview of the methods literature. *Qualitative Report*, *20*(11), 1772–1789. http://nsuworks.nova.edu/tqr/vol20/iss11/5

Glaser, B. (1978). *Theoretical sensitivity*. Mill Valley, California: Sociology Press.

Glaser, B. G., & Strauss, A. L. (1967). *The discovery of grounded theory. Strategies for qualitative research*. Chicago: Aldine.

Groenewald, T. (2004). A phenomenological research design illustrated. *International Journal of Qualitative Methods*, *3*(1), 42–55. https://doi.org/10.1177/160940690400300104

Guest, G., Bunce, A., & Johnson, L. (2006). How many interviews are enough? An Experiment with data saturation and variability. *Field Methods*, *18*(1), 59–82.

Guest, G., Namey, E., & Chen, M. (2020). A simple method to assess and report thematic saturation in qualitative research. *PloS One*, *15*(5), e0232076. https://doi.org/10.1371/journal.pone.0232076

Guetterman, T. C. (2015). Descriptions of sampling practices within five approaches to qualitative research in education and the health sciences. *Forum Qualitative Sozialforschung / Forum: Qualitative Social Research*, *16*(2). https://doi.org/10.17169/fqs-16.2.2290

Harmon, J., Summons, P., & Higgins, I. (2019). Nurses' culturally mediated practices influencing pain care provision for older people in acute care: Ethnographic study. *Applied Nursing Research*, *48*, 22–29.

Hennink, M. M., Kaiser, B. N., & Marconi, V. C. (2017). Code saturation versus meaning saturation: How many interviews are enough? *Qualitative Health Research*, *27*(4), 591–608.

Hood, J. C. (2007). Orthodoxy vs. power: The defining traits of grounded theory. In A. Bryant, & K. Charmaz (Eds.) *The Sage handbook of grounded theory* (pp. 151–164). London: Sage Pub. Ltd.

Liberati, E., Richards, N., Willars, J., Scott, D., Boydell, N., Parker, J., Pinfold, V., Martin, G., Dixon-Woods, M., & Jones, P. B. (2021). A qualitative study of experiences of NHS mental healthcare workers during the Covid-19 pandemic. *BMC Psychiatry*, *21*(1), 250. https://doi.org/10.1186/s12888-021-03261-8

Ligita, T., Harvey, N., Wicking, K., Nurjannah, I., & Francis, K. (2020). A practical example of using theoretical sampling throughout a grounded theory study: A methodological paper. *Qualitative Research Journal*, *20*(1), 116–126.

Low, L. P., Chien, W. T., Lam, L. W., & Wong, K. K. (2017). A qualitative study protocol of ageing carers' caregiving experiences and their planning for continuation of care for their immediate family members with intellectual disability. *BMC Geriatrics*, *17*(1), 81. https://doi.org/10.1186/s12877-017-0473-9

McKeaveney, C., Noble, H., Courtney, A. E., Gill, P., Griffin, S., Johnston, W., Maxwell, A. P., Teasdale, F., & Reid, J. (2020). Understanding the holistic experiences of living with a kidney transplant: An interpretative phenomenological study (protocol). *BMC Nephrology*, *21*(1), 222. https://doi.org/10.1186/s12882-020-01860-3

Morse, J. M. (2003). A review committee's guide for evaluating qualitative proposals. *Qualitative Health Research*, *13*(6), 833–851.

Noon, E. (2018). Interpretive phenomenological analysis: An appropriate methodology for educational research? *Journal of Perspectives in Applied Academic Practice*, *6*. https://doi.org/10.14297/jpaap.v6i1.304

Nyanchoka, L., Tudur-Smith, C., Porcher, R., & Hren, D. (2020). Key stakeholders' perspectives and experiences with defining, identifying and displaying gaps in health research: A qualitative study. *BMJ Open*, *10*(11), e039932. https://doi.org/10.1136/bmjopen-2020-039932

Parahoo, K. (2003). Square pegs in round holes: Reviewing qualitative research proposals. *Journal of Clinical Nursing, 12*, 155–157.

Parahoo, K. (2014). *Nursing research: Principles, process and issues* (3rd ed.). London: Palgrave Macmillan.

Patton, M. Q. (2002). *Qualitative research and evaluation methods* (3rd ed.). Thousand Oaks, CA: Sage Publications.

Patton, M. Q. (2015). *Qualitative research & evaluation methods: Integrating theory and practice* (4th ed.). Thousand Oaks, CA: Sage.

Rashid, M., Hodgson, C. S., & Luig, T. (2019). Ten tips for conducting focused ethnography in medical education research. *Medical Education Online, 24*(1), 1624133. https://doi.org/10.1080/10872981.2019.1624133

Robinson, O. C. (2014). Sampling in interview-based qualitative research: A theoretical and practical guide. *Qualitative Research in Psychology, 11*(1), 25–41.

Sadler, K., Vizard, T., Ford, T., Marcheselli, F., Pearce, N., Mandalia, D., Davis, J., Brodie, E., Forbes, N., Goodman, A., Goodman, R., McManus, S., & Collinson, D. (2018). *Mental health of children and young people in England, 2017.* NHS Digital. https://digital.nhs.uk/data-and-information/publications/statistical/mental-health-of-children-and-young-people-in-england/2017/2017

Saunders, B., Sim, J., Kingstone, T., Baker, S., Waterfield, J., Bartlam, B., Burroughs, H., & Jinks, C. (2018). Saturation in qualitative research: Exploring its conceptualization and operationalization. *Quality & Quantity, 52*(4), 1893–1907.

Sebele-Mpofu, F. Y. (2020). Saturation controversy in qualitative research: complexities and underlying assumptions. A literature review. *Cogent Social Sciences, 6*(1). https://doi.org/10.1080/23311886.2020.1838706

Sim, J., Saunders, J., Waterfield, J., & Kingstone, T. (2018). Can sample size in qualitative research be determined a priori? *International Journal of Social Research Methodology, 21*(5), 619–634.

Strauss, A. L., & Corbin, J. (1990). *Basics of qualitative research: Grounded theory procedures and techniques.* Thousand Oaks, CA: Sage.

Strauss, A. L., & Corbin, J. M. (1998). *Basics of qualitative research: Techniques and procedures for developing grounded theory.* Thousand Oaks, CA: Sage Publications.

Thomson, S. B. (2010). Grounded theory – Sample size. *Journal of Administration and Governance, 5*(1), 45–52. https://ssrn.com/abstract=3037218

van Manen, M. (2014). *Phenomenology of practice: Meaning-giving methods in phenomenological research and writing.* Walnut Creek, CA: Left Coast Press.

Vasileiou, K., Barnett, J., Thorpe, S., & Young, T. (2018). Characterising and justifying sample size sufficiency in interview-based studies: Systematic analysis of qualitative health research over a 15-year period. *BMC Medical Research Methodology, 18*(1), 148. https://doi.org/10.1186/s12874-018-0594-7

13

ETHICAL ISSUES IN STUDY DESIGN AND PROPOSALS

∎ ∎ ∎ ∎ ∎ ∎ ∎ ∎ ∎ ∎ ∎ ∎ ∎ ∎ ∎ ∎ ∎ ∎

INTRODUCTION

There are a number of ethical issues to consider when designing a study, from the time that research questions are developed to well after the study has been completed. However, researchers should be mindful that unforeseen ethical issues and challenges may arise at any time. In research proposals, researchers have to highlight the key ethical issues they are aware of (specific to their proposed study) and those they anticipate, and explain how they will address them.

There are four main areas or aspects of a study that researchers can reflect upon when assessing how ethical principles will be followed when designing a study: the research topic or questions, the types of participants, the design and methods to be used, and the researchers conducting the study. In the rest of this chapter, we will look closely at these four areas and discuss the ethical issues that may arise in relation to each of them.

Nursing, health and social care researchers collect data mainly, but not exclusively, from people who are quite often their patients, clients, students or colleagues. Apart from participants' verbal or written responses (and data collected through observations), researchers also undertake physical, psychological, physiological, biomedical and biological measurements. Demographic and other social data are collected directly or indirectly. Patients' and clients' notes are often used for research purposes. The actions of researchers when collecting and analysing these data can be intrusive and potentially harmful to those taking part in a study. Researchers have the responsibility to ensure that the wellbeing, safety and rights of participants are safeguarded at all times throughout the research process and subsequently. This responsibility lies with the principal investigator, who must ensure that everyone involved in the study behaves ethically. The idea that researchers are responsible for the ethical conduct of their studies applies to researchers worldwide, no matter what legal, structural or organisational policies are, or are not, in place in the countries where the studies are carried out. The wellbeing, safety and rights of participants always take precedence over the research study.

Ethical principles have been developed to guide researchers. There are also of course ethical principles for policy and practice (for an example, see Varkey, 2021, 'Principles of clinical ethics and their application to practice'). The Belmont Report (US Department of Health and Human Services, 1978) is perhaps the most referred to guidance for the ethical conduct of research. The report lists three 'basic ethical principles': respect for persons, beneficence and justice. Most research ethical guidelines are based on these principles. For example, the UK Economic and Social Research Council (ESRC, 2022) lists six core principles for the conduct of ethical research:

- *Research should aim to maximise benefit for individuals and society and minimise risk and harm;*
- *The rights and dignity of individuals and groups should be respected;*
- *Wherever possible, participation should be voluntary and appropriately informed;*
- *Research should be conducted with integrity and transparency;*
- *Lines of responsibility and accountability should be clearly defined; and*
- *Independence of research should be maintained and where conflicts of interest cannot be avoided they should be made explicit.*

(p. 1)

These principles can be used to reflect upon and address, where possible, the specific ethical issues arising from the proposed research.

Of the Belmont Report principles, the concept of beneficence is perhaps the most fundamental, because a study should not be carried out if one cannot demonstrate what benefit it will bring. There are a number of safeguards for the conduct of research that is ethically and methodologically sound and feasible. In-house ethics committees (e.g. set up in hospitals or universities) or national independent committees (such as the Research Ethics Committees in the UK and the Institutional Review Board in the USA) look at the feasibility, benefits and the potential harm of studies. However, the assessment of risks starts at the design stage of a study. This exercise is best conducted by the research team, which should include users as much as possible (see Chapter 15). At this early stage of the design, it is only possible to make educated guesses of the type, level and extent of ethical risks that the study poses. By reviewing previous, similar studies one can identify some of the potential risks. However, it is not always possible to predict what may happen while the study is being conducted.

ETHICAL ISSUES RELATED TO THE RESEARCH TOPIC OR QUESTION

Any topic for research requires sensitivity in the way the study is conducted. The degree of sensitivity depends on a number of factors including the research question, the setting, the methodology, the cultural context and who is undertaking the data collection. A study exploring the experience of women survivors of domestic abuse is likely to be more sensitive than one exploring social workers' perception of domestic abuse and how it can be prevented. Interviewing patients in hospitals about the care they are receiving is likely to be more sensitive than if they were interviewed in their own homes after discharge. In focus group interviews it may be more difficult to handle personal disclosures than in one-to-one interviews on a similar topic, due to the presence of other participants when disclosures are made.

Culturally, there are some topics or practices that participants may not want to discuss. People may not want to talk about religious beliefs or politics, or reveal what they do or earn. This may be compounded by who asks the question. For example, a man asking women about breastfeeding practices is not appropriate in many cultures. Therefore, researchers should consider the topic as well as these factors (question, setting, methodology, culture and researcher) when assessing the potential risks.

In the design of a study, there are some research topics that are known to be particularly sensitive. Lee (1993) listed sensitive topics as 'illegal behaviour', 'private, stressful or sacred' topics and those that pose a political threat. The ESRC Framework for Research Ethics (ESRC, 2015) listed some of the main sensitive topics as: research involving participants' sexual behaviour; illegal or political behaviour; experience of violence, abuse or exploitation; mental health; participants' personal or family lives; or their gender or ethnic status. Below are some examples of studies involving sensitive topics and how researchers have dealt with the sensitive issues that arise. These studies provide useful insights into the complexity of these issues.

- Fahie (2014), 'Doing sensitive research sensitively: ethical and methodological issues in researching workplace bullying'.
- Ellsberg and Heise (2005), 'Researching violence against women: a practical guide for researchers and activists'.
- Rodriguez (2018), 'Methodological challenges of sensitive topic research with adolescents'.

In a proposal for a qualitative study of 'the realities of middle and front-line management work in health care', Buchanan et al. (2013) anticipated that some participants may share 'information about work experiences that they may have found difficult and/or distressing' (p. 128). They also think that such disclosure, although voluntary 'could nevertheless lead to personal discomfort' (p. 128). Buchanan et al. (2013) decided to address this by pointing out to prospective participants, in the information sheet, that such a situation might arise and that the prospective participants should take this into account when deciding whether or not to take part. Buchanan et al. (2013) also stated that if such a situation did arise in a group discussion or interview, the researcher would 'terminate the conversation immediately' and offer a 'private debriefing, off the record' (p. 128).

One can see that Buchanan et al. (2013) used three steps in dealing with this sensitive topic in their proposal: anticipate what could happen, think about how this might impact on participants, and then explain the strategies that would be used to prevent and deal with the situation if it arose. For another example showing how others deal with a sensitive topic in a proposal, see Fiori et al. (2019) in Research Example 13.1. Although sensitive topics carry additional responsibility for researchers, 'the decision to avoid research on sensitive topics could be seen by some researchers as evasion of responsibility (Dickson-Swift et al., 2008, p. 6).

ETHICAL ISSUES RELATED TO PARTICIPANTS

All research participants can potentially be vulnerable to harm because of the unequal relationship between the researchers and participants as the balance of power is nearly always in favour of

---

RESEARCH EXAMPLE 13.1

REPORTING SENSITIVE AND ETHICAL ISSUES IN A RESEARCH PROPOSAL

Fiori et al. (2019), 'Exploring patients' and healthcare professionals' experiences of patient-witnessed resuscitation: a qualitative proposal'.

COMMENTS

1. This study received ethical approval from the relevant committees and organisations. The proposal gave details about the measures to be taken to ensure confidentiality and anonymity. The authors recognised that 'witnessed resuscitation may be a sensitive topic for participants to discuss' (p. 210). Fiori et al. (2019) listed a number of strategies they proposed to use before, during and after the interview to support participants if they were upset or unsettled.

2. The authors also recognised that the study might pose risks to the researchers as well. The measures they proposed to take include arrangements for the researcher conducting the interviews to be debriefed with an experienced researcher.

3. One can see evidence at the design phase of the study and in the proposal that these researchers anticipated the potential implications of researching a sensitive topic (witnessing resuscitation) and who might be affected (participants and researchers). They have thought of a number of strategies to prevent, and to cope with, the possible risks that this study poses.

---

the researchers. 'They can, potentially, put' pressure on, and exploit, participants to reveal information about themselves that is then outside the participants' control in terms of how it is used.

Vulnerability is a concept that has been used to refer to participants who are particularly susceptible or exposed to the risks of being harmed, exploited or simply made uncomfortable in research. The term 'vulnerable' population or participants has been used mainly to designate those groups that are particularly at risk of harm (e.g. through disclosure, discomfort, exploitation, etc.), due to their age and their conditions (illness, impairment, cognitive state, etc.). Hence children, older people and individuals with mental illness or learning disability are believed to be vulnerable in a research context. Classifying these groups as vulnerable can be seen as unnecessary stereotyping since not everyone in these groups will consider themselves as vulnerable or requiring 'special protection' when taking part in a study. According to Gordon (2020), 'a more accurate approach is to consider vulnerability as occurring along a spectrum of seriousness and as a consequence of situations and context' (p. 34).

Although the concept of vulnerability has been central to research ethics guidance, 'there is considerable disagreement in the scholarly literature about the meaning and delineation of vulnerability, stemming from a perceived lack of guidance within ethics standards' (Bracken-Roche et al., 2017, p. 1). Bracken-Roche et al. (2017), who reviewed the concept of vulnerability in research ethics policies and guidelines, found that the concept of vulnerability is vague and 'very few define it' (p. 15). Bracken-Roche et al. (2017) acknowledged that there was widespread agreement that some research participants may be particularly vulnerable and in need of special protection. They also found that the policies and guidelines they reviewed offer a 'richer and more complex' perspective of vulnerability to include 'sources of vulnerability that are both individual and situational' (p. 15). This means that age, for example, does not by itself make people vulnerable but the condition they may have (e.g. dementia), and what they are asked to do and in what circumstances, may make them vulnerable in a research context.

Designating groups of people as vulnerable can, in some circumstances, do more harm than good. Snipstad (2022), referring to people with intellectual disability, explained that they are 'not necessarily more vulnerable than others in all areas of life but, like everyone else, experience many social contexts that may or may not place them in vulnerable positions' (p. 107). He believes that 'the negative attitudes often related to the label intellectual disability and vulnerability affect the decisions and views of the researchers' (p. 107). The latter may exclude those labelled 'vulnerable' from research because of the perception that it may require more work. The exclusion of 'vulnerable' groups in studies evaluating the effectiveness of interventions, for example, means that the benefits or harm of those interventions will not be known for the excluded population. According to US Food and Drug Administration (2018), 'it is important to consider on a case-by-case basis whether such exclusions are truly necessary' (p. 2). Exclusion from research studies on grounds of vulnerability may itself be unethical. Over recent decades, ethical guidelines for research have been tightened to protect vulnerable groups and it would be ironic if this had the effect of such groups not being involved in research. The literature is rich on ethical issues for groups considered to be 'vulnerable'. Below are useful articles on this topic:

- Götzelmann et al. (2021), 'The full spectrum of ethical issues in dementia research: findings of a systematic qualitative review'.
- Low et al. (2017), 'A qualitative study protocol of ageing carers' caregiving experiences and their planning for continuation of care for their immediate family members with intellectual disability'.
- Chetty-Mhlanga et al. (2018), 'A prospective cohort study of school-going children investigating reproductive and neurobehavioral health effects due to environmental pesticide exposure in the Western Cape, South Africa: study protocol'.
- Choudhry and Ghosh (2020), 'Ethical considerations of mental health research amidst COVID-19 pandemic: mitigating the challenges'.
- Hilário and Augusto (2020), 'Practical and ethical dilemmas in researching sensitive topics with populations considered vulnerable'. Hilário and Augusto explain that this publication 'integrates several articles that explore a wide range of challenges and dilemmas relating to the development of social research and, particularly, to the vulnerability of the participants involved and the sensitivity of the topics covered' (p. xiii).

Seeking Access and Consent

At the design phase of a study, researchers should identify who the prospective participants are, how they can be accessed and who the gatekeepers are, and make contact with them. This process can be time-consuming. Therefore, it is best to make enquiries while the study is being designed. Obtaining assurances from the gatekeepers and reporting this in the proposal will show that the researcher has undertaken preliminary investigations.

Accessing patients' or clients' notes without their permission can be unethical, even if researchers intend to keep the patients or clients anonymous. Health and social care services and hospitals normally have their own policies (research governance) regarding who can access these notes. Where such policies do not exist, researchers should not access these notes without seeking permission from those responsible for protecting patients' and clients' data, and from the prospective participants themselves. The ESRC Framework for Research Ethics (ESRC, 2015) explained that census data and personal data provided for administrative and clinical purposes can be used for research, provided researchers abide by the legal and policy requirements in order to use such information. Data from a primary study can be used as secondary data for further research. The ESRC (2015) reminded us that even though the primary (original) study had obtained ethical approval, there might be ethical issues related to the reuse of data.

Once access to patients and clients is granted, researchers must seek informed consent from them. All research involves some degree of discomfort for the participants as they have to find time and effort to give information about themselves and others. There may be physical and mental discomfort depending on what they are required to do (e.g. give blood specimens or undergo psychometric testing). However, it is up to participants to decide whether they agree to take part in research studies. They require all the relevant information about the proposed study so that they can, of their own free will, make this decision. Informed consent has two interrelated components: information and consent.

There are two main aspects to giving information to prospective participants. The first relates to the content of the information and the second to their understanding of it. The key relevant information to be given to prospective participants is as follows:

- an explanation of the study, its aims, why it is necessary and what it is expected to achieve;
- the location and duration of the study;
- what is expected of participants (e.g. how many times they will be interviewed and for how long);
- how they were selected and why;
- who is organising, funding and sponsoring the research and who is leading it;
- the benefits of the study to participants and to others;
- the actual and potential risk and/or discomfort to participants;
- expenses and/or incentives;
- how the data will be kept confidential and how participants' anonymity will be safeguarded;
- how the findings of the study will be reported;
- how they are required to give consent (e.g. orally or by signing a consent form) – their consent is voluntary and they can withdraw consent at any time without having to give reasons;
- who they should contact if they have a complaint or need further information and clarification.

There are countless participant information sheets (PISs) online and it is advisable to consult existing PISs before developing new ones. However, the information sheet should fit the particular study being designed. For examples of guidance on how to develop a PIS see:

- University College London (n.d.), 'Guidance on completing a participant information sheet'.
- University of Oxford (2020), 'Informed consent: information and guidance for researchers'.

The second component of informed consent relates to the participants' decision on whether or not to take part. This decision relies on how the information is presented to them and how they understand it. Central to the concept of informed consent is the notion that their agreement or consent is of their own free will, free from any form of pressure. Any relationship between the researcher seeking consent and the participants should not in any way influence the participants' decision to take part in a study.

Putting pressure, overt or subtle, on people to participate in a study is unethical. Sometimes researchers are also be care providers. In such circumstances the two roles (researcher and care provider) should be separated. Measures should be put in place to avoid and deal with conflicts of interest. This may involve setting up a steering group or committee to ensure that patients or clients are protected, and that all professional guidance is followed.

Incentives (see also Chapter 11) may also put undue pressure on participants to take part in a study. Research ethics committees will look closely at this practice. For further discussion on the ethics of incentives, see:

- Halpern et al. (2021), 'Effectiveness and ethics of incentives for research participation. 2: Randomized clinical trials'.
- Zutlevics (2016), 'Could providing financial incentives to research participants be ultimately self-defeating?'
- Manríquez Roa and Biller-Andorno (2022), 'Financial incentives for participants in health research; when are they ethical?'

Giving information about a research study to lay people can be challenging. Research terms such as 'placebo', 'randomised', 'control groups' or 'ethnographic' can mean little to non-researchers. Lay people's comprehension may differ according to their cognitive levels. Therefore, information, both written and verbal, should be presented at the reading level of the prospective participants. Giving time for them to read, digest and talk with family members or carers, before deciding on participation, is crucial. Researchers should not rush prospective participants in making decisions. Providing opportunities for explanation and discussion is crucial to obtaining informed consent.

Some groups such as children, people with an intellectual disability and individuals with dementia require particular effort on the part of researchers in terms of how best the information can be conveyed. This may require using formats such as drawings and video clips. For further information on this topic, see:

- Santovito et al. (2021), 'To draw or not to draw: informed consent dilemma'.
- Fanaroff et al. (2018), 'An observational study of the association of video- versus text-based informed consent with multicenter trial enrollment'.

Guidelines and tips for making scientific, medical or research information comprehensible to lay people are available on the internet (especially on universities' websites). For example, Johns Hopkins University has a page on how to prepare readable consent forms for different populations (Johns Hopkins University, n.d.). The tips include: keep words to three syllables or fewer, write short and direct sentences, keep paragraphs short and limited to one idea, use active verbs, etc. The European Commission (European Commission, n.d.) has recommended that 'information for children five years and under should be predominantly pictorial' (p. 4). The latter's guidance also stated that informed consent is required when research involves patients, children, incapacitated persons, healthy volunteers, immigrants and some other groups (e.g. prisoners).

A number of tools have been used to validate reading levels of informed consent forms. These include the Flesch Reading Ease, the Flesch Kincaid Grade level, the Clear Communication Index and the Suitability Assessment of Materials. For a review of these and other tools, see O'Sullivan et al. (2020). See also:

- Foe and Larson (2016), 'Reading level and comprehension of research consent forms: an integrative review'.
- Hadden et al. (2017), 'Improving readability of informed consents for research at an academic medical institution'.

The World Health Organization (WHO, 2022), pointed out that 'children are an exceptional population with specific ethical clinical concerns' and that the 'vulnerable nature of this population must be considered when balancing the risks of research with the need for safe and validated therapies'. Parents or guardians should be fully informed of the nature of the study and its risks and benefits. They may be required by law to give consent when the children are minors, and the latter may also have to give their assent after hearing the study explained to them (WHO, 2022). The National Society for the Prevention of Cruelty to Children (NSPCC, 2020) has provided information about what researchers need to consider when conducting research with children. The information includes how to manage the risk of harm to participants, how to obtain informed consent, and what to do if researchers are concerned that a child is experiencing or at risk of abuse (NSPCC, 2020).

The Mental Capacity Act 2005 (Health Research Authority, 2021) in the UK, 'provides a comprehensive framework for decision making on behalf of adults aged 16 and over who are unable to make decisions for themselves'. These decisions include those of people taking part in research. The core principles of the Mental Capacity Act 2005 can guide researchers when seeking consent from those unable to decide for themselves. These principles (Health Research Authority, 2021) are as follows:

- *a person must be assumed to have capacity unless established otherwise*
- *individuals should be helped to make their own decisions as far as practicable*
- *a person is not to be treated as unable to make a decision merely because he makes an unwise decision*
- *all decisions and actions must be in the best interests of the person lacking capacity*
- *all decisions and actions must be the least restrictive of the person's rights and freedom of action.*

Researchers are advised to abide by the legal human rights legislation in their own countries. However, the principles mentioned above have universal application.

People with a learning disability sometimes lack the capacity to consent to participation in research. This is one reason why they are occasionally excluded from research that could provide the much-needed evidence to improve their lives. A number of researchers have explained the challenges of recruiting people with learning disability in their studies and the strategies they have used. Goldsmith and Skirton (2015) discussed the methodological challenges and ethical issues involved in the recruitment of people with a learning disability to their study 'exploring the information needs of people with learning disabilities with respect to consent for genomic tests' (p. 435). Ho et al. (2018) reflected on the challenges in gaining consent from people with intellectual disability for their study investigating falls in this population. For an excellent example of a completed PIS, in a study on 'improving hearing services for people with learning disabilities', see The University of Manchester (2021).

Researchers recruiting people with dementia into their studies also face issues similar to those described above. As Thorogood et al. (2018) explained, 'researchers seeking consent from persons with dementia confront ethical and legal uncertainty, such as when and how to assess capacity to consent' (p. 1335). According to them, decision making can be helped by making forms simpler and by using visual or memory aids in an interactive process that allows discussion, clarification and explanation. In their proposal for a study on 'Reminiscence groups for people with dementia and their family carers', Woods et al. (2009, p. 5) described the 'risks and benefits for trial participants' and the 'arrangements' they would put in place to address the issues that might arise. They also explained in detail how informed consent would be sought, including the involvement of 'a family member or other supporter' in the consent process. For further information on this topic, see Chandra et al.'s (2021) review of ethical issues in dementia.

The three groups mentioned above (children, people with intellectual disability and individuals with dementia) were chosen as examples of challenges that researchers may face when they consider the ethical implications at the design stage and during their study. These groups are, however, by no means the only ones that require careful ethical considerations. There is a large volume of literature dealing with the issue of obtaining informed consent from a range of population groups. You are not alone as long as you can access this literature.

ETHICAL ISSUES RELATED TO DESIGNS AND METHODS

All research designs and data collection methods have ethical implications. However, each has its own implications that researchers should be aware of. Whereas issues such as informed consent and confidentiality apply to all research, there are other issues that are pertinent to particular research designs.

Intervention studies involve doing something to participants, while surveys only require participants to respond orally or in writing to questions that they may choose to answer. While both trials and surveys have ethical implications, the former can have a direct effect on participants' health and behaviour. Trials also tend to involve several collaborators such as clinicians, data collectors and others, thereby creating a context that may give rise to its own particular ethical issues. For a more detailed discussion of issues in randomised controlled trials, see Colli et al. (2014). Other useful references include:

- Grote (2022), 'Randomised controlled trials in medical AI: ethical considerations'.
- Nix and Weijer (2021), 'Uses of equipoise in discussions of the ethics of randomized controlled trials of COVID-19 therapies'.
- Gewandter et al. (2015), 'Research design considerations for chronic pain prevention clinical trials: IMMPACT recommendations'.

Other designs such as ethnography and those involving longitudinal data collection have specific ethical issues. Longitudinal studies can raise issues such as building relationships and trust and re-obtaining informed consent at each phase of the project. Ethnographic studies may require researchers to get immersed in the lives and practices of participants, in the latter's own settings. This may present researchers with dilemmas that they may not have foreseen. In an ethnographic study into how people with dementia in care settings manage 'personal appearance' (the Hair and Care project), Ward et al. (2016) used a mix of qualitative methods including observation and filming as well as in situ interviewing aimed at exploring what goes on in a care-based hairdressing salon. In such circumstances, ethical dilemmas can arise at any time during the study and researchers should be prepared to address ongoing and unexpected issues.

Methods of data collection such as qualitative interviews, observations (qualitative and quantitative) and online interviews have some ethical implications that are specific to these methods. For example, the nature and process of qualitative interviews are such that there is no anonymity, because the interviewer knows who the interviewee is, but how the researchers deal with confidentiality can be challenging. Managing and reporting intimate disclosure can be difficult. The interview is often stressful for the researcher and the interviewee. Researchers intending to use such data collection methods should be aware that this can happen and have a plan to deal with it.

When interviewing young men who were potentially suicidal, Jordan et al. (2012) predicted that the questions asked might trigger a depressive reaction in respondents. To deal with this, the researchers arranged for interviewers to have mental health nursing backgrounds and for support, including counselling sessions, to be available after the interviews for participants. Similarly, Braden et al. (2010) surveyed heroin users and were faced with the fact that they were interviewing individuals who were involved in an illegal activity. This raised issues of informed consent and access and distress, which were addressed by interviewer training and pre-interview agreements between respondents and researchers.

The literature on the issue of distress in interviews can provide some guidance to what can be done. For example, Haigh and Witham (2015) have developed a 'distress protocol for qualitative data collection' that gives examples of the types of distress that may occur and what responses the interviewer can offer. Wright et al. (2020), in their proposal for a grounded theory study of 'mental health recovery for survivors of modern slavery', explained that 'distress protocols' would be put in place to 'protect the research participants, the researcher undertaking the interviews, interpreters and transcribers'. They explained further that:

The researcher will receive relevant training to ensure that they have the skills required. They will also receive monthly clinical supervision to assist with the processing of any difficult material or interviews. Participants will be made aware that if they make disclosures which indicate they are at risk this may need to be escalated to the appropriate authorities. Signposting materials to support organisations will also be available to participants should these be required.

(p. 3)

Observations can pose particular dilemmas for researchers. For example, researchers may not know how to handle situations such as witnessing accidents, abuse or neglect when observing in clinical or other similar settings. The issue of consent can also be magnified, as researchers sometimes have no control over who enters the observation sites. For example, while observing interactions between patients and clinicians, other health professionals or even relatives may walk in. There are also other issues related to covert observations, including the privacy of the individuals being observed, recording (including video recording) of what is taking place as well as reporting of the findings. For more information on this topic, see:

- Johnson et al. (2011), 'The challenges and benefits of using participant observation to understand the social interaction of adults with intellectual disabilities'.
- Parry et al. (2016), 'Acceptability and design of video-based research on healthcare communication: evidence and recommendations'.
- Podschuweit (2021), 'How ethical challenges of covert observations can be met in practice.'
- Watts (2011), 'Ethical and practical challenges of participant observation in sensitive health research'.

With the increase in online research, we need to be aware of the particular legal and ethical implications of this new approach. Online research usually involves the use of questionnaires, interviews or focus groups. There are also a lot of data already available on the web for researchers to retrieve and analyse. Researchers need to rethink how informed consent, anonymity and confidentiality and other ethical issues in online research can be handled sensitively, ethically and legally. There is a growing body of literature on the topic. For more information, see:

- Sipes et al. (2020), 'Ethical considerations when using online research methods to study sensitive topics'.
- Sugiura et al. (2017), 'Ethical challenges in online research: public/private perceptions'.
- British Psychological Society (2021), 'Ethics guidelines for internet-mediated research'.
- Norwegian National Research Ethics Committees (2019), 'A guide to internet research ethics'.
- Ford et al. (2021), 'Toward an ethical framework for the text mining of social media for health research: a systematic review'.
- Cilliers and Viljoen (2021), 'A framework of ethical issues to consider when conducting internet-based research'.

For an example of how ethical issues are reported in a research proposal involving an online survey, see Gaikwad et al. (2016). The University of Edinburgh (2020) provided a resource for its staff and students to consider and deal with potential ethical issues that may arise when undertaking online interviews. This document adds to the growing literature on the topic of online research.

The examples given above are to show that there are specific ethical issues that are related to research design and methods. It is beyond the scope of this book to detail the specific ethical and legal issues related to each one of them.

RESEARCHER-RELATED ETHICAL ISSUES

Research has the potential to harm researchers as well as participants. This can happen during data collection or afterwards when the data are analysed and reported. Qualitative research, in particular, can present risks in a number of forms to researchers. Stahlke (2018), drawing from her experience in conducting research on 'nursing work', listed the unexpected ethical challenges that she faced. These included 'hearing and responding to disagreeable participant statements, listening to distressing stories, managing the high expectations of research participants in terms of purpose and outcomes of the research', and facing 'potential professional marginalisation because of the political nature' of the research (Stahlke, 2018, p. 1). The UK Social Research Association (2022), in its 'Code of practice for the safety of social researchers', listed five different types of risks that 'social researchers may face when involved in close social interaction':

- *risk of physical threat or abuse*
- *risk of psychological trauma, as a result of actual or threatened violence or the nature of what is disclosed during the interaction*
- *risk of being in a comprising situation, in which there might be accusations of improper behaviour*
- *increased exposure to risks of everyday life and social interaction, such as road accidents and infectious illness*
- *risk of causing psychological or physical harm to others.*

(p. 1)

The document explains how researcher safety can be built into the design of proposals and provides a checklist of questions to ask when 'assessing risk in the fieldwork site'. The list includes, among others, an 'assessment of local tensions to be aware of', 'meeting local community leaders to explain the research and gain their endorsement' and 'awareness of transport to get to and return from the research site'. Most universities' websites offer guidance for lone researchers.

Sensitive topics and/or researching vulnerable populations can potentially cause distress to researchers. According to Fenge et al. (2019, p. 1), such research 'can expose researchers to emotionally disturbing situations throughout data collection and analysis, which can be emotionally challenging'. For useful information on how research can have a negative impact on researchers and strategies to use in order to avoid or minimise it, see:

- Fenge et al. (2019), 'The impact of sensitive research on the researcher: preparedness and positionality'.
- Mallon and Elliott (2019), 'The emotional risks of turning stories into data: an exploration of the experiences of qualitative researchers working on sensitive topics'.

Finally, while all potential legal and ethical issues should be considered at the design stage of the study, there is no obligation to report this in great detail in the proposal. Only report what is relevant and pertinent to the proposed study. As a rule of thumb, think about the questions that members of a research ethics committee may ask and issues related to your study that they may be concerned about.

It may also be relevant to include any information that may give ethics committee review panel members the assurance that you and your team have the necessary experience and training to carry out the proposed study in an ethical manner. In their proposal for a study to develop 'an intervention to support the reproductive health of Cambodian women who seek medical abortion', Oreglia et al. (2020) highlighted the expertise and training of researchers in the team with regards to the ethical conduct of the study:

> *Ethical considerations, including informed consent procedures, measures to protect confidentiality, and potential risks and benefits to participants, are considered by participant type, as follows. For all participants, the PIs [principal investigators] will be responsible for the overall informed consent procedures for the project. CS undertook the Introduction to Good Clinical Practice course in May 2012 and has experience in recruiting women seeking abortion services for the Mobile Technology for Improved Family Planning study in Cambodia. EO has experience in undertaking ethnographic research with garment factory workers in China and completed the Ethics in Social and Behavioral Sciences course at SOAS in January 2016.*

(p. 6)

Checklist for items to include in proposals regarding ethical issues:
1. Is the research topic sensitive? What are the ethical issues and how will they be addressed?
2. Is the population for the study considered to be vulnerable? What issues may arise and how will they be addressed?
3. Are there specific ethical issues relating to the setting (e.g. clinical area, prison, nursing home, etc.)? What are the issues and how will they be addressed?
4. Are there specific design-related ethical issues? What are they and how will they be addressed?
5. How will informed consent be sought? Does the informed consent form contain all the relevant information?
6. Are incentives to be offered for participation? Are these incentives likely to influence the decision to participate?
7. Is data collection likely to cause distress? What strategies will be used to prevent or minimise distress?
8. Are there any risks to researchers? What are these risks and how will they be addressed?

SUMMARY AND CONCLUSIONS

In this chapter, the ethical issues that researchers need to consider when designing a study have been highlighted. These issues are mostly related to four aspects of a study: topic, population, methodology and researchers. Using this framework can help researchers to think about the actual and potential ethical and sensitive issues that they may face before, during and after the study. Throughout this chapter, examples of how other researchers have completed the section on ethical issues in their study proposals have been given. A checklist of potential items to include in proposals has also been provided.

REFERENCES

Bracken-Roche, D., Bell, E., Macdonald, M. E., & Racine, E. (2017). The concept of 'vulnerability' in research ethics: An in-depth analysis of policies and guidelines. *Health Research Policy and Systems*, *15*(1), 8. https://doi.org/10.1186/s12961-016-0164-6

Braden, M., McGowan, I. W., McLaughlin, D. F., McKenna, H. P., Keeney, S. R., & Quinn, B. (2010). Users, carers and professionals experiences of treatment and care for heroin dependency: Implications for practice. A preliminary study. *Journal of Substance Use*, *16*(6), 452–463.

British Psychological Society. (2021). *Ethics guidelines internet-mediated research*. https://www.bps.org.uk/guideline/ethics-guidelines-internet-mediated-research. Retrieved on 31/01/2024.

Buchanan, D. A., Denyer, D., Jaina, J., Kelliher, C., Moore, C., Parry, E., & Pilbeam, C. (2013). How do they manage? A qualitative study of the realities of middle and front-line management work in health care. *Health Services and Delivery Research*, *1*(4). https://www.ncbi.nlm.nih.gov/books/NBK259397/pdf/Bookshelf_NBK259397.pdf

Chandra, M., Harbishettar, V., Sawhney, H., & Amanullah, S. (2021). Ethical issues in dementia research. *Indian Journal of Psychological Medicine*, *43*(5_suppl), S25–S30.

Chetty-Mhlanga, S., Basera, W., Fuhrimann, S., Probst-Hensch, N., Delport, S., Mugari, M., Van Wyk, J., Röösli, M., & Dalvie, M. A. (2018). A prospective cohort study of school-going children investigating reproductive and neurobehavioral health effects due to environmental pesticide exposure in the Western Cape, South Africa: Study protocol. *BMC Public Health*, *218*(1), 857. https://doi.org/10.1186/s12889-018-5783-0

Choudhury, S., Ghosh, A. (2020). Ethical considerations of mental health research amidst COVID-19 pandemic: Mitigating the challenges. *Indian Journal of Psychological Medicine*, *42*(4), 379–381.

Cilliers, L., & Viljoen, K. (2021). A framework of ethical issues to consider when conducting internet-based research. *South African Journal of Information Management*, *23*(1), 1–9.

Colli, A., Pagliaro, L., & Duca, P. (2014). The ethical problem of randomization. *Internal and Emergency Medicine*, *9*, 799–804.

Dickson-Swift, V., James, E., & Liamputtong, P. (2008). *Undertaking sensitive research in the health and social sciences: Managing boundaries, emotions and risks*. Cambridge: Cambridge University Press. http://assets.cambridge.org/97805217/18233/excerpt/9780521718233_excerpt.pdf

Ellsberg, M., & Heise, L. (2005). *Researching violence against women: A practical guide for researchers and activists*. Washington DC, United States: World Health Organization, PATH.

ESRC. (2015). *Framework for research ethics*. Updated January. https://esrc.ukri.org/files/funding/guidance-for-applicants/esrc-framework-for-research-ethics-2015/

ESRC. (2022). *Framework for research ethics*. https://www.ukri.org/councils/esrc/guidance-for applicants/research-ethics-guidance/framework-for-research-ethics/our-core-principles/#contents-list

European Commission. (n.d.). *Guidance for APPLICATIONS for obtaining informed consent*. https://ec.europa.eu/research/participants/data/ref/fp7/89807/informed-consent_en.pdf

Fahie, D. (2014). Doing sensitive research sensitively: Ethical and methodological issues in researching workplace bullying. *International Journal of Qualitative Methods*, *13*(1), 19–36.

Fanaroff, A. C., Li, S., Webb, L. E., Miller, V., Navar, A. M., Peterson, E. D., & Wang, T. Y. (2018). An observational study of the association of video- versus text-based informed consent with multicenter trial enrollment. *Circulation: Cardiovascular Quality and Outcomes*, *11*, e004675.

Fenge, L. A., Oakley, L., Taylor, B., & Beer, S. (2019). The impact of sensitive research on the researcher: Preparedness and positionality. *International Journal of Qualitative Methods*, *18*, 1–8.

Fiori, M., Endacott, R., & Latour, J. M. (2019). Exploring patients' and healthcare professionals' experiences of patient witnessed resuscitation: A qualitative study protocol. *Journal of Advanced Nursing*, *75*, 205–214.

Foe, G., & Larson, E. L. (2016). Reading level and comprehension of research consent forms: An integrative review. *Journal of Empirical Research on Human Research Ethics: An International Journal, 11*(1), 31–46. https://www.jstor.org/stable/90012114

Food and Drug Administration. (2018). *Public workshop: Evaluating inclusion and exclusion criteria in clinical trials*. https://www.fda.gov/media/134754/download

Ford, E., Shepherd, S., Jones, K., & Hassan, L. (2021). Toward an ethical framework for the text mining of social media for health research: A systematic review. *Frontiers in Digital Health, 2*, 592237. https://doi.org/10.3389/fdgth.2020.592237

Gaikwad, M., Vanlint, S., Moseley, G. L., Mittinty, M. N., & Stocks, N. (2016). Understanding patient perspectives on management of their chronic pain - online survey protocol. *Journal of Pain Research, 10*, 31–35.

Gewandter, J. S., Dworkin, R. H., Turk, D. C., Farrar, J. T., Fillingim, R. B., Gilron, I., Markman, J. D., Oaklander, A. L., Polydefkis, M. J., Raja, S. N., Robinson, J. P., Woolf, C. J., Ziegler, D., Ashburn, M. A., Burke, L. B., Cowan, P., George, S. Z., Goli, V., Graff, O. X., ... Walco, G. A. (2015). Research design considerations for chronic pain prevention clinical trials: IMMPACT recommendations. *Pain, 156*(7), 1184–1197.

Goldsmith, L., & Skirton, H. (2015). Research involving people with a learning disability – methodological challenges and ethical considerations. *Journal of Research in Nursing, 20*(6), 435–446.

Gordon, B. G. (2020). Vulnerability in research: basic ethical concepts and general approach to review. *Ochsner Journal, 20*(1), 34–38.

Götzelmann, T. G., Strech, D., & Kahrass, H. (2021). The full spectrum of ethical issues in dementia research: Findings of a systematic qualitative review. *BMC Medical Ethics, 22*, 32. https://doi.org/10.1186/s12910-020-00572-5

Grote, T. (2022). Randomised controlled trials in medical AI: Ethical considerations. *Journal of Medical Ethics, 48*(11), 899–906.

Hadden, K. B., Prince, L. Y., Moore, T. D., James, L. P., Holland, J. R., & Trudeau, C. R. (2017). Improving readability of informed consents for research at an academic medical institution. *Journal of Clinical and Translational Science, 1*(6), 361–365. https://doi.org/10.1017/cts.2017.312

Haigh, C., & Witham, G. (2015). *Distress protocol for qualitative data collection*. https://www.mmu.ac.uk/media/mmuacuk/content/documents/rke/Advisory-Distress-Protocol.pdf

Halpern, S. D., Chowdhury, M., Bayes, B., Cooney, E., Hitsman, B. L., Schnoll, R. A., Lubitz, S. F., Reyes, C., Patel, M. S., Greysen, S. R., Mercede, A., Reale, C., Barg, F. K., Volpp, K. G., Karlawish, J., & Stephens-Shields, A. J. (2021). Effectiveness and ethics of incentives for research participation. 2: Randomized clinical trials. *JAMA Internal Medicine, 181*(11), 1479–1488.

Health Research Authority. (2021). *Mental Capacity Act*. https://www.hra.nhs.uk/planning-and-improving-research/policies-standards-legislation/mental-capacity-act/

Hilário, A. P., & Augusto, F. R. (2020). *Practical and ethical dilemmas in researching sensitive topics with populations considered vulnerable*. MDPI - Multidisciplinary Digital Publishing Institute. https://www.mdpi.com/books/book/3052-practical-and-ethical-dilemmas-in-researching-sensitive-topics-with-populations-considered

Ho, P., Downs, J., Bulsara, C., Patman, S., & Hill, A. M. (2018). Addressing challenges in gaining informed consent for a research study investigating falls in people with intellectual disability. *British Journal of Learning Disabilities, 46*, 92–100.

Johns Hopkins University. (n.d.). *Consent forms*. https://publichealth.jhu.edu/offices-and-services/institutional-review-board-irb/forms/consent-forms

Johnson, H., Douglas, J., Bigby, C., & Iacono, T. (2011). The challenges and benefits of using participant observation to understand the social interaction of adults with intellectual disabilities. *Augmentative and Alternative Communication, 27*(4), 267–278.

Jordan, J., McKenna, H., Keeney, S., Cutcliffe, J., Stevenson, C., Slater, P., & McGowan, I. (2012). Providing meaningful care: Learning from the experiences of suicidal young men. *Qualitative Health Research, 22*(9), 1207–1219.

Lee, R. M. (1993). *Doing research on sensitive topics*. Sage Publications, Inc.

Low, L. P., Chien, W. T., Lam, L. W., & Wong K. K. (2017). A qualitative study protocol of ageing carers' caregiving experiences and their planning for continuation of care for their immediate family members with intellectual disability. *BMC Geriatrics, 17*, 81. https://doi.org/10.1186/s12877-017-0473-9

Mallon, S., & Elliott, I. (2019). The emotional risks of turning stories into data: An exploration of the experiences of qualitative researchers working on sensitive topics. *Societies, 9*(3), 62. https://doi.org/10.3390/soc9030062

Manríquez Roa, T., & Biller-Andorno, N. (2022). Financial incentives for participants in health research: When are they ethical? *Swiss Medical Weekly, 152*, w30166. https://doi.org/10.4414/smw.2022.w30166

Nix, H. P., & Weijer, C. (2021). Uses of equipoise in discussions of the ethics of randomized controlled trials of COVID-19 therapies. *BMC Medical Ethics, 22*, 143.

Norwegian National Research Ethics Committees. (2019). *A guide to internet research ethics.* https://www.forskningsetikk.no/en/guidelines/social-sciences-humanities-law-and-theology/a-guide-to-internet-research-ethics/

NSPCC. (2020). *Research with children: Ethics, safety and avoiding harm.* https://learning.nspcc.org.uk/research-resources/briefings/research-with-children-ethics-safety-avoiding-harm

Oreglia, E., Ly, S., Tijamo, C., Ou, A., Free, C., & Smith, C. (2020). Development of an intervention to support the reproductive health of Cambodian women who seek medical abortion: Research protocol. *JMIR Research Protocols, 9*(7), e17779. https://doi.org/10.2196/17779

O'Sullivan, L., Sukumar, P., Crowley, R., McAuliffe, E., & Doran, P. (2020). Readability and understandability of clinical research patient information leaflets and consent forms in Ireland and the UK: A retrospective quantitative analysis. *BMJ Open, 10*, e037994. https://doi.org/10.1136/bmjopen-2020-037994

Parry, R., Pino, M., Faull, C., & Feathers, L. (2016). Acceptability and design of video-based research on healthcare communication: Evidence and recommendations. *Patient Education and Counseling, 99*(8), 1271–1284.

Podschuweit, N. (2021). How ethical challenges of covert observations can be met in practice. *Research Ethics, 17*(3), 309–327.

Rodriguez, L. (2018). Methodological challenges of sensitive topic research with adolescents. *Qualitative Research Journal, 18*(1), 22–32.

Santovito, D., Cena, G., Tattoli, L., Di Vella, G., & Bosco, C. (2021). To draw or not to draw: Informed consent dilemma. *Health Primary Care, 5*, 1–6. https://doi.org/10.15761/HPC.1000211

Sipes, J. B., Mullan, B., & Roberts, L. D. (2020). Ethical considerations when using online research methods to study sensitive topics. *Translational Issues in Psychological Science, 6*(3), 235–239.

Snipstad, Ø. I. M. (2022). Concerns regarding the use of the vulnerability concept in research on people with intellectual disability. *British Journal of Learning Disabilities, 50*(1), 107–114.

Social Research Association. (2022). *A code of practice for the safety of social researchers.* https://the-sra.org.uk/common/Uploaded%20files/SRA-safety-code-of-practice.pdf

Stahlke, S. (2018). Expanding on notions of ethical risks to qualitative researchers. *International Journal of Qualitative Methods, 17*, 1–9.

Sugiura, L., Wiles, R., & Pope, C. (2017). Ethical challenges in online research: Public/private perceptions. *Research Ethics, 13*(3-4), 184–199.

The University of Manchester. (2021). *Improving hearing services for people with learning disabilities.* https://documents.manchester.ac.uk/display.aspx?DocID557000. Retrieved on 30/01/2024.

Thorogood, A., Mäki-Petäjä-Leinonen, A., Brodaty, H., Dalpé, G., Gastmans, C., Gauthier, S., Gove, D., Harding, R., Knoppers, B. M., Rossor, M., Bobrow, M., & Global Alliance for Genomics and Health, Ageing and Dementia Task Team. (2018). Consent recommendations for research and international data sharing involving persons with dementia. *Alzheimer's & Dementia: the journal of the Alzheimer's Association, 14*(10), 1334–1343.

University College London. (n.d.). *Guidance on completing a participant information sheet.* https://ethics.grad.ucl.ac.uk/forms/model-participant-information-sheet-and-guidance.pdf

University of Edinburgh. (2020). *Some ethical considerations when rethinking research projects in light of COVID-19 situation.* https://www.ed.ac.uk/files/atoms/files/rethinking_research_projects_in_light_of_covid-19_situation_ethical_considerations_final_version_4.pdf

University of Oxford. (2020). *Informed consent: information and guidance for researchers.* https://researchsupport.admin.ox.ac.uk/ctrg/conduct/consent

US Department of Health and Human Services. (1978). *Ethical principles and guidelines for the protection of human subjects of research (Belmont Report).* Bethesda, MD: The Commission.

Varkey, B. (2021). Principles of clinical ethics and their application to practice. *Medical Principles and Practice, 30,* 17–28.

Ward, R., Campbell, S., & Keady, J. (2016). Assembling the salon: Learning from alternative forms of body work in dementia care. *Sociology of Health & Illness, 38*(8), 1287–1302.

Watts, J. H. (2011). Ethical and practical challenges of participant observation in sensitive health research. *International Journal of Social Research Methodology, 14*(4), 301–312.

WHO. (2022). *Clinical trials in children.* https://www.who.int/clinical-trials-registry-platform/clinical-trials-in-children

Woods, R. T., Bruce, E., Edwards, R. T., Hounsome, B., Keady, J., Moniz-Cook, E. D., Orrell, M., & Russell, I. T. (2009). Reminiscence groups for people with dementia and their family carers: Pragmatic eight-centre randomised trial of joint reminiscence and maintenance versus usual treatment: A protocol. *Trials, 10,* 64. https://doi.org/10.1186/1745-6215-10-64

Wright, N., Hadziosmanovic, E., Dang, M., Bales, K., Brookes, C., Jordan, M., Slade, M., & Lived Experience Research Advisory Board. (2020). Mental health recovery for survivors of modern slavery: Grounded theory study protocol. *BMJ Open, 10*(11), e038583. https://doi.org/10.1136/bmjopen-2020-038583

Zutlevics, T. (2016). Could providing financial incentives to research participants be ultimately self-defeating? *Research Ethics, 12*(3), 137–148.

14

RESEARCH IMPACT IN PROPOSALS

INTRODUCTION

The focus on research impact has been growing in the last two decades. Researchers are expected to demonstrate in their proposals the impact their study can potentially make to the economy and to the wellbeing of people in society. In this chapter, we will look briefly at the background to this increasing interest in research impact, what researchers can do at the design stage of their study regarding impact and the information they should include in their research proposals.

BRIEF BACKGROUND TO THE RISE OF 'RESEARCH IMPACT'

Although there is no need to revisit the arguments in the centuries-old debate over 'basic' versus 'applied' research, we need to look at differences between these two terms to understand the current focus on research impact. Basic research (also known as fundamental, blue-sky or curiosity-driven research) aims to increase our understanding of phenomena around us. It can change the way we understand our world. Hence Newton's discovery of the laws of gravity led to a number of applications such as how to make planes fly without falling to the ground. The problem with basic research is that it may take years before the benefits are realised. Research such as the discovery of the structure of DNA is ground breaking and has great significance as it changes the way we think about phenomena. Scientific progress depends on basic research.

Applied research, as the term suggests, is aimed at finding solutions to current practice or policy problems. For example, applied research is conducted to develop and test an intervention to empower people to exercise more. Evaluation and action research are forms of applied research because they aim to provide research data to make changes to existing services or policies, where appropriate. Research in nursing, health and social care is mostly applied research. While basic research can still be undertaken, there are issues and problems in nursing, health and social care that cannot wait.

Another reason for focusing on research impact is that those who fund research projects (governments, charities, foundations etc.) want to see the benefits of their investment. Research funders have their own local, national and international priorities that they believe should be addressed. To drive their own agenda, funders have become more prescriptive (or targeted) both in the topics or questions that they want researchers to study, as well as the information they require (regarding impact) that researchers should provide in research proposals. For example, in the UK the Warry Report (Department for Business Education and Skills, 2006) addressed the leadership role of UK Research Councils in the knowledge transfer agenda, their role in influencing the knowledge transfer behaviour of UK universities and their engagement with user organisations. Following the Warry Report, researchers were expected to include an impact plan within all grant applications from 2009 onwards (Morton, 2012). Another response to the report was the introduction of 'impact' as one of three components in 2014 and 2021 UK Research Excellence Frameworks (periodic assessments of research quality, impact and research environment in UK universities).

Every country wants to be economically competitive, and they expect their investment in research to make an impact on the economy and society. The UK government is by no means the only one to implement a research impact agenda. For example, the Hong Kong University Grants Committee (2022) has set up a Research Impact Fund to encourage local academics to maximise the impact potential of their research and to encourage more research in collaboration with government departments, the business sector, industries and research institutes. Ireland has recently published its Research and Innovation Strategy: Impact 2030 (Government of Ireland, 2022). Proposals to the US National Institutes of Health are given 'impact/priority' scores to determine which projects are to be funded.

The Australian Research Council (2022) has developed its Research Impact Principles and Framework and expects researchers applying for funding to use a Research Impact Pathway Table to demonstrate both the expected outcomes and benefits over time, in the impact statement. This document sums up succinctly the aim of the research impact agenda in countries around the world:

> There is an increasing focus on showcasing or measuring the societal benefits from research, and a need for better coordination in reporting and promoting the impact of these research outcomes. This will become increasingly important in a tight fiscal government environment where returns on investment in research will need to be demonstrated in terms of environmental, economic and social impact. For these reasons and others, key stakeholders including government, industry and the community require more information on the benefits derived from investment in Australian research activities.

(p. 1)

WHAT IS RESEARCH IMPACT?

There are many definitions of research impact. For example, the Economic and Social Research Council (ESRC, 2022) defines impact as the 'demonstrable contribution that excellent research makes to society and economy' (p. 1). It includes academic, economic and societal impact. According to the ESRC (2022) impact can be 'instrumental', 'conceptual' or 'capacity building'.

It seems that the ESRC definition refers to the impact of both basic and applied research. Impact, for the purpose of the UK Research Excellence Frameworks is defined as an 'effect on, change or benefit to the economy, society, culture, public policy or services, health, the environment or quality of life, beyond academia' (UK Research and Innovation [UKRI], 2022, p. 1). Reed et al. (2021) explain that impact can be subjective and that it may be difficult to show causal relationships between 'research' and 'impact'. They define research impact as 'demonstrable and/or perceptible benefits to individuals, groups, organisations and society (including human and non-human entities in the present and future) that are causally linked (necessarily or sufficiently) to research' (Reed et al., 2021, p. 3).

The ESRC (2021) fully recognises 'the non-linear, emergent and diffuse nature of the research' that they fund and the effects it has, and understands that 'impact cannot be predicted or guaranteed' (p. 1). For example, no matter how much impact we think our newly developed intervention can make, that impact will not be realised if the randomised controlled trial shows that it is not as effective as we predicted. Of course, the study should be published even if the results are negative as there is much to be learnt from such an experience.

There is a significant body of literature to show that research utilisation or knowledge transfer in policy and practice is not as straightforward as one thinks. There are also a number of models and frameworks that have been developed to facilitate research utilisation (see the examples from Bailey and Mouton, 2005; Kim et al., 2018; Konwar, 2018; Cordier, 2021). It would be fair to say that researchers normally have control over their research studies while practitioners have control over their practice. For research impact to be achieved both researchers and users should work together. As Morton (2012) explains, 'research impact cannot be achieved from the research production side alone'. She added that 'the ways in which research is taken up and used, discussed, shared and applied in different policy, practice and wider settings is complex' (p. 33). According to Morton (2012), users in the different roles should play an active part if research is to be implemented. Researchers have the responsibility to identify key professionals who are in a position to authorise change. They should discuss, in advance of the study, how change (if appropriate), will be facilitated. The ESRC (2021) also recognises that 'doing effective knowledge exchange with non-academic communities takes time, skills, confidence and money' (p. 1).

The measurement and evaluation of impact can also be complex and problematic. Williams and Lewis (2021) point out that 'existing research evaluation practices include an assortment of concepts and methods that largely fail to capture the breadth of impact' (p. 556). They go on to say that 'much discussion of research impact lacks an understanding of the engagement necessary to generate impact, rests on naïve notions of what the measurement can actually reveal, and is ignorant of the different pathways through which research contributes to society' (p. 556). Reed et al. (2021) conducted an analysis of research evaluation frameworks drawn from cross-disciplinary peer-reviewed and grey literature. They developed a 'methodological framework for evaluating research impact' that researchers, funders, and other stakeholders from a range of disciplines can use 'to design more effective evaluations to evidence the impact of research' (p. 12).

Researchers should make every effort to facilitate the utilisation of their research. Whether their study is funded or unfunded, at the very least they have the moral responsibility to share their acquired knowledge with other researchers and those for whom the research has relevance and potential benefit. Before the introduction of 'impact pathways' in proposals, the publication of findings and other research-related aspects of studies were too often left at the discretion of researchers. It was not uncommon to find that many research projects, although completed, were never published.

From 2006 onwards, the UKRI expected researchers applying for funding from UK Research Councils to complete two sections related to impact in their proposal: 'Pathways to impact' and 'Impact summary'. However, from April 2020, researchers were no longer required to do so. Instead, the overall approach 'is that impact has now become centrally embedded into the application and assessment process' (Livingstone-Banks, 2020, p. 1). According to the UKRI, impact is still important and needs to be addressed throughout the proposal.

Livingstone-Banks (2020), who has examined all the UK Research Councils' websites, found a 'range of differences' in what each Research Council requires from applications for funding and the criteria each uses to assess applications. It is therefore wise to pay particular attention to your prospective funder's requirement. Information about impact can also be included in the 'Case for support' section, as appropriate. Activities leading to impact will still need to be costed in the proposal. Livingstone-Banks (2020) concluded that the change from 'Pathways to impact' to 'embedding impact' in the proposal means that 'rather than people slotting engagement or impact into another box, the new-found freedom of researchers to build in engagement activities into their case for support will hopefully result in more relevant and meaningful activities that are well-planned' (p. 1). Those who do not want to include impact in their proposal will not feel pressurised to do so.

STRATEGIES AND ACTIVITIES TO FACILITATE IMPACT

At the Design Stage

Not all studies require a detailed impact pathway. It is not appropriate for students undertaking a small study or writing a research proposal as a course assignment to do so. In such circumstances, one cannot, with time and resources limitations, engage with users and stakeholders to plan an impact strategy. However, all research studies must identify the gap in knowledge that their study seeks to fill and the benefits that it may bring and to whom. They can be expected to have a dissemination plan, but one cannot expect much more for a small unfunded project or proposal. For studies seeking funding support, researchers should identify the potential impact of the study and the particular contribution (e.g. conceptual, instrumental, methodological, etc.) that they hope to make. This itself requires preparatory work in terms of finding the current policy or practice they want to change and the economic, health or other benefits that the study can potentially bring.

For example, if the study's aim is to develop and test a practice guideline (such as a guideline to facilitate the delivery of a sexual health promotion intervention if one does not exist or needs replacing), one could say that the guideline is an outcome of the study. For impact to happen, this guideline will have to be tested in terms of, for example, the frequency of use and satisfaction of health professionals in the use of the guideline. The satisfaction of patients or clients with the sexual health service they receive due to the implementation of the guideline is another impact that could be measured. If positive results are obtained, one can claim that the study has had an impact on practice. For a higher level of impact to be achieved one has to assess whether the change in patients' behaviour (as a result of health professionals using the guideline) has resulted in a less frequent use of health services or better sexual health wellbeing for the patients. This could be one study in different phases, or two or three studies. Achieving impact on such a topic may require a well-funded programme of work that may last a number of years. Researchers should be realistic and resist promising an impact they cannot achieve in the lifetime of the study.

In their proposal for a study on stroke management by nurses and physiotherapists, in a hospital in Zambia, Katowa-Mukwato et al. (2021) explain that they 'hoped' the study's findings would be used as a basis for recommending a streamlined role for nurses and physiotherapists in both acute care and rehabilitation. They added that 'the information can also be used as a basis for developing teaching materials for nursing and physiotherapy students, staff and stroke patients with a potential for improved care and compliance to treatment respectively' (p. 31). According to them, the findings can be used to advocate for better services for stroke patients. In this case, it seems that although they have a clear dissemination plan for their findings, they do not have strategies to facilitate the impact that they described above. This is probably because there is little research on this topic in Zambia and they may not have the resources for engagement with health professionals to take this work further, in terms of impact.

The group or population who may benefit from the study should also be clearly identified at the design stage. In the above study, nurses and physiotherapists who work with stroke patients are the first line of beneficiaries as the study's findings, if positive, are likely to enhance their practice. Stroke patients are ultimately the ones to benefit as they will potentially receive improved care.

Involving Users and Beneficiaries in the Project

The first step to achieve impact is to involve users and public representatives in the design of the study. Public involvement in research projects is explored in detail in the next chapter. To maximise impact, it is important that those likely to use research in their practice or policy are invited at the design stage. Selecting who to invite often depends on the researchers' existing network of collaborators in the practice setting. Building relationships with practitioners and policy makers takes time and effort. For some researchers who may already have links with professionals in the practice sector it will be straightforward, although there are many factors such as time commitment and availability that may decide who can participate. Someone in a senior position (or their nominated representative) who has enough time and interest to be involved is ideal, because it is likely that any subsequent change in practice will have to be approved and facilitated by them.

Researchers should be specific about who is involved and what their role will be in the project, their time commitment and the contribution they will make towards impact. It is also helpful to give a brief description of their expertise and what they bring to the project in the biographical section of the proposal. For researchers with little or no network of practice collaborators, the process of recruiting users and potential beneficiaries may take longer and will require persuasion and negotiating skills. There may also be cost implications that need to be taken into account.

The rationale for including users' and beneficiaries' representatives in a meaningful way in the design of the project is because they are more aware of the issues and problems that need to be addressed. They can potentially help researchers to develop practice-relevant research questions. They may also help with identifying patient/client outcomes.

Pathways or Routes to Impact

Even when there is no requirement to complete a 'pathways to impact' section in a proposal, researchers should describe the approach (strategy) and the activities they will use to facilitate impact. From the outset it is important to understand that the pathways or routes to impact do not in themselves constitute impact; they are activities that researchers will engage in to facilitate impact. The National Co-ordinating Centre for Public Engagement (NCCPE) has a number of useful tips on how to develop pathways to impact. They recommend 'a combination of dissemination and more active engagement' with relevant users and beneficiaries (NCCPE, 2022, p. 1).

Publishing studies in peer-reviewed journals is the usual route that researchers (in particular those in universities) use to disseminate their findings. In academic circles, such publications are valuable to both researchers and their universities and are considered as outcomes of studies. In research proposals, researchers should explain what they will publish, when and where. They should also explain other dissemination 'routes' they will use. In their proposal for 'an ethnographic study of the retention problem in emergency medicine in the UK', Darbyshire et al. (2020) explain that they will disseminate the findings through lectures, seminars, conference presentations and academic publications. They add that:

> *Dissemination to the public will be facilitated by presentations at knowledge translation events and by engaging with local media and research translation services such as The Conversation. Policy briefs summarising the findings will be provided for key audiences such as NHS England, Health Education England and the Royal College of Emergency Medicine.*

(p. 6)

The temptation to over-promise should be resisted. Research funders can hold researchers accountable for what they put in their proposals. For example, the National Institute of Health and Care Research (NIHR) in the UK, a major health and social care research funder, collects information on the research activities that are undertaken by its award holders using Researchfish, a digital platform that uses technology and algorithms to collect outcomes and outputs of research from the web, external data sources and the researchers themselves. The NIHR explains that 'on an annual basis, holders of NIHR-funded research and personal awards are asked to submit data about their outputs, outcomes and impacts' (NIHR, 2019a, p. 1).

Research funders look for impact beyond publications. Dissemination is a necessary route to impact but is not sufficient for impact to happen. Presenting at academic conferences is another traditional route for researchers to communicate their studies. Summaries of research studies in professional, practice-based journals and presentations at health and social care professionals' conferences, in a non-academic language, would make it easier for the findings to be understood by practitioners and policy makers. Identifying, and meeting with, key relevant individuals and groups would also be another way to disseminate the findings directly to potential users. Engaging with users and beneficiaries is vital in order that research findings reach the relevant people who can utilise them. Impact-related activities should be coherent and together they should reflect the overall strategy for facilitating impact.

There are different ways in which research can be communicated. The literature on the use of social media for transferring knowledge is growing rapidly. However, according to Elliott et al. (2020), 'a gap exists around best practices in establishing, implementing, and evaluating an effective social media knowledge translation (KT) and exchange strategies' (p. 1). For an insight into good practices in how social media can be used to transfer knowledge, see the scoping review by Chan et al. (2020) on 'social media in knowledge translation and education for physicians and trainees'. Elliott et al. (2020) make a number of recommendations for researchers when they develop their social media knowledge strategy. These include: 'set a clear goal and identify a theory, framework or model that aligns with the project goals and objectives'; 'understand the intended audience'; 'choose a platform or platforms that meet the needs of the intended audience and align well with the research team's capabilities'; 'tailor messages to meet user needs and platform requirements'; 'consider the timing, frequency, and duration of messaging as well as the nature of interactions'; 'ensure that adequate resources and personnel are available'; 'develop an evaluation plan a priori driven by goals and types of data available'; and 'consider the ethical approvals needed' (p.1–2).

In their proposal for a 'randomised controlled trial evaluating the effectiveness of strengths model case management (SMCM) with Chinese mental health service users in Hong Kong', Tse et al. (2019) explain that their approach to knowledge translation will target service users and their families by working with the local community and the media. They add that:

> *Healthcare professionals will benefit from the study's contribution to workforce training and professional meetings. We will disseminate our findings to researchers both locally and internationally through conference presentations and publications in peer-reviewed journals. Our results will also be disseminated through seminars organised by the PI's [principal investigator's] department and the websites of the participating NGOs [non-governmental organisations].*

(p. 8)

Making use of, and referring to, the Concordat for Engaging the Public with Research (UKRI, 2011) will demonstrate awareness of this important document. Referring to specific principles in the Concordat, as appropriate, will help to show that this guidance is being used in a meaningful way and not just as a token gesture.

Proposal Example 14.1 shows how research impact was addressed in a protocol.

PROPOSAL EXAMPLE 14.1
RESEARCH IMPACT IN A PROPOSAL

The NIHR (2019b), in the UK, has produced two detailed case studies to show good practice in how public engagement and impact were described in a proposal. One of them is about how engagement and impact are reported in a proposal on 'Making positive moves: what support do people with Learning Disabilities need to remain living in the community after moving under the Transforming Care Programme? A qualitative longitudinal study' (Louisa Rhodes, Principal Investigator).

Here are some key points (from the case study) to illustrate some of the issues highlighted in this chapter:

1. The 'good mix of frontline operational expertise and those who know how to make change happen' (p. 1) made it a balanced team. This impressed the funder, especially as there were two non-researchers as co-applicants. A local authority professional was selected to chair the advisory group for the project. The funder stated that it was 'good to have a non-academic as a chair to encourage ongoing engagement' (p. 2).

2. One of the outcomes was to be the co-production (with users and carers) of a website to 'disseminate findings nationally in real time Transforming Care Teams, commissioners as well as directly to people with learning disabilities, carers and the public' (p. 3). NHS England awarded £40,000 for the website development.

3. In this proposal the target audience and the outcomes are clearly identified. The proposal also gives examples of previous studies to show a track record and 'provides documentary evidence of previous success in reaching the right people' (p. 5). The team also included one academic individual with expertise in knowledge transfer.

4. There was evidence that the team already had relationships with key relevant people in NHS England and the Association of Directors of Adult Social Services and Local Authority prior to developing this proposal.

5. Dissemination routes included a website, webinars and a national conference to bring together a relevant audience including service users, carers, care providers, social workers, etc.

6. The proposal outlines a long-term plan (5–10 years after the study). This includes implementing and embedding the best practice guidelines and training packages produced by the study in the practice of learning disability teams and community placement providers. This shows that the applicants are fully committed to enhancing the care of people with a learning disability.

Checklist for reporting research impact in a proposal:

1. Has the potential for impact been identified in the proposal? Has evidence of this been supported by the literature and/or other reliable sources?

2. Have potential users and beneficiaries been identified in the proposal?

3. How will representatives of potential users and beneficiaries be involved in designing the study? Is there evidence that contact has been made with them and agreement about their participation sought? What are their roles and time commitment?

4. Has a dissemination and communication plan been described? What is the overall approach/strategy of the plan? Has any particular model/framework been used to underpin the approach?

5. Have the activities to communicate and engage with potential users and beneficiaries been outlined?

6. Are these activities appropriate, varied and coherent?

7. Have impact activities been costed in the proposal?

SUMMARY AND CONCLUSIONS

The focus on research impact is not a passing trend: it is likely to grow as pressure on the economy grows. With or without pressure from governments or research funders, researchers should always maximise the benefits of their research and facilitate others to make use of their research findings.

   Involving representatives of users and beneficiaries in the design of the study from the start will help make the study more relevant to those most likely to use the findings and to those who can potentially benefit from them. Identifying the potential impact of the study in the proposal and how researchers will disseminate the findings and engage with users and beneficiaries are key aspects that funders will assess. Impact pathway plans should be feasible, appropriate, as specific as possible and, above all, coherent. Funders know the limitations of researchers in affecting change in policy and practice. They, and reviewers, do not expect applicants to make precise predictions about impact. However, they expect to see evidence that researchers have carefully thought out the strategy and activities that will facilitate knowledge transfer.

REFERENCES

Australian Research Council. (2022). *Research impact principles and framework.* https://www.arc.gov.au/about-arc/strategies/research-impact-principles-and-framework

Bailey, T., & Mouton, J. (2005). *The production and utilisation of knowledge in higher education institutions in South Africa (Volume 1).* South Africa: Centre for Research on Science & Technology. Stellenbosch University. https://core.ac.uk/download/pdf/188225673.pdf

Chan, T. M., Dzara, K., Dimeo, S. P., Bhalerao, A., & Maggio, L. A. (2020). Social media in knowledge translation and education for physicians and trainees: A scoping review. *Perspectives on Medical Education, 9*(1), 20–30.

Cordier, R. (2021). The research challenges we face: Identifying and minimising research waste. *Australian Occupational Therapy Journal, 68,* 1–2.

Darbyshire, D., Brewster, L., Isba, R., Body, R., & Goodwin, D. (2020). 'Where have all the doctors gone?' A protocol for an ethnographic study of the retention problem in emergency medicine in the UK. *BMJ Open, 10*(11), e038229. https://doi.org/10.1136/bmjopen-2020-038229

Elliott, S. A., Dyson, M. P., Wilkes, G. V., Zimmermann, G. L., Chambers, C. T., Wittmeier, K. D., Russell, D. J., Scott, S. D., Thomson, D., & Hartling, L. (2020). Considerations for health researchers using social media for knowledge translation: Multiple case study. *Journal of Medical Internet Research, 22*(7), e15121. https://doi.org/10.2196/15121

ESRC. (2021). *How to demonstrate support for impact.* https://www.ukri.org/councils/esrc/impact-toolkit-for-economic-and-social-sciences/how-to-demonstrate-support-for-impact/

ESRC. (2022). *Defining research impact.* https://www.ukri.org/councils/esrc/impact-toolkit-for-economic-and-social-sciences/defining-impact/#:,:text=The%20Economic%20and%20Social%20Research,to%20society%20and%20the%20economy

Government of Ireland. (2022). *Impact 2030: Research and innovation strategy.* https://www.gov.ie/en/publication/27c78-impact-2030-irelands-new-research-and-innovation-strategy/

Katowa-Mukwato, P., Banda, M., Kanyanta, M., Musenge, E., Phiri, P., Mwiinga-Kalusopa, V., Chapima, F., Simpamba, M., Kapenda, C., & Shula, H. (2021). Study protocol on stroke management: Role of nurses and physiotherapists at the Adult University Teaching Hospital, Lusaka Zambia. *Journal of Biosciences and Medicines, 9,* 25–37.

Kim, C., Wilcher, R., Petruney, T., Krueger, K., Wynne, L., & Zan, T. (2018). A research utilisation framework for informing global health and development policies and programmes. *Health Research Policy and Systems*, *16*(1), 9. https://doi.org/10.1186/s12961-018-0284-2

Konwar, G. (2018). A review on challenges and barriers: implementation of the existing nursing research findings. *International Journal of Advanced Research*, *6*, 1556–1560. https://doi.org/10.21474/IJAR01/6389

Livingstone-Banks, M. (2020). *No more pathways to impact: How impact is being embedded into research grant proposals.* https://www.mpls.ox.ac.uk/public-engagement/latest/no-more-pathways-to-impact-how-impact-is-being-embedded-into-research-grant-proposals#mrc

Morton, C. (2012). *Exploring and assessing social research impact: A case study of a research partnership's impacts on policy and practice.* PhD thesis. Scotland: University of Edinburgh. https://era.ed.ac.uk/bitstream/handle/1842/9940/Morton2012.pdf?sequence=2&isAllowed=y

NCCPE. (2022). *Pathways to impact.* https://www.publicengagement.ac.uk/do-engagement/funding/pathways-impact

NIHR. (2019a). *NIHR Researchfish guidance.* https://www.nihr.ac.uk/documents/nihr-researchfish-guidance/12294

NIHR. (2019b). *Example of an engagement and impact plan – Making positive moves.* https://www.nihr.ac.uk/documents/example-of-an-engagement-and-impact-plan-nihr-research-for-patient-benefit-programme/12300

Reed, M. S., Ferré, M., Martin-Ortega, J., Blanche, R., Lawford-Rolfe, R., Dallimer, M., & Holden, J. (2021). Evaluating impact from research: A methodological framework. *Research Policy, 50*, 104147. https://doi.org/10.1016/j.respol.2020.104147

Tse, S., Ng, S., Yuen, W., Fukui, S., Goscha, R. J., & Lo, W. (2019). Study protocol for a randomised controlled trial evaluating the effectiveness of strengths model case management (SMCM) with Chinese mental health service users in Hong Kong. *BMJ Open, 9*(5), e026399. https://doi.org/10.1136/bmjopen-2018-026399

UKRI. (2011). *Concordat for engaging the public with research.* https://www.ukri.org/publications/concordat-for-engaging-the-public-with-research/

UKRI. (2022). *How Research England supports research excellence.* https://www.ukri.org/about-us/research-england/research-excellence/ref-impact/#:,:text=The%20Research%20Excellence%20Framework%20(REF,of%20life%2C%20beyond%20academia'

University Grants Committee. (2022). *Research impact fund.* https://www.ugc.edu.hk/eng/rgc/funding_opport/rif/

Department for Business Education and Skills. (2006). *Increasing the economic impact of research councils: Advice to the Director General of Science and Innovation, DTI from the Research Council Economic Impact Group. The Warry Report.* London: Department for Business, Innovation and Skills.

Williams, K., & Lewis, J. M. (2021). Understanding, measuring, and encouraging public policy research impact. *Australian Journal of Public Administration, 80*, 554–564.

15 INVOLVING USERS, PATIENTS AND THE PUBLIC IN RESEARCH

INTRODUCTION

In Chapter 14, we focused on the issue of impact in research designs and proposals. We pointed out that engagement with potential users and beneficiaries is crucial to maximising impact. The aim of this chapter is to examine, in more detail, the rationale for involving patients and the public in research studies, how this can be done and the resources that are available for researchers, patients and the public to support such endeavours. We will highlight some of the benefits, impact and challenges that have been reported in studies evaluating the involvement of patients and the public in research studies. We will also provide examples of how patient and public involvement (PPI) has been reported in research proposals.

BACKGROUND TO PPI IN NURSING, HEALTH AND SOCIAL CARE RESEARCH

Over the last two decades, international recognition of the importance and benefits of involving patients and the public in health and social care has increased at a great pace (McCoy et al., 2019). PPI can be described as researchers, patients and members of the public working, as partners, to design and conduct research studies. It is research being carried out 'with' or 'by' members of the public rather than 'to', 'about' or 'for' them (NIHR, 2021).

Patient participation in research is not new. Participatory action research, described as research involving 'researchers and participants working together to understand a problematic situation and change it for the better' has been conducted since the 1940s (Institute of Development Studies, 2022). What is new is how PPI has been vigorously advocated by policy makers and research funders. As a result, PPI-related policy documents and the international literature on the topic 'has more than tripled in the last 10 years' (Boivin et al., 2018, p. 1). Two new journals, *Research Involvement and Engagement* (2015) and *Research for All* (2017), dedicated to this topic, have been created. More and more researchers have embraced the practice, not least because some funders have made it mandatory for researchers to provide information about PPI in their proposals.

PPI is part of a wider movement or policy involving ordinary people and local communities in the planning, commissioning, delivery and evaluation of the health and social care services they receive (Department of Health 2022). The overall aim is to increase accountability, transparency and the democratic participation of citizens in decision making, and thereby make services more relevant to their needs. Stephens and Staniszewska (2015) explain that 'such involvement also reflects a wider intention, of ensuring a democratic accountability for research, much of which is paid for from public monies, whether by taxation or by donation' (p. 1). According to Boivin et al. (2018), 'PPI is justified by two lines of argument: one on the basis of ethical principles, the other on the assumption that it may improve the quality, relevance, and uptake of research' (p. 1).

Staley (2013) conducted a series of case studies to explore the impact of service user and carer involvement on research. These case studies appear to show, for example, that involvement:

- *ensures research addresses the issues that service users and carers identify as being important and relevant – to ensure services better meet their needs, and questions about their treatment and care are answered.*
- *ensures that service users' and carers' questions are addressed through the project design, developing valuable lines of enquiry that might not have otherwise been considered.*
- *keeps the project grounded in reality so expectations of participants are reasonable, and the practical arrangements for participation reflect the interests and concerns of service users and carers.*
- *brings a wide range of skills to a project in addition to people's lived experience – as service users and carers also bring knowledge and expertise from their professional lives;*
- *ensures any intervention that is developed to benefit service users and carers is better designed to reflect their genuine interests and needs.*
- *ensures research findings are more likely to be translated into action, to bring about change and make a difference to people's lives.*

(pp. 56–57)

These case studies and others, for example those reported by Cancer Research UK (CRUK, 2023a), demonstrate the many benefits that PPI has brought to research projects and researchers, as well as patients and public contributors. Examples of benefits to projects include providing insights into what matters to patients rather than focusing on what researchers think is important to patients. Staley (2013) explains that in one intervention study involving the use of statins in the management of cardiovascular risk, patients involved in the project suggested more emphasis on the communication between the clinician and the service user, because they wanted an opportunity to have a discussion with the clinician rather than be told to take the drug.

In a study by Sihre et al. (2019), on the 'lived experiences of severe postnatal psychiatric illnesses in English speaking South Asian women living in the UK', a South Asian patient was able to provide views and opinions about the methodology and the research materials (letter of invitation to participant, participant information sheet, interview schedule, etc.). Some of the terms used in the materials and interview schedule were rephrased as a result of the review by the patient. PPI is not just an exercise to obtain different perspectives; these are the perspectives of those about whom and for whom the studies are carried out. Therefore, they are all the more necessary and important, otherwise the findings may have little relevance to the reality of these people's lives. For more PPI case studies, see CRUK (2023a).

While these case studies clearly demonstrate the benefits of PPI, measuring its impact beyond the time span of the project is more problematic because of the involvement of other confounding factors and the time it takes for an impact to happen. Some of these benefits are conceptual and cognitive and may not be subject to quantitative measurements. However, as Boivin ct al. (2018, p. 1) explain, 'if we are serious about involvement, we need to be equally serious about evaluation'. In a systematic review investigating the impact of PPI on rates of enrolment and retention in clinical trials, Crocker et al. (2018) concluded that while 'the findings for retention were inconclusive owing to the paucity of eligible studies', the 'involvement of people with lived experience of the condition under study was significantly associated with improved enrolment' (p. 1). Boivin et al. (2018) emphasised the importance of these findings as 'recruitment difficulties can reduce trial validity, add costs, and increase the risk of studies being abandoned or not reported' (p. 1).

PPI is not, however, without its challenges. Staley et al. (2013), who carried out an evaluation of projects adopted by the National Institute of Health Research (now the National Institute of Health and Care Research; NIHR) Mental Health Research Network in the UK, listed some of the challenges researchers faced. These included organisational barriers to PPI, a lack of training for researchers as part of their early career development and a lack of induction processes or ongoing professional development. They also reported that many researchers have much narrower expectations of involvement. Brett et al. (2014), who conducted a systematic review of the impact of PPI on service users, researchers and communities, reported that some service users reported 'being empowered and valued' (p. 387) while others reported a lack of preparation and training that led some service users to feel unable to contribute to the research. Other service users and communities reported feeling overburdened with the work involved. Brett et al. (2014) also reported that researchers faced difficulties in incorporating PPI in meaningful ways due to lack of money and time.

There can also be power relationship issues between researchers and patient and public contributors (Green and Johns, 2019). The literature gives the impression that some researchers are not convinced of the benefits of PPI, particularly when weighed against what they perceive as the additional 'burden' on their project. Reviewing progress in public involvement in NIHR-funded research, Staniszewska et al. (2018) reported that some researchers were sceptical about the value of PPI and some felt confused and anxious about how to involve patients and public contributors in their projects 'in a way that demonstrated a positive impact' (p. 7). Overall, Staniszewska et al. (2018) identified 'a range of barriers including limited awareness of opportunities, lack of diversity, resistant attitudes to involvement, inconsistent levels of resources, systems that work in different ways, patchy training and support and variable organisational implementation' (p. 10).

A paradigm shift towards more recognition that patients and the public have valuable experience to offer to research is required as 'research without evidence of public involvement would be considered flawed' (Stephens and Staniszewska, 2015, p. 2). Organisational support, training, funding and a change in researchers' perceptions of the value of PPI may help to foster more positive attitudes towards it.

CLARIFICATION OF PPI TERMS

The PPI movement has spawned its own vocabulary. Some of the terms are used loosely and interchangeably, which has the potential to cause confusion. These terms include 'patient', 'public', 'user', 'involvement', 'participation', 'partnership' and 'engagement', but this list is by no means exhaustive. The PPI movement has given its own meaning to some of these terms.

The term 'patient' is used to designate anyone who has a lived experience of an illness or condition (e.g. diabetes). Their perceptions and expertise can be valuable for some studies on diabetes. The NIHR (2023) describes 'public' as 'patients, potential patients, carers and people who use health and social care services as well as people from organisations that represent people who use services'. Bagley et al. (2016) point out that patients and members of the public who are involved in research are sometimes 'referred to as PPI representatives' (p. 12), implying that they are representing the views of patients and members of the public. This is rarely the case, even when they are members of patient groups. Bagley et al. (2016) prefer the term 'public contributor'.

'User' refers to those who use research findings in their policies and practice. They are mostly health and social care professionals. 'Involvement' in research 'is an active partnership between patients, carers and members of the public with researchers that influences and shapes research' (NIHR, 2023). 'Participation' in research is when patients or members of the public take part in research as participants who provide data for a study (e.g. when they complete a questionnaire or respond to interview questions). 'Engagement' is a term mostly used when researchers and those involved in research raise awareness of research, share knowledge or engage and create a dialogue with the public (NIHR, 2021). Therefore 'engagement' is a term mostly used, in research circles, to describe the activities in the dissemination and impact phase of a study (see Chapter 14). However, it is not unusual for 'involvement' and 'engagement' to be used interchangeably. For example, in the 'aims and scope' section of *Research for All*, the journal explains that:

> *Engagement with research goes further than participation in it. Engaged individuals and communities initiate research, advise, challenge, or collaborate with researchers. Their involvement is always active and they have a crucial influence on the conduct of the research – on its design or methods, products, dissemination or use.*

Research for All (2022)

What is called 'engagement' here is what others may term 'involvement'.

There are different types of involvement in research, such as consultation, collaboration and partnership. 'Consultation' is when patients and members of the public are asked their views and opinions on a particular aspect of the study but are not involved in the study's design or conduct. 'Collaboration' involves being part of the study team and being recognised as such on the proposal. 'Partnership' is a term used to describe what type of collaboration it is. Partnership is a form of collaboration where the extent of ownership of, and responsibility for, the project is known in advance (e.g. as an equal, dormant or minor partner). In research terms, partnership may be a case where the patient or public contributor is a co-applicant or co-researcher on the proposal. Someone once said that 'all partners are collaborators but not all collaborators are partners'. These two terms are, however, often used interchangeably. Terms are also joined together, as in 'collaborative partnership' (Masotti et al., 2006) or 'collaborative involvement' (Stephens and Staniszewska, 2015). As usual it is more important to describe in detail what is done than to focus on getting the right label.

The extent of involvement can be on a continuum from 'consultancy' (as an individual consultant/advisor or part of a steering committee) to 'equal partnership' (taking part in every aspect of a study, from design to post-study completion). PPI can also be characterised as 'peripheral', 'partial' or 'integral'. An example of 'peripheral' involvement comes from Sihre et al. (2019). In their proposal for a study of the 'lived experiences of severe postnatal psychiatric illnesses in English speaking South Asian women, living in the UK', Sihre et al. (2019) explained that they informally approached patients on a unit to seek their views and opinions about their research study. One patient volunteered and she was presented with a brief overview of the proposal and asked for her views on 'the appropriateness of the research methods in obtaining information about experiences of postnatal psychiatric illness' (p. 3). She also reviewed research materials (patient consent form, etc.) and changes were made following her feedback. The involvement of this patient was useful but peripheral, as she seems to have taken no further part in the study. This type of involvement is usually undertaken in the pilot phase of a study, but there is no patient or public involvement thereafter.

An example of partial involvement is from a proposal, by AshaRani et al. (2020), for a nationwide 'Knowledge, Attitudes and Practices (KAP) survey on diabetes in Singapore's general population'. Patients and members of the public were involved in developing the questionnaire and selecting the outcome measures. The content and wording of the questionnaire were reviewed by people with diabetes and members of the public. However, as they stated, 'there was no patient/public involvement in the recruitment and conduct of the study' (AshaRani et al., 2020, p. 3).

An example of PPI being integral to the study is from a proposal by O'Keefe et al. (2022) for a pilot randomised controlled trial of 'a tailored occupational therapist-led vocational intervention for people with stroke'. They sought the views of people with lived experience of a stroke from the 'inception of the trial, including during a review of the funding application and protocol and selection of the primary outcome' (p. 3). They also explained that patients would be part of an expert panel 'who will have oversight across the lifetime of the research' (p. 3). This panel would meet at least three times a year 'to provide input into the trial processes, documents, and intervention resources' (p. 3). The panel would also review the findings and advise on dissemination strategies.

For more information and clarification on PPI-related terms and vocabulary, see NIHR (2023), Hoddinott et al. (2018) and Nyström et al. (2018).

PPI BEFORE, DURING AND AFTER THE STUDY

Researchers should reflect upon, or assess, the need for PPI and the potential contribution that patients and public contributors can make to the proposed study. Needs may change as the study proceeds, and more or different users, patients or members of the public could be invited to contribute accordingly. There are many aspects of a study that they can contribute to. These include discussing an idea for research, designing the study, writing or reviewing the proposal, collecting and analysing data and disseminating the findings.

The degree of involvement is likely to be influenced by the input required from users, patients or members of the public, and the nature of the project (e.g. the more patient focused the topic, the more substantial the contribution is likely to be), the specific needs of the project, and the skills and expertise already in the research team. Other factors that can potentially affect the type and degree of involvement are related to the researchers initiating the study (e.g. their attitudes, skills, training and perceptions of and previous experience with PPI). The setting or organisation where the study will be based (e.g. the support available for PPI in terms of structures and policies regarding PPI, finance and flexibility) will also be a deciding factor. The patient/public-related factors include the availability of potential contributors, access to them, what they have to offer to the different needs of the project and their commitment, including time.

The potential for involvement can be at the planning and design stage (prior to the study), at the delivery stage (during the study) and at the dissemination and impact stage (after completion of the study).

At the Planning and Design Stage

In Chapter 1, we explained how research starts with an idea that is then turned into research questions. In nursing, health and social care, ideas can come from practitioners or researchers. The idea and the research questions would benefit from the expertise and experience of users, patients or the public, in order to make the study relevant to the needs of those most likely to benefit from it. Researchers, on the other hand, should be able to develop the idea into research questions, objectives or a hypothesis. We can see that working together to discuss issues, problems or topics of relevance to patients can be turned into answerable research questions.

At the planning and design stage, concepts are clarified and operationally defined. Researchers may bring an academic slant to the concept, but patients are more likely to ground the concept in the reality of people's experience. For example, Lajoie et al. (2020), referring to 'vulnerability', explain that 'despite scholarly debates, the descriptive and normative meanings ascribed to the concept have remained disengaged from the perspective of users of the concept and those concerned by its use' (p. 128). Staley et al. (2013) conducted a small-scale evaluation of 45 projects (a third of which were just starting, a third were about mid-way and a third were near completion). A small number of researchers in the studies reported that the research questions had been identified by service users. Staley et al. (2013) also reported that researchers undertaking these projects used various approaches, including focus groups, a pilot study or a service user reference group to identify ideas or questions for research.

At this early stage of the study, there are opportunities for researchers, users and patients to discuss the need for, and the feasibility of, the study and identify potential sources of research funding. Patients and users can also help with making preliminary contact with stakeholders for research sites and access to potential participants.

PPI can also make a valuable contribution to the methodology of the study. Patient and public contributors can ensure that patient-centred data collection tools and outcomes are selected. They can contribute towards the development of questionnaires, interview schedules and other tools. They can advise on the practicalities of the study and identify potential barriers and challenges. In the study by Staley et al. (2013), 61% of the 45 studies reported that PPI made an impact on the design of the study, 22% reported that it had an impact on conceptual elements and 27% on practicalities. In their proposal for a trial on the clinical effectiveness, efficacy and cost effectiveness of splints for symptomatic thumb base osteoarthritis (OA), Adams et al. (2019) explained that 'two patient and public group meetings were carried out with eight patient partners living with hand OA to listen to patient experiences of living with hand OA, explore intervention components of the trial and help to inform co-design a placebo splint design' (p. 2). They added that patient partners discussed which splint they found more credible. Adams et al. (2019) concluded that:

> *this involvement at an early stage ensured that clinicians felt that they had contributed and had ownership in the trial design and patient input ensured that patients' perspectives had been integral to the study design, hopefully making the trial relevant and appealing to prospective patients.*

> *(p. 2)*

After the study has been designed, patients and public contributors can also get involved in writing or reviewing the proposal, especially if funding is applied for. Assessors are likely to view proposals favourably if users, patients or public contributors are identified on the proposal and their role clearly specified. Out of her seven case studies, Staley (2013) reported that five involved patient/public contributors in their funding applications. The NIHR (2018) has developed three online interactive modules on PPI. Module 1 is an introduction to the NIHR and PPI in research, module 2 is on 'Public reviewing roles and useful skills', and module 3 is about 'How to review research documents from a patient and public point of view'.

The Delivery Phase

At this stage, the researchers start the process of collecting data. This includes accessing and recruiting participants, selecting (or developing) and refining data collection tools, applying for ethical approval, collecting data (e.g. via questionnaires or interviews), analysing the data and interpreting the findings. As this is the 'conducting research' phase, there are a number of tasks that can benefit from patient and public contribution. The main task that they are invited by researchers to contribute to seems to be writing or reviewing materials (e.g. consent forms, questionnaires, etc.) to make them participant friendly. Earlier in this chapter, the impact of PPI on participant recruitment was reported. Reviewing the impact of PPI on a survey of patients taking part in the early phase of clinical trials, CRUK (2023a) reported that the response rate in that study was extremely high (80%). The researchers believe that PPI shortened the questionnaire, made the questions more relevant for patients and increased recruitment.

Patients and public contributors can also be involved in the development of interventions in order to make them more patient centred. The case studies in Staley (2013) provide numerous examples of how researchers have benefited from such input. Although data collection, data analysis and interpretation of findings can be perceived as being mainly researchers' tasks, patients and public contributors can also be involved. In the Staley (2013) study, patient or public contributors were involved in data collection in three out of seven studies and in data analysis in four out of seven studies. In one case study, researchers found that the service users' interpretation of findings was more grounded in reality (Staley, 2013).

Dissemination and Impact Stage

There are many opportunities for PPI after the study has been completed. These include participation in the dissemination of findings and engagement with users and other potential beneficiaries. Examples of proposals that identify the role of users, patients and members of the public in dissemination include those by O'Keefe et al. (2022) and Jong et al. (2022). They explain in the proposals how users, patients and public contributors will be engaged in the dissemination of findings. O'Keefe et al. (2022) aimed to set up an expert panel comprising stroke survivors with lived experience who would be invited to review the preliminary findings at the completion of data collection and would inform strategies based on the findings. Jong et al. (2022), in their proposal, stated that PPI is an integrative part of all study phases, including the dissemination of the results. They aimed to involve different groups including users (health professionals and outdoor instructors) and patients to meet the different needs of their project (evaluating a wilderness programme for adults and young adult cancer survivors), and all of them would be involved in the interpretation and dissemination of findings.

Dissemination is mostly in the form of a publication of papers from the study and oral and poster presentations at conferences and other meetings with potential users and beneficiaries. In one of the case studies by Staley (2013), service users were found to be helpful in reaching groups that researchers were not in everyday contact with, and also in designing a conference and contributing to it.

The post-study period is also a time when users, patients and public contributors may begin to think of taking the research further or getting involved in new studies. In a proposal by Mitchell et al. (2018) for a 'qualitative interview study to investigate the healthcare experiences and preferences of children and young people with life-limiting and life-threatening conditions and their families', they explain that they intend to work with the PPI group 'to plan innovative, accessible outputs for patients, the public and commissioners which will include infographics and film-based reports' (p. 9) outlining their recommendations. They state that PPI has been integral to the design and conduct of the study. They list future plans including conducting a survey (as co-researchers) to investigate the meaning of palliative care for children and young people and health professionals (Mitchell et al., 2018).

ROLES AND STATUS OF USERS, PATIENTS AND PUBLIC CONTRIBUTORS IN RESEARCH TEAMS

The number and type of users and lay people needed in the study depends on the particular needs of the study. Sometimes, one patient may take part in all the stages of the study and get involved in all aspects of the research process. Others may be involved as consultants, advisors or collaborators at specific times in the study, as required. Often more than one collaborator is needed. For example, in their proposal, Jong et al. (2022) describe the different PPI needs of the project and what different contributors will offer. Below is a summary of their roles:

- *Patients/participants: They will be involved in study protocol development, development of the wilderness/holiday programme, risk and safety plan, recruitment of participants, preparation for the train-the-trainer programme.*
- *Wilderness/outdoor instructor: They will work on the development of the programme, advise and assist in the train-the-trainer programme, encourage and motivate participants to move from more urbanisation to going out in nature.*
- *Public health actors: They will advise how to involve participants from different multi-cultural backgrounds, how to motivate participants to move from urbanisation to going out in nature, and how to guarantee sustainability of the wilderness programme.*
- *Healthcare professionals: They will prescribe the necessary study rescue medication, advise regarding the (medical) condition of participants, advise on monitoring of medical safety of participants during the study.*

(p. 6)

Additionally, they all will advise on the interpretation and dissemination of the findings of the study.

As explained earlier, PPI can occur at any or all stages of a project. Roles and expectations should be clarified at the start of the collaboration. In the studies that they reviewed, Staley et al. (2013) identified these three main approaches to involvement: as 'contributors to research design', as 'members of steering groups' and as 'co-researchers'. These roles are not mutually exclusive. The first approach is when patients and public contributors are consulted at the planning stage of study, as described earlier. Researchers should be clear what they expect of PPI, and they should have questions that will guide and get the most out of the involvement.

It is common practice for projects to have a steering group, advisory board or expert panel to oversee the development, progress and completion of the project. Members, drawn from a range of relevant groups and professions, meet a number of times at key points of a project and provide advice designed, among other things, to address issues that may arise. Expert panels are one forum where PPI can be very useful. For example, see O'Keefe et al. (2022), who provided a detailed description in their proposal of how they planned to use an expert panel in a study evaluating a tailored occupational therapist-led vocational intervention for people with stroke.

The third approach, involvement as co-researchers, is when the patient or public contributor becomes a member of the project team. Researchers are familiar with this approach as many of them undertake interdisciplinary research involving experts from different disciplines. In the case of PPI, the patient or public contributor becomes a team member, the same as the others. An effective team is one where members use their individual expertise to make contributions to the project. Each member's contribution is valued according to its own merits. One cannot normally expect a patient to be knowledgeable about research methodology in much the same way as one would not expect researchers to have personal experience of the disease or condition they are researching. Once researchers understand that they are not experts in everything and that others (e.g. statisticians, health economists, epidemiologists, patients, clinicians, etc.) have useful contributions to make, they will realise the benefits of working collaboratively with others. Teamwork is about the division of labour, with clearly identified roles and expectations of team members.

Teamwork is not without its challenges. The most common one is that power may not be equally shared, with the result that some team members may feel undervalued and even overwhelmed in the presence of researchers and other health professionals. If there is an unequal power dynamic, PPI risks being 'tokenistic' (Green and Johns, 2019). Principal investigators should make every effort to maximise the participation of all team members, in particular patient and public contributors. Processes should be put in place to review how PPI is progressing in the project. Their support and training needs should be assessed and met accordingly. It is important that everyone has a sense of ownership of the project. Shared ownership involves shared responsibility and shared rewards.

RECRUITING PATIENTS AND PUBLIC CONTRIBUTORS

The recruitment of users, patients and members of the public for a research project requires careful thought. Identifying the specific needs of the study is the first step in the recruitment process. Matching the needs with potential people, contacting them and meeting with them for preliminary discussion about the project is the next step. It may require the preparation of material regarding the project and the patient/public input needed. INVOLVE and the NIHR have produced a series of PPI tips sheets, including one on 'recruiting members of the public to get involved in research funding and commissioning processes' (INVOLVE, 2012). This covers areas such as planning, advertising, selecting, appointing, supporting and moving on.

PPI is a career-long 'project' for researchers. Relationships with clinicians and other health and social care professionals are built over a long period of time before networks become established. These types of relationship work best when they are reciprocal and all the collaborators benefit. For some researchers who have good 'connections' with policy makers and practitioners, patient/public groups and charities, the task of finding and involving patient and public collaborators may not be too difficult. For others, especially new researchers, it is a learning process. According to Jinks et al. (2013), 'PPI requires a long-term perspective with participation and trust growing over time, and both users and researchers learning what approaches work best' (p. 146).

ETHICAL ISSUES IN PPI

Ethical approval is not needed for PPI in research. However, if PPI results in direct contact with the study participants (e.g. a public contributor interviewing participants), the ethics committee will need to 'check that any patient or member of the public carrying out the research has adequate training, support and supervision appropriate and proportionate to the circumstances in the same way as they do for any other member of the research team' (INVOLVE and the National Research Ethics Service, 2009, p. 3). This is to safeguard the wellbeing and safety of both the patient/public contributor and the participants in the study. The same ethical principles that apply to the patients and clients and to research participants also apply to PPI in research. Hoddinott et al. (2018) listed some of the ethical principles to consider when involving patients/public as consultants, collaborators or co-researchers in research, including:

- *avoiding discrimination, undue persuasion, excessive burden or creating a sense of obligation to be involved in the study*
- *the distribution of power in research*
- *valuing patient contributions and fair financial compensation*
- *conflicts of interest, research integrity and respect for intellectual property*
- *the confidentiality of data and protecting anonymity of research participants*
- *advancing science through honest and accurate reporting.*

(p. 13)

Pandya-Wood et al. (2017), drawing from their experience as advisors to researchers about PPI, observed that researchers' behaviour can sometimes be unintentionally unethical when they involve the public in the design of their studies. Pandya-Wood et al. (2017) used their observations to develop a framework to help researchers avoid unethical practice regarding PPI. The framework listed 10 areas, as follows:

1) Allocating sufficient time for public involvement; 2) Avoiding tokenism; 3) Registering research design stage public involvement work with NHS Research & Development Trust Office at earliest opportunity; 4) Communicating clearly from the outset; 5) Entitling public contributors to stop their involvement for any unstated reasons; 6) Operating fairness of opportunity; 7) Differentiating qualitative research methods and public involvement activities; 8) Working sensitively; 9) Being conscious of confidentiality and 10) Valuing, acknowledging and rewarding public involvement.

(p. 1)

The NIHR (2019) has developed a 'UK standards framework for public involvement' in research. It comprises six standards as follows:

- *Inclusive opportunities*
Offer public involvement opportunities that are accessible and that reach people and groups according to research needs.

■ *Working together*
Work together in a way that values all contributions, and that builds and sustains mutually respectful and productive relationships.
■ *Support and learning*
Offer and promote support and learning opportunities that build confidence and skills for public involvement in research.
■ *Governance*
Involve the public in research management, regulation, leadership and decision making.
■ *Communications*
Use plain language for well-timed and relevant communications, as part of involvement plans and activities.
■ *Impact*
Seek improvement by identifying and sharing the difference that public involvement makes to research.

Some patients and public contributors may be vulnerable to unintentional harm as a result of their involvement in research. Researchers should treat each contributor as an individual and reflect on how they are treated throughout the research process and afterwards. People who are sick may have limited time that they may want to share with those close to them but also to make a contribution to others (through research). This requires careful thought about how their precious time is used by researchers. Young children, people with a learning disability, individuals with dementia and others have valuable experience that they may want to put to good use. At the same time, they may be put in situations that they may not want or where their human rights are overlooked. It is beyond the scope of this chapter to discuss the ethical issues related to the involvement of potentially vulnerable individuals in research. Readers are advised to consult the literature on this topic. Below are some useful references:

- Hersh et al. (2021), 'The ethics of patient and public involvement across the research process: towards partnership with people with aphasia'.
- Parkinson et al. (2021), 'Patient and public involvement for mental health researchers'.
- Gove et al. (2018), 'Alzheimer Europe's position on involving people with dementia in research through PPI (patient and public involvement)'.
- van Schelven et al. (2020), 'Patient and public involvement of young people with a chronic condition in projects in health and social care: a scoping review'.

BUDGETING FOR PPI IN PROPOSALS

Payment is one area where equity and fairness can be demonstrated in PPI. Patients and public contributors may not know what they are entitled to or may not have the confidence to request payment or claim expenses. If this aspect is done properly, it will instil confidence in the contributors that they are being taken seriously and that their involvement is valued. Payments include remuneration and expenses. Involving public contributors in costing their involvement is crucial to making an accurate estimation of their time and potential expenses. Researchers and public contributors can also work together to identify potential sources of funding for preliminary work on the proposal. There is much easy-to-read guidance offering advice on the topic of payments for PPI, including:

■ Mental Health Research Network and INVOLVE (2013), 'Budgeting for involvement: Practical advice on budgeting for actively involving the public in research studies'. This guide provides practical advice on how to budget for involving patients, carers and the public in research. It can be helpful for working out the costs of involvement at any stage of the research process – whether it is a planned focus group in a study already underway or putting together an entire budget for a study. This document also has seven examples of budgeting for PPI in research proposals, with actual costings.
■ NIHR (2022a), 'Payment guidance for members of the public considering involvement in research'. This guide is for patients, carers and members of the public thinking about getting actively involved in research. It explains that expenses and/or payments are being offered for public involvement. It provides answers to some frequently asked questions.
■ NIHR (2022b), 'Payment guidance for researchers and professionals'. This guidance is for researchers, anyone in a professional role, public contributors, research advisors/managers, commissioners of research, reviewers and panel members dealing with costing PPI in research.

TOOLKITS FOR PPI

There are numerous toolkits designed to support researchers, patients and public contributors in PPI. Bagley et al. (2016) gave a useful account how they developed a PPI toolkit 'for meaningful and flexible involvement in clinical trials' (p. 1). A number of national and local organisations have also developed their own toolkits (freely available on the internet). Examples of these include:

■ Health Research Charities Ireland and Trinity College Dublin (2020), 'Making a start: a toolkit for research charities to begin a PPI relationship'.
■ Involving People (2023), 'Patient and public involvement toolkit'.
■ CRUK (2023b), 'Patient involvement toolkit for researchers'.

DESCRIBING PPI IN RESEARCH PROPOSALS

The aim here is to convince anyone reading the proposal that PPI is genuine, appropriate and used to achieve maximum effect. This requires detailed information about key components of the PPI, including why PPI is needed, what contribution (and difference) it is likely to make, who the contributors are, how their experience and expertise match the needs of the project, how they were recruited, what their roles and responsibilities are, the time commitment required of them, the processes and structures that will be put in place to train and support them (as required), who will oversee their involvement and how the PPI is being costed.

Describing all these aspects of PPI within the word limits of a proposal is a skill in itself. Visual displays may be a more succinct way to describe PPI in the proposal. Statements such as 'patients and members of the public have been involved in designing the study' is too broad and may fail to convince assessors that PPI is genuine. Some funding organisations have members of the public on their review panels; they are likely to scrutinise this section of the proposal with care.

Proposal Example 15.1 shows how PPI is integral to a study.

PROPOSAL EXAMPLE 15.1
DESCRIBING PPI IN A PROPOSAL

Saini et al. (2022), COMplex mental health PAThways (COMPAT) Study: a mixed methods study to inform an evidence-based service delivery model for people with complex needs: study protocol.

This study aims to understand 'the profile and history of service users described as having complex needs; the decision-making processes by clinicians that lead to complex needs categorisation; service users and carers experience of service use; and, associated economic impact' (p. 1).

COMMENTS

1. The authors recognise that PPI is 'extremely important' to ensure that their study meets the needs of the target population. They use a table to illustrate the PPI approach they will use. This is a useful way to convey visually the different ways in which PPI will be integrated in the study.
2. The authors state clearly that stakeholder and service users will contribute to every aspect of the study, from the design, analysis and interpretation of the findings to dissemination and implementation.
3. According to the authors, prior consultation with stakeholders informed the study design, the recruitment procedures and the choice of data collection tools.
4. The authors explain that they are engaging with the NHS Trust PPI Groups to set up a Service User Advisory Group for the study. They also give information about how and when the service user group will be used.
5. This proposal shows a genuine attempt towards integrating PPI in a study. The authors have provided adequate information on PPI from pre- to post-study. It is likely that the original proposal has much more detail on PPI than the journal article word limitation allowed.

Checklist for PPI in proposals:

1. Has the need for PPI been identified? What specific areas, issues and questions will PPI address?
2. Who has been selected to provide this input? How have they been selected? What makes them suitable to provide the input (i.e. the experience or expertise they bring to the project)?
3. What has their contribution to the project been so far? Has a brief list of what they have already contributed been provided? Are they included in the proposal?
4. Will they continue to provide an input? If so, what will they do? What will be their role or responsibility (e.g. co-researcher, member of expert panel etc.)?
5. Have their expectations of their involvement been explored with them? If so, how was this done?
6. Have their training or support needs been assessed? If so, who carried out the assessment? How will training or support be provided?
7. Has someone on the research team been named as the person responsible for overseeing the PPI? Why was this person selected (e.g. has previous experience of PPI)?
8. Who will provide feedback regarding their involvement?
9. Has PPI been costed and detailed in the proposal? Was the patient or the public involved in the assessment? Has the hosting organisation provided some funding to support the pre-proposal PPI?
10. How does the process of identifying, recruiting and involving patients or the public measure up to the UK Standards for Public Involvement in Research or similar frameworks?
11. Will patients or the public be engaging with users and beneficiaries for 'impact'? What activities will they be conducting (e.g. oral/poster presentation, helping to organise a conference or workshops)?
12. Are there plans for involving them in writing papers or reports and other materials?
13. Are there plans for future research involving them?

SUMMARY AND CONCLUSIONS

In this chapter, we have outlined the benefits and challenges of PPI and the different ways in which patients and public contributors can get involved in research studies. There is ample qualitative, and some quantitative, evidence that PPI benefits research projects as well as researchers, patients and the general public.

The importance of supportive processes and context for PPI has been emphasised. Throughout this chapter, reference has been made to existing literature, including guidance and toolkits, that researchers and the public can access. The key information relating to PPI that should be provided in proposals has been highlighted, and a checklist has been developed.

The literature, in particular guidance to help researchers and the public to engage in PPI, has grown at a fast pace in the last two decades, led mainly by the NIHR in the UK and other organisations. PPI in nursing, health and social care research has not, however, followed at the same pace. The main reasons for this are that researchers may not perceive it as beneficial but are more likely to see it as difficult and time-consuming to undertake. The lack of training and support may be another reason. The requirement for mandatory evidence of PPI in proposals to funding organisations, as is the case with the NIHR, may help persuade more researchers to adopt a more positive attitude to PPI. Researchers should not think about PPI only when they are about to start a study. Building and maintaining ongoing relationships with users and others in the care sector and relevant patient organisations, including charities, should be part of the portfolio of researchers if PPI is to make research more relevant to people's needs.

REFERENCES

Adams, J., Barratt, P., Arden, N. K., Barbosa Bouças, S., Bradley, S., Doherty, M., Dutton, S., Dziedzic, K., Gooberman-Hill, R., Hislop Lennie, K., Hutt Greenyer, C., Jansen, V., Luengo-Fernandez, R., Meagher, C., White, P., & Williams, M. (2019). The Osteoarthritis Thumb Therapy (OTTER) II trial: A study protocol for a three-arm multi-centre randomised placebo controlled trial of the clinical effectiveness and efficacy and cost-effectiveness of splints for symptomatic thumb base osteoarthritis. *BMJ Open*, *9*(10), e028342. https://doi.org/10.1136/bmjopen-2018-028342

AshaRani, P. V., Abdin, E., Kumarasan, R., Siva Kumar, F. D., Shafie, S., Jeyagurunathan, A., Chua, B. Y., Vaingankar, J. A., Fang, S. C., Lee, E. S., Van Dam, R., Chong, S. A., & Subramaniam, M. (2020). Study protocol for a nationwide Knowledge, Attitudes and Practices (KAP) survey on diabetes in Singapore's general population. *BMJ Open*, *10*(6), e037125. https://doi.org/10.1136/bmjopen-2020-037125

Bagley, H. J., Short, H., Harman, N. L., Hickey, H. R., Gamble, C. L., Woolfall, K., Young, B., & Williamson, P. R. (2016). A patient and public involvement (PPI) toolkit for meaningful and flexible involvement in clinical trials – A work in progress. *Research Involvement and Engagement*, *2*, 15. https://doi.org/10.1186/s40900-016-0029-8

Boivin, A., Richards, T., Forsythe, L., Grégoire, A., L'Espérance, A., Abelson, J., & Carman, K. L. (2018). Evaluating patient and public involvement in research. *BMJ (Clinical research ed.)*, *363*, k5147. https://doi.org/10.1136/bmj.k5147

Brett, J., Staniszewska, S., Mockford, C., Herron-Marx, S., Hughes, J., Tysall, C., & Suleman, R. (2014). A systematic review of the impact of patient and public involvement on service users, researchers and communities. *The Patient*, *7*(4), 387–395.

Crocker, J. C., Ricci-Cabello, I., Parker, A., Hirst, J. A., Chant, A., Petit-Zeman, S., Evans, D., & Rees, S. (2018). Impact of patient and public involvement on enrolment and retention in clinical trials: Systematic review and meta-analysis. *BMJ (Clinical research ed.), 363*, k4738.

CRUK. (2023a). *Involving people affected by cancer in early phase cancer trials.* https://www.cancerresearchuk.org/sites/default/files/clinical_case_study_01.pdf

CRUK. (2023b). *Patient involvement toolkit for researchers.* https://www.cancerresearchuk.org/funding-for-researchers/patient-involvement-toolkit-for-researchers

Gove, D., Diaz-Ponce, A., Georges, J., Moniz-Cook, E., Mountain, G., Chattat, R., Øksnebjerg, L., & European Working Group of People with Dementia. (2018). Alzheimer Europe's position on involving people with dementia in research through PPI (patient and public involvement). *Aging & Mental Health, 22*(6), 723–729.

Green, G., & Johns, T. (2019). Exploring the relationship (and power dynamic) between researchers and public partners working together in applied health research teams. *Frontiers in Sociology, 4*, 20. https://doi.org/10.3389/fsoc.2019.00020

Health Research Charities Ireland and Trinity College Dublin. (2020). *Making a Start: A toolkit for research charities to begin a PPI relationship.* Dublin: HRCI.

Hersh, D., Israel, M., & Shiggins, C. (2021). The ethics of patient and public involvement across the research process: Towards partnership with people with aphasia. *Aphasiology.* https://doi.org/10.1080/02687038.2021.1896870

Hoddinott, P., Pollock, A., O'Cathain, A., Boyer, I., Taylor, J., MacDonald, C., Oliver, S., & Donovan, J. L. (2018). How to incorporate patient and public perspectives into the design and conduct of research. *F1000Research, 7*, 752. https://doi.org/10.12688/f1000research.15162.1

INVOLVE and The National Research Ethics Service. (2009). *Patient and public involvement in research and research ethics committee review.* https://www.invo.org.uk/wp-content/uploads/2016/05/HRA-INVOLVE-updated-statement-2016.pdf

INVOLVE. (2012). *Tips sheet: Recruiting members of the public to get involved in research funding and commissioning processes.* https://www.invo.org.uk/wp-content/uploads/2012/04/Recruitment-tips-sheet.pdf

Involving People. (2023). *Patient and public involvement toolkit.* https://involvingpeople.org/wp-content/uploads/2023/03/Involving-People-PPI-Toolkit-Guide-1.pdf

Jinks, C., Carter, P., Rhodes, C., Beech, R., Dziedzic, K., Hughes, R., Blackburn, S., & Ong, B. N. (2013). Sustaining patient and public involvement in research: A case study of a research centre. *Journal of Care Services Management, 7*(4), 146–154.

Jong, M. C., Mulder, E., Kristoffersen, A. E., Stub, T., Dahlqvist, H., Viitasara, E., Lown, E. A., Schats, W., & Jong, M. (2022). Protocol of a mixed-method randomised controlled pilot study evaluating a wilderness programme for adolescent and young adult cancer survivors: The WAYA study. *BMJ Open, 12*(5), e061502. https://doi.org/10.1136/bmjopen-2022-061502

Lajoie, C., Poleksic, J., Bracken-Roche, D., MacDonald, M. E., & Racine, E. (2020). The concept of vulnerability in mental health research: a mixed methods study on researcher perspectives. *Journal of Empirical Research on Human Research Ethics : JERHRE, 15*(3), 128–142.

Masotti, P., Rivoire, E., Rowe, W., Dahl, M., & Plain, E. (2006). Collaborative partnerships: Managing increased healthcare demand without increasing overall system capacity. *Healthcare Quarterly (Toronto, Ont.), 9*(2), 72–76.

McCoy, M. S., Warsh, J., Rand, L., Parker, M., & Sheehan, M. (2019). Patient and public involvement: Two sides of the same coin or different coins altogether? *Bioethics, 33*(6), 708–715. https://doi.org/10.1111/bioe.12584

Mental Health Research Network and INVOLVE. (2013). *Budgeting for involvement: Practical advice on budgeting for actively involving the public in research studies.* Eastleigh, UK: Mental Health Research Network, London and INVOLVE. https://www.invo.org.uk/wp-content/uploads/2013/07/INVOLVEMHRNBudgeting09Jul2013.pdf

Mitchell, S., Slowther, A. M., Coad, J., & Dale, J. (2018). The journey through care: Study protocol for a longitudinal qualitative interview study to investigate the healthcare experiences and preferences of children and young people with life-limiting and life-threatening conditions and their families in the West Midlands, UK. *BMJ Open, 8*(1), e018266.

NIHR. (2018). *Learning for involvement.* https://www.learningforinvolvement.org.uk/an-interactive-course-for-new-and-experienced-patient-public-reviewers-of-health-and-social-care-research/

NIHR. (2019). *UK standards for public involvement in research.* https://www.nihr.ac.uk/news/nihr-announces-new-standards-for-public-involvement-in-research/23830

NIHR. (2021). '*Briefing notes for researchers – Public involvement in NHS, health and social care research*'. https://www.nihr.ac.uk/documents/briefing-notes-for-researchers-public-involvement-in-nhs-health-and-social-care-research/27371

NIHR. (2022a). *Payment guidance for members of the public considering involvement in research.* https://www.nihr.ac.uk/documents/payment-guidance-for-members-of-the-public-considering-involvement-in-research/27372

NIHR. (2022b). *Payment guidance for researchers and professional.* https://www.nihr.ac.uk/documents/payment-guidance-for-researchers-and-professionals/27392

NIHR. (2023). *Glossary.* https://www.nihr.ac.uk/about-us/glossary.htm?letter=P#SKPostAToZ

Nyström, M. E., Karltun, J., Keller, C., & Andersson Gäre, B. (2018). Collaborative and partnership research for improvement of health and social services: Researcher's experiences from 20 projects. *Health Research Policy and Systems, 16*(1), 46. https://doi.org/10.1186/s12961-018-0322-0

O'Keefe, S., Radford, K., Farrin, A., Oakman, J., Alves-Stein, S., Cloud, G., Douglas, J., Stanley, M., & Lannin, N. A. (2022). A tailored occupational therapist-led vocational intervention for people with stroke: Protocol for a pilot randomized controlled trial. *JMIR Research Protocols, 11*(10), e40548.

Pandya-Wood, R., Barron, D. S., & Elliott, J. (2017). A framework for public involvement at the design stage of NHS health and social care research: Time to develop ethically conscious standards. *Research Involvement and Engagement, 3*, 6. https://doi.org/10.1186/s40900-017-0058-y

Parkinson, B., Lawrence, M., & Booth, J. (2021). Patient and public involvement for mental health researchers. *Mental Health Practice, 24*(6), e1481. https://doi.org/10.7748/mhp.2020.e1481

Research for All. (2022). *Aims and scope.* https://uclpress.scienceopen.com/collection/UCL_RFA

Saini, P., Martin, A., McIntyre, J., Balmer, A., Burton, S., Roks, H., Sambrook, L., Shetty, A., & Nathan, R. (2022). COMplex mental health PAThways (COMPAT) Study: A mixed methods study to inform an evidence-based service delivery model for people with complex needs: Study protocol. *PLoS One, 17*(3), e0264173. https://doi.org/10.1371/journal.pone.0264173

Sihre, H. K., Gill, P., Lindenmeyer, A., McGuiness, M., Berrisford, G., Jankovic, J., Patel, M., Lewin, J., & Fazil, Q. (2019). Understanding the lived experiences of severe postnatal psychiatric illnesses in English speaking South Asian women, living in the UK: A qualitative study protocol. *BMJ Open, 9*(8), e025928. https://doi.org/10.1136/bmjopen-2018-025928

Staley, K. (2013). *A series of case studies illustrating the impact of service user and carer involvement on research.* https://www.twocanassociates.co.uk/wp-content/uploads/2017/05/MHRN_CaseStudiesAugust_2013.pdf

Staley, K., Kabir, T., & Szmukler, G. (2013). Service users as collaborators in mental health research: Less stick, more carrot. *Psychological Medicine, 43*(6), 1121–1125.

Staniszewska, S., Denegri, S., Matthews, R., & Minogue, V. (2018). Reviewing progress in public involvement in NIHR research: Developing and implementing a new vision for the future. *BMJ Open, 8*(7), e017124.

Stephens, R., & Staniszewska, S. (2015). One small step.... *Research Involvement and Engagement, 1*, 1. https://doi.org/10.1186/s40900-015-0005-8

van Schelven, F., Boeije, H., Marín, V., & Rademakers, J. (2020). Patient and public involvement of young people with a chronic condition in projects in health and social care: A scoping review. *Health Expectations: An international journal of public participation in health care and health policy, 23*(4), 789–801.

16 TIMELINE, COSTINGS AND RESEARCH TEAM

. . . .

INTRODUCTION

This book is written mainly for those new to research, including undergraduates doing a research proposal as a course assignment, postgraduate students, including doctoral students doing a dissertation, and others undertaking small research projects. Whether or not researchers will seek funding, they are aware that research studies need resources. In this chapter, we will explore the types of resources required for a study and highlight the necessary information that researchers should provide in research proposals. In particular, we will show how a timeline can be developed and what to include when costing staff time, equipment/facilities and other expenses. We will also highlight some of the key issues that researchers should be aware of when completing the resources section of a proposal.

RESOURCES FOR RESEARCH STUDIES

Resources, in this context, include time, equipment, materials, facilities, expertise (staff) and other expenses (e.g. travelling costs). Although information about resources comes towards the end of a research proposal, resource considerations do not come after the study has been designed; they are part of decision making at every stage of the design process. One does not start buying goods in a shop without being aware of the amount of money one has to spend.

Having an idea for research and designing a study are prerequisites for a research project. Equally important are the resources needed in order to undertake and complete the study. Designing a study and identifying resources are not separate components of a study; they are intertwined. As researchers begin to design a study, they are broadly mindful of the resource parameters within which they are working. For example, doctoral students know they have a limited amount of time to complete their projects and little or no funding to do so. Therefore, they design their study with these limitations in mind. Funding bodies may stipulate the amount of funding available for researchers and the timescale within which they want the projects to be completed. Researchers, applying for these grants, have to operate within these parameters. Decisions about design may be influenced by cost and time constraints; therefore, plans may change. Focus group interviews may be preferred to individual, face-to-face interviews.

However, the implications of basing decisions solely on cost should be carefully considered. The selection of design and data collection tool should be justified, and it is advisable to support these decisions by evidence. For example, Hanbury et al. (2015) evaluated the cost and feasibility of the use of different data collection methods for their study on 'barriers for a behaviour-change intervention'. They found that a single focus group was 'more feasible than conducting individual interviews or administering a questionnaire, with less recruitment challenges experienced, and quicker data collection' (p. 1). However, they suggested that research should be undertaken to compare the 'robustness of the methods in terms of the comprehensiveness of barriers identified' (p. 1). This comment highlights the point that cost and convenience are not the only factors to take into account when selecting designs and methods.

Whether or not they are applying for funding, the exercise of planning a timeline and estimating costs can be beneficial for researchers as well. This provides the first opportunity to break the study into its many parts and find out what exactly needs to be done, how long it will take, who will undertake this and how much (in some detail) the project is likely to cost. The resource section of a proposal is more than just being about time and cost; it is an indication of how well thought out the project is. An underestimation of the time it takes to undertake the study can indicate 'naivety' or inexperience on the part of researchers or their inability to grasp the complexity of the tasks involved.

Sometimes, researchers may not know how much detail to provide. The word limit of a proposal can restrict the amount of information. However, the 'rule of thumb' is to cover the main items (discussed later in this chapter) and provide enough detail for panel assessors or others to decide whether the timeline, costs and personnel show that the project is realistic and feasible, and provides value for money. Researchers are aware that some tasks and activities can take longer than one hopes for. Doctoral students have learnt, by experience, that seeking approval for their study can be a long, time-consuming process. Things do not always go to plan in the life of a project. Researchers rely on others, such as gatekeepers to access potential participants. Sometimes decisions to grant access can change at the last minute.

Applying for funding is a competitive process. However, it is not a bidding process whereby underestimating costs or asking for less funding than is required is an advantage. Funders look for a realistic timeline and costing and want to spend their precious money in the most cost-effective and efficient way. It is wise to bear this in mind when carrying out this exercise.

The amount of time and funding that a project needs depends on its nature and complexity. It may not be as straightforward to calculate the time and resources needed for mixed methods studies, longitudinal surveys or multisite randomised controlled trials (RCTs) as it would be for a single-site RCT or a cross-sectional survey. However, the same consideration should be given to all studies regardless of their complexities. The process of estimating and calculating resources should be carried out by the project team or at least with the input of more than one researcher. The human resources and finance departments of the host institutions and health and social care organisations should be involved, if appropriate.

ESTIMATING AND CALCULATING RESOURCES

Below is a list (by no means exhaustive) of some of the key questions to ask when estimating and calculating resources for a project:

- What is the timescale for the study (i.e. when it will start and finish)?
- What are the tasks (e.g. interviewing) and activities (e.g. meeting with practitioners to disseminate findings) that will be undertaken?
- When will each task or activity be undertaken?
- Who will be responsible for undertaking them or overseeing their completion?
- Does the research team have the necessary experience and expertise to successfully complete this study?
- How much will each task or activity cost (e.g. staff time in terms of recruiting participants, travelling to and from interview sites or impact and dissemination activities)?
- What equipment, facilities and materials will be required for the study?

These are broad questions. Detailed accounts of all tasks, activities and items (facilities, equipment and materials) should be undertaken. Therefore, a detailed plan of resources is required. Researchers may have their own way of approaching planning, identifying and costing what needs to be done, when it will be done and who will be responsible or involved. For those new to planning a study and developing a research proposal, we propose a systematic approach based on the structure of the research process. It consists of three stages, as follows:

- *Stage 1* – list the main tasks/activities (literature review, data collection, sample recruitment etc.).
- *Stage 2* – break each task or activity into its constituent parts (e.g. break data collection into developing instruments, piloting and administering them, etc.). Identify who will undertake these tasks, when they will be undertaken and how much they will cost.
- *Stage 3* – from the information in stage 2, calculate the overall time and cost of the study as well as all the facilities, equipment and materials required. It is mostly the information from stage 3 that will be reported in the research proposal. However, the necessary detail should be provided.

This exercise can be carried out by constructing a normal table with columns and rows, as shown in Table 16.1. This can be done manually but is best done electronically as this can make it more manageable, modifiable and easy to share with others.

This table/spreadsheet is only one example of how this can be carried out. The first question researchers need to ask themselves is why they need to carry out this exercise – it is for the purpose of systematically identifying what needs to be done, who will do it and how much it will cost. The table can have as many columns and rows as required and should be modifiable. For example, researchers can have a column to insert their 'to do tasks' and highlight issues that need to be addressed. This document can become the main reference for discussion at team meetings. Whether staff are named on it depends on the team, but it can be used to make the study as transparent as possible. However, this document is not the one that is included in the

					Preliminary	**Other**	
TABLE 16.1							
Broadsheet for Identifying and Estimating Resources (Including Timelines)							
Key Tasks	**Sub-Tasks**	**Timescale**	**Timeline**	**Staff**	**Costs**	**Expenses**	**Comments**
Literature review	Searching, retrieving and reviewing the literature. Writing a draft of the review and making the necessary changes after discussion with the team	3 months	March 2024 – May 2024	RA	0.25 RA salary	Library services, access to a computer, etc.	Research team/ human resources to discuss appropriate salary for the RA
Data collection							
Recruiting participants							

RA: research assistant.

proposal; from it, the timeline and cost of the study can be developed and then reported in the proposal.

CONSTRUCTING A TIMELINE FOR THE STUDY

Based on the information in the spreadsheet about how long and when the tasks will be undertaken and completed, a timeline for the study can be constructed. The Cambridge Dictionary defines a timeline as 'a plan or a line that shows the different dates when the different stages of an activity or process should be completed'. It is a brief chronological description of tasks within a project and the time by which the deliverables will be completed. The 'timescale' is 'a period of time that is needed to do an activity or process'. An example of a partially completed timeline is given in Table 16.2.

This is only an example of how it can be done. Researchers can develop and present their own timelines for their project. Timelines can be presented graphically to enable readers to grasp what is to be delivered, the delivery period (in weeks or months) and the timescale for this to be achieved. A Gantt chart is one of the most common approach researchers use to show the timeline visually. The Gantt chart website (https://www.gantt.com/) explains that the chart allows readers to see at a glance:

- what the various activities are;
- when each activity begins and ends;
- how long each activity is scheduled to last;
- where activities overlap with other activities, and by how much;
- the start and end dates of the whole project.

TABLE 16.2
Example of a Timescale and Timeline for a Study

Task	Objectives	Timescale	Timeline
Conduct a literature review	■ Search and critique literature ■ Map out studies already carried out on the topic ■ Identify gaps in the literature for a study ■ Discuss preliminary topic selection and agree on a study	3 months	March 2024 – May 2024
Formulate research questions	■ Write research questions for the study ■ Discuss with supervisor and agree final questions	1 month	June 2024
Selecting data collection methods	■ Identify appropriate data collection methods for the study ■ Identify their strengths and weaknesses ■ Select one or more methods (as appropriate) after discussion with supervisor ■ Refine methods (e.g. this will involve selecting an existing questionnaire or developing a new one)	3 months	July 2024 – Spetember 2024
Identify sample population			
Apply for ethical approval			
Collect data			
Analyse data			
Interpret data and report findings			
Write up report			
Submit report			

There are many Gantt chart templates on the internet that researchers can choose from to generate timelines for their projects. Colours can be used to highlight the tasks that have been achieved and those that urgently require attention. Notes can also be inserted as appropriate. Figure 16.1 shows an example of a Gantt chart. For examples of Gantt charts in research proposals, see Swiatek et al. (2016) and Afshar et al. (2019).

There is, however, more to timelines than just showing the tasks and their duration. Researchers still have to make decisions and estimate how long each of the tasks can take. Charts

Task	Months																							
	1	2	3	4	5	6	7	8	9	10	11	12	13	14	15	16	17	18	19	20	21	22	23	24
Complete literature review and write-up	▪	▪	▪																					
Finalise interview schedule			▪																					
Make arrangements to recruit participants			▪	▪																				
Prepare consent documents			▪																					
Prepare and submit ethical approval form				▪	▪																			
Undertake interviews							▪	▪	▪	▪	▪	▪	▪											
Transcribe interviews									▪	▪	▪	▪	▪	▪	▪									
Analyse data											▪	▪	▪	▪	▪	▪	▪							
Write up report																		▪	▪	▪	▪			
Disseminate findings																						▪	▪	▪

Fig. 16.1 ▪ An example of a Gantt chart in a protocol for a 2-year study involving qualitative interviews.

can also be used to track activities and progress. They can be circulated at team meetings to show what has been achieved and to discuss issues or problems that need to be addressed.

COSTING RESOURCES

Identifying, estimating and costing resources are exercises that cannot and should not be undertaken by only one individual. There are at least three groups that should be involved. The research team should be responsible for identifying what needs to be costed. A brainstorming session, based on the master broadsheet described earlier, should facilitate the exercise of determining every resource that is needed, whether or not funding will be applied for, and whether or not all costed items are eligible for external funding. This will show how much the study will cost in its entirety, including dissemination and impact activities.

Second, if funding is to be sought, it is important to know what the potential funder for the study will fund, the funding parameters and what is eligible for funding. Therefore, reading and becoming familiar with the funder's guidelines is crucial. If, after this, there are still ambiguities or confusion, funders can be contacted for clarification. Although they will not be involved in costing resources, they can help researchers request only what is eligible for funding.

The third group that researchers should consult when applying for funding are experts in their own institutions or organisations. The main departments to consult are human resources, the finance office and research support services. Personnel in these departments normally have considerable experience and knowledge of how to cost resources required for research studies. Institutions and organisations such as universities or research institutes or centres also have their own policies and guidelines that staff should follow when applying for external research funding. For example, the University of Reading (2023) advises its staff to contact their 'Research Development Manager' for accurate staff costings in their proposals. Institutions and organisations are also well experienced in costing facilities, equipment, etc., apart from salaries. Some universities stipulate who is eligible to apply for funding as a principal investigator (PI) or co-PI and who is not eligible to do so. For an example, see University of Massachusetts Amherst (2023). Some researchers in the team may be from other organisations, and their own support services should also be involved. All this suggests that time will be required for such consultations. Therefore, one cannot overemphasise the need to start identifying and costing resources well ahead of the submission date of the proposal.

There are a number of terms in connection with costing that new researchers should become familiar with when applying for external funding:

- *Sponsor* – The sponsor is defined as the institution or organisation assuming overall responsibility for the study (Al Shakarchi, 2022). This responsibility includes putting effective arrangements in place to set up, run and report a research project (Health Research Authority [HRA], 2020).
- *Principal investigator* – This is the person who assumes overall responsibility for the project. There can be a co-PI (who may also be based in a different organisation from the PI).
- *Funder* – This is the organisation that provides funding for a project. This funding is sometimes called an 'award' or 'grant'. Individuals (such as philanthropists) can also make funding available for research.
- *Collaborator* – All those contributing to a project can be called research collaborators. Some are part of the team and are costed in the proposals. Some can be consultants to a project and be paid a fee, while others (e.g. gatekeepers facilitating access to participants) may contribute to the project without being paid.
- *Direct costs* – These are expenses or costs that can directly be traced to the project. These costs would not be incurred if the project was not undertaken.
- *Indirect costs* – These are the costs that are incurred by an organisation sponsoring the research study. These costs include, for example, heating rooms or providing library services. Research projects require the support services (such as human resources to recruit participants) and facilities of the organisation where the study is undertaken.
- *Full economic cost* – This is the full cost of a research project, not just the direct costs. It includes indirect costs related to facilities (e.g. laboratories and seminar rooms), equipment (e.g. computers), services (e.g. libraries), etc.

The main items to be costed in a proposal are staff time, facilities, equipment, materials and other expenses including travelling, accommodation (e.g. rooms for a meeting outside one's own organisation) and subsistence when giving presentations (if agreed by funders). By far the most expensive item in a research proposal is usually staff expertise and labour.

Staff time is calculated in terms of the number of hours to be spent on the project. However, even before any calculations take place one has to decide whether the grade of staff is appropriate for the task to be undertaken. As explained earlier, if the time of highly paid staff is costed for work that could be done more cheaply, this should be justified. Literature reviews and data collection are activities that do not normally need to be undertaken by highly qualified staff. However, managing a project, supervising and training junior researchers and doing sophisticated data analysis require experience and appropriate expertise. Interviewing vulnerable populations may require staff with prior experience. Therefore, costing an expert interviewer in the proposal may be justified.

If the project spans two or three years, any expected salary increment should be included in the costing, but any potential promotion is not. The hourly rate is based on the current salary of the researcher; if they are employed on a part-time basis, their salaries are converted into full-time equivalents before the hourly rate is determined. Depending on the size of a project and the number of hours required to complete it, one or more new researchers may have to be recruited. If only a few hours of staff time are required (e.g. 100 hours of technical support), there may not be a need to appoint new staff, as recruitment can add to the costs. A currently employed technician may be released to do this work. Secretarial support is another item to be taken into consideration. Recruiting staff to projects includes costs related to advertising and job interviews. Other staffing costs include the employer's contributions to pensions and employees' contribution to national insurance, if applicable. Sometimes redundancy costs can also be included depending on funders' policy and guidelines. The time and contribution of practice staff, patients and lay persons involved in the project should also be included.

Facilities include such items as furniture (e.g. chairs and desks), rooms, lecture halls, toilets, cafeterias, etc. These are used for multiple purposes including teaching, research, meetings, conferences and other functions. Each project only makes use of part of these facilities. Consumables and equipment and other items that should be costed in proposals include placebos, stationery, photocopying, printing, postal costs of questionnaires (including reminders), telephone calls and translating and transcribing interview scripts. If researchers require new equipment to be used specifically in the project, they need to provide quotations from sellers and the price should include relevant taxes. Equipment may need installation, maintenance and repairs. These can be carried out in-house or by external contractors. Either way, they have to be properly costed and supported by quotations from the suppliers of these services.

Researchers may want to include the cost of computers in their proposal. Normally, a case has to be made to explain why the computers provided by the sponsoring institution are not adequate for undertaking the project. It could be that the demands of the project require specific computers and software (e.g. if the project is about computer games, the average workplace computer may not be adequate). Travel costs are another item that should be listed in some detail. This should include the number of journeys and their purpose, the mileage rate and the number of nights for subsistence, if applicable. Costs in relation to attending meetings and to presenting and disseminating findings should also be included.

These are the main costs that are generally incurred in an average project. Multisite RCTs, longitudinal surveys, intervention studies with multiple groups and interdisciplinary projects can be complicated to cost. This is why it is important to involve the relevant people in this exercise. While estimating cost is not without its difficulties, it is even more problematic when one cannot know, in advance, what can go wrong with a project. For example, although one can calculate the size of the sample for a survey or RCT, one cannot guarantee that it will be possible to recruit the number of participants required or that they will remain for the duration of the study. In a systematic review of 125 RCTs, Raftery et al. (2015) reported that 'on average, trials needed about twice as many centres as planned to complete the study, reflecting the difficulties in recruiting' (p. 47). This highlights the need to do preparatory work to estimate the number of potential participants and their willingness to take part and to remain in the study.

Feasibility studies, prior to the main trial, can give a more accurate estimation of the potential target population and reveal the issues and challenges related to sample recruitment. Consulting with local clinical research networks, stakeholders and gatekeepers can make recruitment estimates more realistic. In their review, Raftery et al. (2015) reported that estimates of recruitment were 'almost always overoptimistic' (p. 108). For some information on how to cost interviews and clinical trials, see Schwab (2022) and Speich et al. (2018a, 2018b), respectively.

It is a mistake when estimating resources to promise more than can be delivered within the budget requested in the proposal. Equally, one should not under-cost the resources required for a research study. It is also important to trace every item costed to other parts of the proposal. For example, if 20 interviews are costed in the proposal, this should correspond to the number of interviews listed in the data collection section. Researchers should ensure that the sums add up and that their organisation is involved and agrees with the costings. For an example of full economic costings, see University of Birmingham (2023).

THE RESEARCH TEAM

Selecting Team Members

Researchers are the most valuable resource for a research study. Putting together a strong, well-motivated research team is one of the first requirements when designing a study. This involves contacting potential team members and negotiating their participation in the proposed study. Although the formation of a research team can come naturally, as researchers may already have their own network of collaborators, it is crucial that the right team is assembled. The criteria for selection depend on, among others, the specific skills and expertise required to successfully complete the study, the time commitment of potential team members, the particular contribution they can make and, ideally, their experience and track record on the topic being investigated.

It is likely that researchers for the project will be recruited internally. This is sometimes preferable (as opposed to external collaboration) as it can make the project more manageable in terms of less travelling and more opportunities to meet formally and informally. However, external expertise may be sought if the sponsoring institution does not have researchers with some of the specific skills that the study requires. Therefore, it is quite common to seek external collaborators nationally (or internationally, if the project has global significance). External potential team members may come from one's own network of collaborators, built over time. A literature search can also reveal the key researchers in the field and they can then be contacted.

Sometimes the project requires an interdisciplinary or multidisciplinary team. Interdisciplinary research occurs when members of different disciplines bring their perspectives and theories to study a particular topic. It involves the cross-fertilisation of ideas and the synthesis of perspectives (Bruce et al., 2004). Multidisciplinary research is when researchers from various disciplines investigate the same issue or topic from their own perspectives without cross-fertilisation or synthesis of the findings from these disciplines (Bruce et al., 2004). The selection of team members for interdisciplinary or multidisciplinary projects depends on the research questions, the specific disciplines capable of answering the research questions and, if possible, their previous experience in interdisciplinary or multidisciplinary research, as appropriate.

The aim of a careful selection is to put together a balanced and coherent team capable of answering the research questions, led by an experienced chief or principal investigator. If the person in charge of the project is a new researcher (some funding is specifically aimed at new researchers), there should be a named, experienced researcher in the team who can provide supervision and training. In their proposal for a qualitative study 'exploring the beliefs and experiences of older Irish adults and family carers during the novel coronavirus (COVID-19) pandemic', Robinson et al. (2020) mentioned that one of the team members was a 'novice qualitative researcher' who would be supported and supervised by an experienced researcher in this methodology.

The strength of the team relates to their experience in investigating this topic and how their skills and expertise match the needs of the project. Robinson et al. (2020), in their proposal, describe the experience of each team member. For example, they describe one of the team members as a senior lecturer in occupational therapy, with a PhD in anthropology, who 'has conducted research on mental health and psychosocial support during the "People's war" in Nepal and is an experienced qualitative researcher' (p. 4). It is clear that with such experience, she will be able to bring useful insights into the beliefs and experiences of older Irish adults and family carers during the COVID-19 pandemic.

Although some funders do not specify a limit on the number of applicants on a proposal, there should not be too much overlap in the skills and expertise that they bring. If this happens, a justification should be provided. There can sometimes be 'political' reasons to include colleagues or the boss on proposals. This should be avoided as much as possible, especially if they are likely to be 'dormant' team members or will only make a token contribution to the proposal and project. On the other hand, if the team does not have someone with a specific skill for a particular task, there should be a plan of how the task will be performed (e.g. by external contractors or by providing training for a team member).

Managing the Team

Team cohesion and performance depend on a number of factors including effective leadership, clarity about agreed roles and responsibilities, clear and realistic deliverables (including agreed timelines) and a sense of project ownership by all team members. The mechanisms for effective management involve two-way communication, coordination of the different parts of the project (in particular by the PI or someone delegated to this role), support and training for staff development and regular feedback on performance.

Clarifying roles and responsibilities at the start of a project will avoid ambiguities and confusion regarding what is expected of team members. Everyone should be aware of what everyone else does on the project. The 'timeline broadsheet' (mentioned earlier) should provide detail on the deliverables. Every team member should also feel that their contribution is valued. This should be transparent in team meetings where everyone has opportunities to talk and be heard. Timely feedback by the PI or the team leader will help team members to get an idea of their performance and is likely to increase their confidence and commitment to the project.

One of the challenges that research teams face is to complete the allocated tasks on time. Sometimes researchers are involved in other projects or activities such as teaching and are unable to deliver on time. Delay in completing a task by one team member can bring the whole project to a standstill. For example, if those involved in the analysis of data do not do this on time, the rest of the project can slow down or stop altogether. Everyone has to understand the interrelatedness of their contribution. Managing multisite projects can be particularly challenging. There is a need to identify someone who will lead the project at each site, under the overall supervision of the chief investigator. This will require effective coordination and a number of regular face-to-face meetings. These arrangements should be described in detail in the proposal.

Managing interdisciplinary or multidisciplinary teams can also be challenging, not least because each discipline has its own research culture and has developed its own norms and practices relating to how research should be carried out. Nancarrow et al. (2013) have developed 10 characteristics of good interdisciplinary teams:

> *positive leadership and management attributes; communication strategies and structures; personal rewards, training and development; appropriate resources and procedures; appropriate skill mix; supportive team climate; individual characteristics that support interdisciplinary team work; clarity of vision; quality and outcomes of care; and respecting and understanding roles'*
>
> *(p.1)*.

These characteristics are more or less the same as those for managing any team. The difference is that members of interdisciplinary research teams have to make more effort to understand and value one another's contribution. This calls for an attitude open to learning from other team members, a preparedness to shift or change one's perspective (when appropriate) and a belief that the topic being investigated can benefit from an interdisciplinary approach. In the case of teams that include users, patients and members of the public, researchers should be aware that the academic environment and language can inhibit rather than encourage collaboration. For a checklist 'for a good interdisciplinary research proposal', see Tait and Lyall (2007).

The role and skills of the chief or principal investigator are crucial to the management of the research team. The mechanisms and structures put in place to achieve the effective and smooth running of the project should also be described. This helps proposal assessors to decide whether the project is likely to be well managed and completed on time and within budget. For an example of teamwork in a research study, see Milford et al. (2017). The Research Design Service London of the National Institute of Health and Care Research (https://www.rds-london.nihr.ac.uk/) also has some guidance on how to form a research team. This is especially useful for researchers who do not already have an established network of collaborators.

THE PROFILE OF RESEARCHERS

The quality of the proposal, up to this point, would have inspired some confidence (or not) in funders that the researchers know what they are doing. However, they need to know more about the experience and expertise of the team members and the contribution that each will make to the project. This is why they require a summary of their research achievements and their roles in the project before they decide to allocate funding. This summary or résumé is a brief statement about the experience and expertise of each team member.

Since the PI and co-PI have the responsibility for the whole project, they are expected to provide information about their research profile as well as previous experience in leading or co-leading large, funded projects. Some information is also required about the host institution, the backgrounds of collaborators (including users, patients, members of the public and visiting researchers, as appropriate) and the particular experience they bring to the project. Various terms have been used to call this summary, including 'short curriculum vitae' (CV), 'shortbio', 'biosketch' and 'résumé for researchers'. In this section, we will use the term 'résumé' to describe the section in a proposal where researchers describe their profiles and how they fit the project.

Usually, funders have their own forms that stipulate the type of information they want. For example, the National Institutes of Health (NIH) in the USA have a number of forms to be completed by applicants, depending on the type of funding applied for (e.g. fellowship or non-fellowship grants). Apart from information on the current position, education and training of the applicants, they are asked to provide a personal statement, a statement of their contribution to science and a list of their scientific appointments and honours. For samples of completed forms, see NIH (2021). Funders also set word limits for this section. Therefore, it requires particular skill to provide as much relevant information as possible within these limits.

Recognised research funders have their own forms and templates (most are online) for the résumés. Although these forms may vary in terms of structure and how researchers should complete them, the information required is basically the same. This has three components. First is a statement of (more or less) verifiable facts relating to their current and past academic positions, their grant acquisition profile, their role in previous projects, their relevant publications and any prizes and awards. This is sometimes referred to as the quantitative aspects of the résumé. Researchers are also expected to describe briefly, in their own words, their research focus or programme of work, how it developed and how this project builds on it. There is an opportunity to mention the methodological experience and skills they have acquired through their previous research. Finally, they are asked to explain the contribution to knowledge and to society that their research has made. These are the qualitative aspects of the résumés. Researchers can mention any extenuating circumstances (such as family-related issues) that may have impacted on their career development, if this is the case.

This résumé is different from a CV for a job application. It should be 'crafted' specifically for the project for which funding is applied. It is not a case of 'cutting and pasting' from an already prepared CV. It requires considerable skill and several drafts before a final version can be produced. In the UK, The Royal Society (2023) has proposed a template for Résumé for Researchers. This has four 'modules' or sections, a personal statement and space for extenuating circumstances, volunteering, etc. The four modules are:

- Module 1: How have you contributed to the generation of knowledge?
- Module 2: How have you contributed to the development of individuals?
- Module 3: How have you contributed to the wider research community?
- Module 4: How have you contributed to broader society?

According to the Royal Society, these questions and the personal statement are aimed at providing 'a concise overview of an individual'. Panel assessors will also be able to see how researchers write and structure their information, and whether they show coherence and logic in their thinking. The narrative format of the résumé gives a voice to researchers to express themselves in the best possible way, so long as the information is relevant to the project. This type of résumé is also called a narrative CV, as it requires information in a descriptive or narrative format.

Checklist for resources in a proposal:
1. Is the timescale for the study clear?
2. Has a timeline been constructed? Has a Gantt chart or similar chart been provided?
3. Are the sponsor, PI, co-PI (if applicable), team members and collaborators identified in the proposal?
4. Are staff time, facilities, equipment, materials and other expenses (if applicable) costed?
5. Is a full economic cost presented?
6. Is a résumé provided for each team member? Is there a description of how their experience, skills and expertise fit the project?
7. Are the team members' roles, responsibilities and deliverables clearly described?
8. Are plans for the effective management of the team described?
9. How will supervision, support and staff development be undertaken?

SUMMARY AND CONCLUSIONS

Resources are vital for the successful completion of a project. In this chapter, we have described the three main types of resource: time, money (for facilities, equipment, etc.) and the researchers themselves. Some ideas on how to develop and present the timeline for a study have been provided. The main items to be costed have been explored and the issues related to the profile of the research team have been discussed. The main types of information to be provided in a researcher's résumé have been highlighted. It is recognised that not everyone who develops a proposal do so for the purpose of seeking funding. However, everyone should construct a timeline and estimate the resources that they would need to complete their study. This information is useful for the researchers themselves, their employers or supervisors.

Developing timelines, costing the study, selecting, supporting and managing research teams and providing résumés for researchers should not be an afterthought when a proposal is developed. These activities require as much attention to detail as one gives to the methodology. All team members should be involved. One cannot also over emphasise the importance of following the guidelines and instructions of potential funders; the success or failure of a proposal can depend on it.

REFERENCES

Afshar, K., Müller-Mundt, G., van Baal, K., Schrader, S., Wiese, B., Bleidorn, J., Stiel, S., & Schneider, N. (2019). Optimal care at the end of life (OPAL): Study protocol of a prospective interventional mixed-methods study with pretest-posttest-design in a primary health care setting considering the view of general practitioners, relatives of deceased patients and health care stakeholders. *BMC Health Services Research, 19*(1), 486. https://doi.org/10.1186/s12913-019-4321-9

Al Shakarchi, J. (2022). How to write a research study protocol. *Journal of Surgical Protocols and Research Methodologies, 2022*(1), snab008. https://doi.org/10.1093/jsprm/snab008

Bruce, A., Lyall, C., Tait, J., & Williams, R. (2004). Interdisciplinary integration in the Fifth Framework Programme. *Futures, 36*(4), 457–470.

Hanbury, A., Farley, K., & Thompson, C. (2015). Cost and feasibility: an exploratory case study comparing use of a literature review method with questionnaires, interviews and focus groups to identify barriers for a behaviour–change intervention. *BMC Health Services Research, 15*, 211. https://doi.org/10.1186/s12913-015-0877-1

HRA. (2020). *UK policy framework for health and social care research.* https://www.hra.nhs.uk/planning-and-improving-research/policies-standards-legislation/uk-policy-framework-health-social-care-research/

Milford, C., Kriel, Y., Njau, I., Nkole, T., Gichangi, P., Cordero, J. P., Smit, J. A., & Steyn, P. S. (2017). Teamwork in qualitative research: Descriptions of a multicountry team approach. *International Journal of Qualitative Methods, 16*(1), 160940691772718. https://doi.org/10.1177/1609406917727189

Nancarrow, S. A., Booth, A., Ariss, S., Smith, T., Enderby, P., & Roots, A. (2013). Ten principles of good interdisciplinary team work. *Human Resources for Health, 11*, 19. https://doi.org/10.1186/1478-4491-11-19

NIH. (2021). *Biosketch format pages, instructions and samples.* https://grants.nih.gov/grants/forms/biosketch.htm

Raftery, J., Young, A., Stanton, L., Milne, R., Cook, A., Turner, D., & Davidson, P. (2015). Clinical trial metadata: Defining and extracting metadata on the design, conduct, results and costs of 125 randomised clinical trials funded by the National Institute for Health Research Health Technology Assessment programme. *Health Technology Assessment (Winchester, England), 19*(11), 1–138.

Robinson, K., O'Neill, A., Conneely, M., Morrissey, A., Leahy, S., Meskell, P., Pettigrew, J., & Galvin, R. (2020). Exploring the beliefs and experiences of older Irish adults and family carers during the novel coronavirus (COVID-19) pandemic: A qualitative study protocol. *HRB Open Research, 3*, 16. https://doi.org/10.12688/hrbopenres.13031.1

The Royal Society. (2023). *Résumé for researchers.* https://royalsociety.org/topics-policy/projects/research-culture/tools-for-support/resume-for-researchers/

Schwab, P. N. (2022). *Qualitative interviews in B2B: What is the budget?* https://www.intotheminds.com/blog/en/qualitative-interviews-b2b-budget/

Speich, B., von Niederhäusern, B., Blum, C. A., Keiser, J., Schur, N., Fürst, T., Kasenda, B., Christ-Crain, M., Hemkens, L. G., Pauli-Magnus, C., Schwenkglenks, M., Briel, M., & MAking Randomized Trials Affordable (MARTA) Group. (2018b). Retrospective assessment of resource use and costs in two investigator-initiated randomized trials exemplified a comprehensive cost item list. *Journal of Clinical Epidemiology, 96*, 73–83.

Speich, B., von Niederhäusern, B., Schur, N., Hemkens, L. G., Fürst, T., Bhatnagar, N., Alturki, R., Agarwal, A., Kasenda, B., Pauli-Magnus, C., Schwenkglenks, M., Briel, M., & MAking Randomized Trials Affordable (MARTA) Group. (2018a). Systematic review on costs and resource use of randomized clinical trials shows a lack of transparent and comprehensive data. *Journal of Clinical Epidemiology, 96*, 1–11.

Swiatek, P. R., Chung, K. C., & Mahmoudi, E. (2016). Surgery and research: A practical approach to managing the research process. *Plastic and Reconstructive Surgery, 137*(1), 361–366.

Tait, J., & Lyall, C. (2007). *Short guide to developing interdisciplinary research proposals.* https://jlesc.github.io/downloads/docs/ISSTI_Briefing_Note_1-Writing_Interdisciplinary_Research_Proposals.pdf

University of Birmingham. (2023). *Example of a full economic costing.* https://intranet.birmingham.ac.uk/finance/fec/costing/example.aspx

University of Massachusetts Amherst. (2023). *What is a principal investigator (PI) and who is eligible?* https://www.umass.edu/research/what-principal-investigator-pi-and-who-eligible

University of Reading. (2023). *Costing a proposal.* https://www.reading.ac.uk/research-services/costing-a-proposal#:~:text=When%20costing%20your%20proposal%20you,writing%20project%20reports%20and%20papers

17 TIPS FOR SUCCESSFUL RESEARCH PROPOSALS

INTRODUCTION

In this concluding chapter, we will explore what researchers can do to enhance their chances of success when applying for funding. Even those not seeking financial help for their studies should attempt to write a clear, succinct and well-structured plan for their intended study. There is a lot that can be done to avoid common mistakes and learn from the successes of others.

The process of developing proposals can, for the sake of clarity, be categorised into three phases: pre-proposal, the proposal and post-submission. The previous chapters have focused on the second phase – developing proposals – particularly on how to design studies and what to include in the proposal itself. In this chapter, we will focus on what should happen before the proposal is written and after it is submitted. Equally important is how the proposal is presented in terms of structure, format, language, grammar, punctuation, fonts and other aspects that can enhance or hinder clarity and understanding of the text. The success or failure of proposals can depend on these aspects as much as on their 'scientific' content. If readers cannot make sense of what is written, they will be frustrated and unlikely to rate it highly.

PRE-DEVELOPMENT PHASE

Much can be done before the actual writing starts. The preparation in the pre-development phase will help determine how smoothly the development of the proposal proceeds. However, even before the proposal is thought of, researchers should take steps to create their research profile, which will ultimately put them in a good position to compete for research funding. Doing preliminary work on the topic will go a long way to convince proposal assessors that researchers are serious about the topic as it will show that they have started work on it already. This preliminary work in the form of a literature review should ideally be published or 'in press' by the time the proposal is submitted. A lot of work goes into reviewing, writing and presenting the literature in a proposal. Yet what goes into the proposal is only a summary of the review (see Chapter 2). However, having done all the work (searching and reviewing, etc.), the opportunity to publish the full review should not be missed. One of the (often unintended) outcomes of a literature review is that it can reveal key researchers who have published on the topic. This can be useful when seeking advice or looking for collaborators to join the research team.

Undertaking a small-scale project and carrying out a pilot study on the topic are other activities that can start the creation of a research profile. Lack of time and funding can make a literature review a less costly option as it is a desk-based exercise. The importance of publishing preliminary work should not be overlooked. Identifying and talking with other researchers who have a similar interest in the topic can lead to opportunities for joining others in their projects, if only for training and mentoring purposes. This may lead to being part of any subsequent publication. Reading examples of successful proposals also gives prospective applicants an idea of the magnitude of the task ahead of them and these can serve as templates for future proposals.

New researchers should not feel that they must compete with seasoned, experienced teams when applying for funding. Funding organisations, in particular research councils, are aware of the need to support the development of new researchers. There are funding schemes that specifically address these needs. For those who intend to apply for post-doctoral and other fellowships, it is recommended that they consult their targeted funding bodies for advice on how to proceed and what is required of them. Realistically, new researchers should aim for small grants from charitable organisations and local sources before applying for funding for larger projects.

Time is of the essence when developing and submitting proposals. Applying to research councils and other significant funding organisations will take no less than 3 full months. One major 'beast' that researchers face is the 'date for submission'. There is no shortcut to developing a strong proposal; therefore, it makes sense to start working on it a long time before the deadline. Some universities have put in place a policy whereby prospective applicants should notify their research office or similar departments of the intention to submit a proposal. This sets in motion a number of activities such as identifying the needs of the applicants and alerting those (e.g. human resources, finance departments, etc.) who can provide the support and setting timelines for the various activities and tasks to be completed (see Chapter 16).

A time-consuming but essential task is to read the details of the particular call for proposals and understand what the funders' requirements are. No proposal should be submitted until the applicants are sure that it meets the funder's criteria in terms of the research to be undertaken and who is eligible to apply. Failure to comply with their requirements is almost likely to lead to rejection. Funders' guidance is developed for the purpose of guiding applicants. Therefore, researchers should take time to read them carefully and, when in doubt, should contact the person responsible for the specific call and ask for clarification. An email or telephone call can prevent researchers from submitting proposals that may not 'fit' the call and thereby save the time and effort that they would have otherwise wasted.

Time is also needed in the pre-proposal development phase to assemble a credible team for the project and for agreeing deadlines with support services and potential pre-submission reviewers. Some funders have an established pattern regarding the frequency and timing of their calls. Some may do this yearly or every 2 years, usually at the same time of the year. Therefore, anticipating calls for proposals can give researchers the time to do some preliminary work that can be useful when the actual call is made. One of the drawbacks of this is that an already developed proposal may not fit neatly into the new call. Researchers should be careful not to force the work they have already done previously into what they 'think' funders are looking for.

When estimating the time to prepare a proposal, one has to consider that not everything will go as smoothly as planned. People and computers can be unreliable. Therefore, allowance should be made for 'unpredictables'. It is well known that proposal submission 'goes to the wire'; therefore, such crucial tasks as giving reviewers enough time to provide feedback and for applicants to make the necessary changes rarely happen. Yet researchers know that reviews can make a difference to the proposal. Careful planning and the commitment to do whatever it takes to submit a quality proposal can result in a realistic chance of success. A poor proposal is a waste of time for everyone concerned.

PROPOSAL PRESENTATION

Funders normally provide detailed instructions on what the proposal should look like. These instructions or guidance relate to word limit, font type and size, margins, page limits, use or non-use of URLs (Uniform Resource Locator), letters and appendices (what is or is not permitted), etc. Proposals can be rejected outright if these requirements are not met.

Uploading proposals onto the funder's website, although helpful in terms of their software accepting only what is permitted (e.g. if word limits are reached, the online form will not accept more text), can have its own problems. Getting used to digital online submission requires time. Consulting and enlisting the help of those experienced in online submission is strongly recommended. Last-minute computer problems can ruin months of hard work if the deadline is missed. Deadlines should be strictly adhered to.

The proposal may be scientifically sound, but if it does not make sense to readers and assessors, it will not achieve its aim. Therefore, attention should be paid to how the text is structured and written. Different writing styles in a proposal can be distracting. While every team member should contribute to the proposal, it is best if only one person writes it. For example, if one team member focuses on the background and literature review sections (after discussion with the team), the person writing the whole proposal can use what is written and 'convert' it, if necessary, into their own style. Ambiguities and inconsistencies relating to writing styles and language can thus be avoided.

It is recommended that the text is written in the first person. For example, it is better to write 'we will recruit 25 participants who are waiting for a hip replacement' than '25 participants waiting for a hip replacement will be recruited'. While writing styles may be a matter of personal preference, writing in the third person can sometimes seem impersonal. However, whatever style is used, it should be consistent throughout the text. Mixing styles can be frustrating for readers of the proposal.

Verbs should be in the future tense as the applicants are describing what they will do. Of course, if some tasks have already been completed as part of the development of the proposal, it is right to use past tense. For example, if stakeholders have been contacted and they have agreed to provide access to participants, it is accurate to state this using the past tense.

The structure of a proposal (e.g. sections and headings) may be stipulated by the funding organisation one is submitting the proposal to. However, subheadings can normally be selected by applicants. It is advisable to follow closely the funding organisation's instructions regarding the format of the proposal. Long sentences and long paragraphs should be avoided; they are sometimes an indication of a 'rambling', long-winded style. The National Institute for Health Research (now the National Institute for Health and Care Research; NIHR) warned that 'the use of long passages of dense, unstructured text should be avoided' (2021a, p. 1). This sentence was printed in bold type, indicating perhaps the frustration of reading incomprehensible material.

Italics, bold, underlining and bullet points can all enhance the presentation of the text by highlighting words or key messages to draw the attention of readers. Inappropriate, inconsistent and overuse of these tools can defeat their purpose if everything is highlighted. However, these tools can create full and lasting impressions if they are used purposefully, appropriately and sparingly.

Abbreviations can help to prevent repetition of words and save space in the text, especially when one is trying to be economical with words. However, too many abbreviations can confuse readers as they have to constantly remember them, or turn back the pages to refresh themselves in terms of the meaning of these abbreviations. More than one abbreviation in a sentence makes it awkward to read. It is advisable to keep abbreviations to a minimum. Contractions of words (e.g. 'don't' instead of 'do not') are frowned upon in academic writing, except when they are part of a quote; therefore, this should not be used in academic papers and proposals. Sentences should also not start with numbers. For example, starting a sentence with '75 participants agreed with statement x' should be replaced by 'Seventy-five participants agreed with statement x'.

Tables, figures and graphics are particularly helpful in conveying information in a format that can help readers to grasp key information at a glance. They are particularly good for timelines and flowcharts, and can show trends and patterns. They are also useful in organising materials that are too complicated to express in words (Slutsky, 2014). However, they should not be too 'packed' with data and too complicated to understand and interpret. Tables and figures should be self-contained (i.e. understood on their own without having to consult to text) but they should be referred to in the text. They should also complement what is in the text; not repeat what is already expressed in words. References and appendices should be kept to a minimum. Assessors should be able to understand the text without having to read appendices. The latter should not be used as a strategy to meet the word limit. Examples of items in appendices include letters from stakeholders agreeing to facilitate the project, ethical approval statements, participant consent forms and questionnaires developed for the project.

The title of a proposal is what catches readers' attention first. Therefore, it is worth spending time and effort to agree a title with the project team. It should be short, concise, written in plain English and able to summarise the proposal. The aim of the project conveyed in the title should be the same as the aim of the project in the main text. Below is an example of a title that contains the main information in the proposal:

Protocol for a feasibility study and process evaluation of a psychosocially modelled diabetes education programme for young people with type 1 diabetes: the Youth Empowerment Skills (YES) programme.

(Kariyawasam et al., 2022)

This title shows that it is a feasibility study of a psychosocial programme with young people with type 1 diabetes. It also gives an acronym of the programme (YES). An acronym is a smart abbreviation of keywords to make them into a word itself. In the above example, the authors used the first letter of three keywords – 'youth', 'empowerment' and 'skills' – to make the new word (YES). It is a useful strategy to publicise or 'market' the project. Not all proposals, however, need an acronym.

Abstracts and Summaries

All proposals should have a 'scientific' abstract. Most funders also expect applicants to provide a lay or plain English summary. These abstracts or lay summaries are the sections that assessors may read before delving into the proposal itself. 'Scientific' abstracts are normally aimed at the research community and the language tends to be academic. The structure of the abstract and its content are fairly 'prescribed' in that it should contain information on the importance of, and need for, the study, the research questions to be answered, the proposed methodology of the study (design, sampling, data collection and analysis methods), the implications of the study and the potential impact of the findings (see, for example, Andrade, 2011).

The scientific abstract in a proposal is similar to the abstract in published studies; the difference is that the former is written in the future tense and there are no findings to report (as the study is yet to be undertaken). Although written in an academic style, the scientific abstract should be easy to read and understand. The importance of writing clear abstracts cannot be overemphasised. According to Plavén-Sigray et al. (2017), 'clarity and accuracy of reporting are fundamental to the scientific process' (p. 1). They reviewed 709,577 abstracts published between 1881 and 2015 from 123 scientific journals and showed that 'the readability of science was steadily decreasing' (p. 1). Graf-Vlachy (2022) reported similar findings when they reviewed abstracts in management research. For advice on how to write a scientific abstract, see Nagda (2013). For examples of abstracts in proposals, see Studdard et al. (2020) and Lindsay et al. (2021).

Lay abstracts or plain English summaries are aimed at members of the public who may not have a knowledge of research. The information in these summaries focuses more on the importance of the study, the problems or issues it addresses and the benefits it can potentially bring than on the methodology of the study. The methods should be explained briefly, without research jargon. This summary is best written by patients and members of the public involved in the study or, at the very least, with their help. A draft of the summary should be reviewed by a lay person not involved in the study. For an example of a plain English summary, see Kirkpatrick et al. (2017). Guidance is available online for writing plain English summaries. Examples include:

- NIHR (2021b), Plain English summaries.
- University of Oxford (2023), Guidance for researchers on writing lay summaries.

Readability tools, such as the Flesch Reading Ease Readability Formula (2022), can also help in writing plain English summaries. New tools aimed at making texts clear and readable are being developed at great pace.

PRE-SUBMISSION REVIEW

One of the strategies seldom used to enhance the quality of proposals (and identify obvious errors and omission) is getting the proposal reviewed prior to submission. The reasons given for not doing so are often the 'lack of time' and the possibility that reviewers may 'borrow' ideas from the proposal to submit their own. Selecting reviewers from one's own network can help to allay these fears. Reviewers internal to the organisation, as well as external experts, can be invited to do such reviews. A small financial token of appreciation can facilitate a quick 'turn around' of reviews although potential reviewers should be given enough notice and time for undertaking a thorough review.

To get the best out of the reviewers, one can allocate them different tasks or objectives. For example, one can be asked to focus only on the presentation of the proposal, in particular the English and the readability of the text. Another reviewer, with appropriate experience, can focus on the methodology or science. A third reviewer may be asked to look at issues related to the management of the project, including the justification for the resources requested and the suitability of, and skill mix among, the research team. If this approach is adopted, the task of reviewing is shared.

FUNDERS' CRITERIA

Most funding organisations use four broad criteria for deciding whether to fund a project or not:

1. how the project fits within the organisation's priorities and agenda;
2. the significance of the problem or research questions, and the potential contribution that the study can make in terms of wellbeing, economy, etc.;
3. the scientific quality of the proposal;
4. the ability of the research team to successfully complete the project within the timeframe and budget specified in the proposal.

As explained earlier, proposals can fail even before they are sent to a reviewer's panel. The NIHR (2023) published the success rates of proposals for its Public Health Research Programme. These rates (for all submitted applications) varied from 12.3% in 2017/18 to 28.4% in 2020/21. More revealing were figures showing the number of applications that were not considered by their advisory groups. This varied from 11.8% in 2020/21 to 28.7% in 2017/18. Thirty-five out of 122 applications in 2017/18 were not referred to the NIHR's advisory groups. These 35 projects that did not, presumably, pass the screening stage represent the work of a large number of researchers. The purpose of research is to advance knowledge that can be used to make a difference to people in society. Funders will ask 'What question(s) will this study answer?' and (in nursing, health and social care sectors) 'How can it potentially change policy and practice?' Therefore, it is incumbent on the authors of proposals to make a strong case for the significance of the study and to follow closely the funders' guidance'.

The scientific quality of the proposal, in particular the appropriateness of the methodology, is a key criterion for funding a project. This book has provided detailed checklists of what should be reported in every aspect of the proposal. These checklists can be used to ensure that all key information regarding the methodology is reported. Equally important is the provision of adequate justification for the methodological decisions made. Innovative and creative approaches are other aspects that reviewers and funders look for in proposals.

The ability of the team to complete the project on time and within budget is another important consideration for the panel of reviewers. A checklist for reporting this as well as advice on how to deal with issues that may arise have been provided in Chapter 16. Finally, review panels are likely to have an overall view of whether the project represents value for money.

Beyond the above criteria, there are specific ones tailored to the needs of the funding organisations. According to Shailes (2017) 'funding agencies use many different criteria and peer review strategies to assess grant proposals' (p. 1). This is why researchers should pay particular attention to what their targeted funders require in proposals and the strategies they use to review proposals. The weight that funders give to review criteria can vary. For example, in a review of criteria used by research organisations in Australia in prioritising health research projects for funding, Tuffaha et al. (2018) reported that the most commonly used criteria were research team quality and capability (94%), research plan clarity (94%), scientific quality (92%) and research impact (92%). Value for money was down the list (14%). For an example of criteria used by advisory committees or assessment panels, see NIHR (2019).

The US National Institutes of Health (NIH, 2023) have proposed reviewing the five criteria they currently use (significance, investigators, innovation, approach and environment) and reorganising them into three factors: 'importance of the research', 'feasibility and rigor' and 'expertise and resources'. Each of these factors will be individually scored to form an overall score for the proposal.

COMMON REASONS FOR PROPOSAL REJECTION

Perhaps the first reason for rejection is because the proposed project is not what funders are looking for. Therefore, the research plan or quality of the proposal may not even be assessed. Another reason for early rejection is that the proposal does not adhere to the format and style that the funder expects, especially if clear instructions regarding presentation have been provided. Proposals with these deficiencies may not enter the review process. They can be rejected outright through the screening process initiated in-house by the administrators or project officers in charge of the call. Both these failures are highly preventable through contact with funding organisations' personnel and careful adherence to what is required.

If proposals pass through this screening stage successfully, they are then assessed by experts invited to offer their comments on the significance of the project, the feasibility of the research plan, the scientific methodology (including innovative approaches), the resources (including the research team) and the environment where the research will be carried out. For an example of reasons for proposal rejection, see UK Research and Innovation (UKRI, 2022).

REJECTION, REFLECTION, REVISION AND RESUBMISSION

Applying for funding is a competitive process. Even an excellent proposal can be rejected; therefore, the chance of the rejection is even greater for poor proposals. The UKRI (2021) explains that they 'expect all proposals entering the peer review process to have been carefully planned and written by applicants and quality assured by institutions, so that when they are submitted they are highly competitive, with a genuine prospect of being funded' (p. 1). Rejection is likely to cause initial hurt and may be taken personally. Hopefully, in time, researchers are able to look at the experience rationally and reflect on it once feedback has been received and digested.

Success rates can vary between organisations; on average one can expect that approximately 65% of proposals will be rejected. This depends on the number of factors including available funding, the prestige attached to the award or the number and quality of applications. It is important not to see funders as 'obstructors', preventing researchers from getting a grant. Quite the opposite: one should treat them as allies on the journey that may lead to eventual success. The aim of funding organisations is to allocate funds to projects appropriately, effectively and fairly.

After the period of hurt, there should be some reflection on what was good with the proposal and what did not meet the standards of funders (as listed in the feedback). This is a useful learning process with lessons likely to last the researchers' lifetime. If seen as a learning experience, the impact of rejection and hurt can be softened. Engaging everyone in the team in this reflective process can also be useful in deciding what to do next. There is some evidence and anecdotal observation that the success rate of resubmitted proposals can be higher than for first-time applications. However, review panels would look for genuine changes and a better quality proposal than the one submitted before. Some organisations do not allow resubmission unless specially requested to do so. Therefore, asking funders before resubmission is crucial. Revised proposals can also be submitted to other organisations. However, applicants should ensure that the project is within the scope of targeted funders. Careful editing should be undertaken to ensure the new potential funder does not detect that the proposal was previously submitted elsewhere.

SUMMARY AND CONCLUSIONS

In this chapter we have learned that there are many aspects of the proposal that are important apart from the methodology of the study. Successful research proposals require preparation that includes developing a research profile. Equally important is how the proposal is written, structured and presented. The need to follow closely funders' guidelines and instructions should not be understated. There is also value in having the proposal reviewed prior to submission. All these activities and strategies require a special ingredient: time. If the proposal is unsuccessful, the work done should not go to waste. There are opportunities to reflect on the reasons for rejection and make changes before resubmitting it (if this is allowed by funders). In any case, the work done could form the basis of another proposal.

It is acknowledged that students will not normally be required to submit proposals for funding. However, some may go on to become researchers or may want to apply for funding in their future jobs. This book has shown that writing proposals requires careful planning, time, a good team and, above all, attention to detail. The checklists can remind researchers what should be reported in each of the many sections of a proposal. The examples from real proposals, provided throughout the text, show how others have done this. Writing a high-quality proposal depends on a well-designed study and much more. 'This book has provided some guidance on how to do this'.

REFERENCES

Andrade, C. (2011). How to write a good abstract for a scientific paper or conference presentation. *Indian Journal of Psychiatry*, *53*(2), 172–175.

Flesch Reading Ease Readability Formula. (2022). https://www.readabilityformulas.com/flesch-reading-ease-readability-formula.php

Graf-Vlachy, L. (2022). Is the readability of abstracts decreasing in management research? *Review of Managerial Science*, *16*, 1063–1084. https://doi.org/10.1007/s11846-021-00468-7

Kariyawasam, D., Soukup, T., Parsons, J., Sevdalis, N., Baldellou Lopez, M., Forde, R., Ismail, K., Jones, M., Ford-Adams, M., Yemane, N., Pender, S., Thomas, S., Murrells, T., Silverstien, A., & Forbes, A. (2022). Protocol for a feasibility study and process evaluation of a psychosocially modelled diabetes education programme for young people with type 1 diabetes: The Youth Empowerment Skills (YES) programme. *BMJ Open*, *12*(6), e062971. https://doi.org/10.1136/bmjopen-2022-062971

Kirkpatrick, E., Gaisford, W., Williams, E., Brindley, E., Tembo, D., & Wright, D. (2017). Understanding Plain English summaries. A comparison of two approaches to improve the quality of Plain English summaries in research reports. *Research Involvement and Engagement*, *3*, 17. https://doi.org/10.1186/s40900-017-0064-0

Lindsay, S., Kosareva, P., Sukhai, M., Thomson, N., & Stinson, J. (2021). Online self-determination toolkit for youth with disabilities: Protocol for a mixed methods evaluation study. *JMIR Research Protocols*, *10*(1), e20463. https://doi.org/10.2196/20463

Nagda, S. (2013). How to write a scientific abstract. *Journal of the Indian Prosthodontic Society*, *13*(3), 382–383.

NIH. (2023). *A proposed simplified framework for NIH peer review criteria.* https://grants.nih.gov/policy/peer/Proposed-Framework/index.htm#:,:text=Applications%20are%20evaluated%20based%20on,criterion%20score%20from%20assigned%20reviewers

NIHR. (2019). *General criteria used by advisory committees when assessing applications.* https://www.nihr.ac.uk/documents/general-assessment-criteria/12097

NIHR. (2021a). *Template stage one standard application form.* https://www.nihr.ac.uk/documents/funding/cross-programme/NIHR-Template-Application-Form-stage-1.docx

NIHR. (2021b). *Plain English summaries.* https://www.nihr.ac.uk/documents/plain-english-summaries/27363

NIHR. (2023). *Application success rates for the Public Health Research (PHR) Programme.* https://www.nihr.ac.uk/documents/phr-programme-success-rates/23176

Plavén-Sigray, P., Matheson, G. J., Schiffler, B. C., & Thompson, W. H. (2017). The readability of scientific texts is decreasing over time. *eLife*, *6*, e27725. https://doi.org/10.7554/eLife.27725

Shailes, S. (2017). To fund or not to fund? *eLife*, *6*, e32015. https://doi.org/10.7554/eLife.32015

Slutsky, D. J. (2014). The effective use of graphs. *Journal of Wrist Surgery*, *3*(2), 67–68.

Tuffaha, H. W., El Saifi, N., Chambers, S. K., & Scuffham, P. A. (2018). Directing research funds to the right research projects: A review of criteria used by research organisations in Australia in prioritising health research projects for funding. *BMJ Open*, *8*, e026207. https://doi.org/10.1136/bmjopen-2018-026207

UKRI. (2021). *How to submit your proposal.* https://www.ukri.org/councils/esrc/guidance-for-applicants/how-to-submit-your-proposal/

UKRI. (2022). *Common causes of proposal rejection.* https://www.ukri.org/councils/nerc/guidance-for-applicants/what-to-include-in-your-proposal/common-causes-of-proposal-rejection/

University of Oxford. (2023). *Guidance for researchers on writing lay summaries.* https://researchsupport.admin.ox.ac.uk/ctrg/resources/lay-summaries

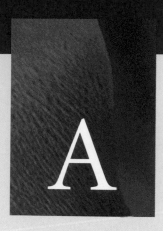

CHECKLIST FOR REPORTING QUANTITATIVE DESCRIPTIVE AND CORRELATIONAL STUDIES (SURVEY, COHORT AND CASE-CONTROL) IN RESEARCH PROPOSALS

RESEARCH QUESTIONS/AIMS AND OBJECTIVES/HYPOTHESES

- Are the questions/hypotheses/objectives clear, unambiguous and complete?
- Are the questions feasible and ethical?

INTRODUCTION AND BACKGROUND

- Has the gap in research and policy/practice been identified?
- Has a strong case (rationale) for this study been made? Has the rationale included reference to any relevant policy/strategy?
- How impactful is this study likely to be in terms of policy/practice, etc.?
- Has up-to-date literature been used to make a compelling case for the study?
- Has a brief summary of a review of previous studies on this topic been provided? Does the review clearly lead to the research questions and to the chosen methodology?

CONCEPTUAL FRAMEWORK

- Is a conceptual framework (or more) used or does this study aim to develop one?
- If a framework is selected, is a rationale/justification for choice given in the proposal? Is this framework new or widely used in other, similar studies?
- Is a brief summary or overview of the framework given in the proposal? Is it based on one or more theories (or part of a theory)?
- How does the framework underpin the study (e.g. to guide research questions, design or data analysis, or is it used throughout the study)?

DESIGN

- Has a particular design (e.g. survey or cohort) been identified?
- Why is this design appropriate for answering the research questions for this study? For example, is there a consensus in the literature that this type of research question is best answered by the chosen design?

- If the selected design is to be modified or adapted, is a rationale or explanation given?
- How will rigour be ensured for the study?

DATA COLLECTION AND ANALYSIS

- Are the data collection methods clearly described? How are they aligned/matched to each of the research questions/objectives?
- Are the methods of data collection appropriate for answering the research questions? Are they suitable for the target population?
- Is a justification for the choice of data collection methods given?
- Are existing questionnaires/scales to be used in the proposed study? If so, how widely are they used in previous studies? Are they valid and reliable? If a number of tools exist for the same outcome, is a justification given for the one(s) selected?
- If modifications/adaptations are to be made to existing tools, how will the reliability and validity of the modified tool be tested?
- Will the existing tool require translation into another language? Is this process briefly described? How will the reliability and validity of the translated tool be tested?
- If new tools are to be developed for the study, is a rationale/justification given for this decision?
- How are the tools to be developed (process)? How will their reliability and validity be tested?
- Will the development of a new questionnaire/tool be carried out before the proposal is submitted (as part of pre-proposal preparation)?
- How will the tools be administered (e.g. face to face, online or via the telephone)? Is a justification given for choice of delivery mode?
- For clinical outcomes, are the measurement tools/techniques the most appropriate, reliable and valid? Who will carry out the measurements/recordings (clinical staff, researchers specially trained for this task, etc.)?
- What is the process for the recording and analysis of data?
- Who will analyse the data and how will rigour be ensured?
- What statistical calculations will be carried out? Are they appropriate and justified?
- What data analysis/management software will be used? Is the choice appropriate and justified?
- How will the data be managed and by whom? How will the security and protection of data be ensured?

SAMPLE AND SAMPLING

- Has the target population been identified and defined? Has an estimation of its size been made? What are the inclusion and exclusion criteria? Are they justified in the proposal?
- What type of sampling will be used (e.g. stratified sampling) and has the rationale for this choice been given?
- How will participants be accessed? Will gatekeepers be involved? Who are they and has initial contact with the gatekeepers been made? What records, if any, will be used? What setting(s) (e.g. community, hospitals, schools, etc.) will be involved?

- What strategies will be used to enhance recruitment, attrition and retention? If incentives are to be used, what are they and are they justified and ethical?

ETHICAL ISSUES/IMPLICATIONS

- Are there ethical issues with the study and how will they be addressed?
- Is the population for the study considered to be vulnerable? What issues may arise and how will they be addressed?
- Are there specific ethical issues relating to the setting (e.g. clinical area, prison, nursing home, etc.)? What are the issues and how will they be addressed?
- Are there specific design-related ethical issues? What are they and how will they be addressed?
- How will informed consent be sought? Does the informed consent form contain all the necessary information? (see the section on 'Seeking Access and Consent' in Chapter 13 for a list of items to include in informed consent forms)
- Are incentives to be offered for participation? Are these incentives likely to influence the decision to participate?
- Is the data collection likely to cause distress? What strategies will be used to prevent or minimise distress?
- Are there any risks to researchers? What are these risks and how will they be addressed?

PATIENT/PUBLIC INVOLVEMENT

- Has the need for patient and public involvement (PPI) been identified? What specific areas/issues/questions will PPI address?
- Who has been selected to provide this input? How have they been selected? What makes them suitable to provide the input (i.e. the experience/expertise they bring to the project)?
- What has their contribution to the project been so far? Has a brief list of what they have already contributed been provided? Are they included in the proposal?
- Will they continue to provide an input? If so, what will they do? What will be their role/responsibility (e.g. co-researcher, member of expert panel, etc.)?
- Have their expectations of their involvement been explored with them? If so, how was this done?
- Have their training/support needs regarding PPI been assessed? If so, who carried out the assessment? How will training/support be provided?
- Has someone on the research team been named as the person responsible for overseeing PPI? Why was this person selected (e.g. they have previous experience of PPI)?
- Who will provide feedback on their involvement?
- Has PPI been costed and detailed in the proposal? Was the patient/public involved in the assessment? Has the hosting organisation provided some funding to support pre-proposal PPI?
- How does the process of identifying, recruiting and involving patients/the public measure up to the UK Standards for Public Involvement in research or similar frameworks?

- Will patients/the public be engaging with users and beneficiaries for 'impact'? What activities will they be conducting (e.g. oral/poster presentation, helping to organise conference/workshops)?
- Are there plans for involving them in writing papers/reports and other materials?
- Are there plans for future research involving them?

RESOURCES

- Is the timescale for the study clear?
- Has a timeline been constructed? Has a Gantt chart or similar chart been provided?
- Are the sponsor, principal investigator (PI), co-PI (if applicable), team members and collaborators identified in the proposal?
- Are staff time, facilities, equipment, materials and other expenses (if applicable) costed?
- Is a full economic cost presented?
- Is a résumé of the profile of each team member provided? Is there a description of how their experience, skills and expertise fit the project?
- Are the team members' roles, responsibilities and deliverables clearly described?
- Are plans for the effective management of the team described?
- How will supervision, support and staff development be undertaken?

IMPACT

- Has the potential for impact been identified in the proposal? Has evidence of this been supported by the literature and/or other reliable sources?
- Have potential users and beneficiaries been identified in the proposal?
- How will representatives of potential users and beneficiaries be involved in the study? Is there evidence that contact has been made with them and agreement about their participation sought? What are their roles and time commitment?
- Has a dissemination and communication plan been described? What is the overall approach/strategy of the plan? Has any particular model/framework been used to underpin the approach?
- Have the activities to communicate and engage with potential users and beneficiaries been outlined?
- Are these activities appropriate, varied and coherent?
- Have impact activities been costed in the proposal?

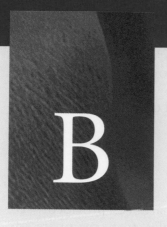

B CHECKLIST FOR REPORTING TRIALS IN RESEARCH PROPOSALS

RESEARCH QUESTIONS/HYPOTHESES

- Are the questions/hypotheses/objectives clear, unambiguous and complete?
- Are the questions feasible and ethical?

INTRODUCTION AND BACKGROUND

- Has the gap in research and policy/practice been identified?
- Has a strong case (rationale) for this study been made? Has the rationale included reference to any relevant policy/strategy?
- How impactful is this study likely to be in terms of policy/practice, etc.?
- Has up-to-date literature been used to make a compelling case for the study?
- Has a brief summary of a review of previous studies on this topic been provided? Does the review clearly lead to the research questions and to the chosen methodology?

CONCEPTUAL FRAMEWORK

- Is a conceptual framework (or more) used or does this study aim to develop one?
- If a framework is selected, is a rationale/justification for the choice given in the proposal? Is this framework new or widely used in other studies?
- Is a brief summary or overview of the framework given in the proposal? Is it based on one or more theories (or part of a theory)?
- How does the framework underpin the study (e.g. to guide research questions, design or data analysis, or is it used throughout the study)?
- If an intervention is to be developed as part of the proposal, is the development of the intervention based on a conceptual framework?
- If the proposal is on the evaluation of an intervention, will a specific framework (or a combination of frameworks) be used in the study? And how?

DESIGN

- Has a trial design (e.g. parallel or quasi-experimental) been identified?
- Has a rationale been provided for the choice of design? (e.g. If the design is quasi-experimental, why is a controlled trial not feasible?)
- If it is quasi-experimental, what type of quasi-experiment is it? Have the strengths, limitations and challenges been identified?
- Has a particular guideline (e.g. the SPIRIT checklist) been used to inform the reporting of items?
- Have the experimental and control groups been described? What will each receive? What implications will this have for the participants, health professionals involved in their care and others in the setting?
- What are the outcomes and how will they be measured? Why are these particular outcomes selected?
- How will rigour be ensured in the study?

DATA COLLECTION AND ANALYSIS

- Are the data collection methods clearly described? How are they aligned/matched to each of the research questions/objectives?
- Are the methods of data collection appropriate for answering the research questions? Are they suitable for the target population?
- Is a justification for the choice of data collection methods given?
- Are existing questionnaires/scales to be used in the proposed study? If so, how widely are they used in previous studies? Are they valid and reliable? If a number of tools exist for the same outcome, is a justification given for the one(s) selected?
- If modifications/adaptations are to be made to existing tools, how will the reliability and validity of the modified tool be tested?
- Will the existing tool require translation into another language? Is this process briefly described? How will the reliability and validity of the translated tool be tested?
- If new tools are to be developed for the study, is a rationale/justification given for this decision?
- How are the tools to be developed (process)? How will their reliability and validity be tested?
- Will the development of a new questionnaire/tool be carried out before the proposal is submitted (as part of pre-proposal preparation)?
- How will the tools be administered (e.g. face to face, online or via the telephone)? Is a justification given for choice of delivery mode?
- For clinical outcomes, are the measurement tools/techniques the most appropriate, reliable and valid? Who will carry out the measurements/recordings (clinical staff, researchers specially trained for this task, etc.)?
- What is the process for the recording and analysis of data?
- Who will analyse the data and how will rigour be ensured?

- What statistical calculations will be carried out? Are they appropriate and justified?
- What data analysis/management software will be used? Is the choice appropriate and justified?
- How will the data be managed and by whom? How will the security and protection of data be ensured? In the case of clinical samples, where will these be stored? And for how long? Who will have access to them?

SAMPLING/RANDOMISATION

- Has the target population been identified and defined? Has an estimation of its size been made? What are the inclusion and exclusion criteria? Are they justified in the proposal?
- Is the sample size for each group (control, experimental, etc.) calculated? Is the minimal clinically important difference taken into account in the calculation of effect size?
- Have the sequence generation and concealment processes been described? Have the sampling and randomisation processes been included in a CONSORT or CONSORT-type flow chart?
- What type of sampling will be used (e.g. block or cluster randomisation) and is the rationale for this choice given?
- How will participants be accessed? Will gatekeepers be involved? Who are they and has initial contact with gatekeepers been made? What records, if any, will be used? What setting(s) will be involved?
- What strategies will be used to enhance recruitment, attrition and retention? If incentives are to be used, what are they and are they justified and ethical?

ETHICAL ISSUES/IMPLICATIONS

- Are there ethical issues with the study and how will they be addressed?
- Is the population for the study considered to be vulnerable? What issues may arise and how will they be addressed?
- Are there specific ethical issues relating to the setting (e.g. clinical area, nursing home, etc.)? What are the issues and how will they be addressed?
- Are there specific design-related ethical issues? What are they and how will they be addressed?
- How will informed consent be sought? Does the informed consent form contain all the necessary information? (see the section on 'Seeking Access and Consent' in Chapter 13 for a list of items to include in informed consent forms)
- Are incentives to be offered for participation? Are these incentives likely to influence the decision to participate?
- Is the data collection likely to cause distress? What strategies will be used to prevent or minimise distress?
- Are there any risks to researchers? What are these risks and how will they be addressed?

PATIENT/PUBLIC INVOLVEMENT

- Has the need for patient and public involvement (PPI) in the study been identified? What specific areas/issues/questions will PPI address?
- Who has been selected to provide this input? How have they been selected? What makes them suitable to provide the input (i.e. the experience/expertise they bring to the project)?
- What has their contribution to the project been so far? Has a brief list of what they have already contributed been provided? Are they included in the proposal?
- Will they continue to provide an input? If so, what will they do? What will be their role/responsibility (e.g., co-researcher, member of expert panel, etc.)?
- Have their expectations of their involvement been explored with them? If so, how was this done?
- Have their training/support needs regarding PPI been assessed? If so, who carried out the assessment? How will training/support be provided?
- Has someone on the research team been named as the person responsible for overseeing PPI? Why was this person selected (e.g. they have previous experience of PPI)?
- Who will provide feedback to their involvement?
- Has PPI been costed and detailed in the proposal? Was the patient/public involved in the assessment? Has the hosting organisation provided some funding to support pre-proposal PPI?
- How does the process of identifying, recruiting and involving patients/the public measure up to the UK Standards for Public Involvement in Research or similar frameworks?
- Will patients/the public be engaging with users and beneficiaries for 'impact'? What activities will they be conducting (e.g. oral/poster presentation, help to organise conference/workshops)?
- Are there plans for involving them in writing papers/reports and other materials?
- Are there plans for future research involving them?

RESOURCES

- Is the timescale for the study clear?
- Has a timeline been constructed? Has a Gantt chart or similar chart been provided?
- Are the sponsor, principal investigator (PI), co-PI (if applicable), team members and collaborators identified in the proposal?
- Are staff time, facilities, equipment, materials and other expenses (if applicable) costed?
- Is a full economic cost presented?
- Is a résumé of each team member's profile provided? Is there a description of how their experience, skills and expertise fit the project?
- Are the team members' roles, responsibilities and deliverables clearly described?
- Are plans for the effective management of the team described?
- How will supervision, support and staff development be undertaken?

IMPACT

- Has the potential for impact been identified in the proposal? Has evidence of this been supported by the literature and/or other reliable sources?
- Have potential users and beneficiaries been identified in the proposal?
- How will representatives of potential users and beneficiaries be involved in the study? Is there evidence that contact has been made with them and agreement about their participation sought? What are their roles and time commitment?
- Has a dissemination and communication plan been described? What is the overall approach/strategy of the plan? Has any particular model/framework been used to underpin the approach?
- Have the activities to communicate and engage with potential users and beneficiaries been outlined?
- Are these activities appropriate, varied and coherent?
- Has impact activities been costed in the proposal?

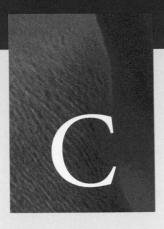

C CHECKLIST FOR REPORTING QUALITATIVE STUDIES IN PROPOSALS

RESEARCH QUESTIONS/AIMS AND OBJECTIVES

- Are the questions or aims and objectives clear, unambiguous and complete?
- Are the questions feasible and ethical?

INTRODUCTION AND BACKGROUND

- Has the gap in research and policy/practice been identified?
- Has a strong case (rationale) for this study been made? Has the rationale included reference to any relevant policy/strategy?
- How impactful is this study likely to be in terms of policy/practice, etc.?
- Has up-to-date literature been used to make a compelling case for the study?
- Has a brief summary of a review of previous studies on this topic been provided? Does the review clearly lead to the research questions and to the chosen methodology?

CONCEPTUAL FRAMEWORK

- Is a conceptual framework (or more) used or does this study aim to develop one?
- If a framework is selected, is a rationale/justification for choice given in the proposal? Is this framework new or widely used in other studies?
- Is a brief summary or overview of the framework given in the proposal? Is it based on one or more theories (or part of a theory)?
- How does the framework underpin the study (e.g. to guide research questions, design or data analysis, or is it used throughout the study)?

DESIGN

- Is qualitative research appropriate to answer your research questions? Has a justification been provided?
- Is a specific approach (e.g. grounded theory) selected for this study?

- Has the rationale for the choice of this design/approach been provided?
- How is the selected approach used to underpin the study (e.g. data collection, data analysis, etc.)?
- How will rigour be ensured for the study?

DATA COLLECTION AND ANALYSIS

- Are the data collection methods clearly described?
- Are the methods of data collection appropriate for answering the research questions? Are they suitable for the target population?
- Is a justification for the choice of data collection methods given?
- How will data be collected (e.g. face to face, online or via the telephone)? Is justification given for this choice?
- What is the process for the recording and analysis of data?
- Who will analyse the data and how will rigour be ensured?
- What data analysis framework will be used? Is it appropriate and justified?
- What data analysis/management software will be used? Is the choice appropriate and justified?
- How will the data be managed and by whom? How will the security and protection of data be ensured?

SAMPLE AND SAMPLING

- Has the target population been identified and defined? Has an estimation of its size been made? What are the inclusion and exclusion criteria? Are they justified in the proposal?
- What type of sampling will be used (e.g. convenience sampling) and is the rationale for his choice given?
- How will participants be accessed? Will gatekeepers be involved? Who are they and has initial contact with gatekeepers been made? What setting(s) will be involved?
- What strategies will be used to enhance recruitment, attrition and retention? If incentives are to be used, what are they and are they justified and ethical?

ETHICAL ISSUES/IMPLICATIONS

- Are there ethical issues with the study and how will they be addressed?
- Is the population for the study considered to be vulnerable? What issues may arise and how will they be addressed?
- Are there specific ethical issues relating to the setting (e.g. clinical area, nursing home, etc.)? What are the issues and how will they be addressed?
- Are there specific design-related ethical issues (e.g. privacy issues related to the ethnographic issues)? What are they and how will they be addressed?
- How will informed consent be sought? Does the informed consent form contain all the necessary information? (see the section on 'Seeking Access and Consent' in Chapter13 for a list of items to include in informed consent forms)

- Are incentives to be offered for participation? Are these incentives likely to influence the decision to participate?
- Is data collection likely to cause distress? What strategies will be used to prevent or minimise distress?
- Are there any risks to researchers? What are these risks and how will they be addressed?

PATIENT/PUBLIC INVOLVEMENT

- Has the need for patient and public involvement (PPI) been identified? What specific areas/issues/questions will PPI address?
- Who has been selected to provide this input? How have they been selected? What makes them suitable to provide the input (i.e. the experience/expertise they bring to the project)?
- What has their contribution to the project been so far? Has a brief list of what they have already contributed been provided? Are they included in the proposal?
- Will they continue to provide an input? If so, what will they do? What will be their role/responsibility (e.g., co-researcher, member of expert panel, etc.)?
- Have their expectations of their involvement been explored with them? If so, how was this done?
- Have their training/support needs regarding PPI been assessed? If so, who carried out the assessment? How will training/support be provided?
- Has someone on the research team been named as the person responsible for overseeing PPI? Why was this person selected (e.g. they have previous experience of PPI)?
- Who will provide feedback to their involvement?
- Has PPI been costed and detailed in the proposal? Was the patient/public involved in the assessment? Has the hosting organisation provided some funding to support pre-proposal PPI?
- How does the process of identifying, recruiting and involving patients/the public measure up to the UK Standards for Public Involvement in Research or similar frameworks?
- Will patients/the public be engaging with users and beneficiaries for 'impact'? What activities will they be conducting (e.g. oral/poster presentation, helping to organise conference/workshops)?
- Are there plans for involving them in writing papers/reports and other materials?
- Are there plans for future research involving them?

RESOURCES

- Is the timescale for the study clear?
- Has a timeline been constructed? Has a Gantt chart or similar chart been provided?
- Are the sponsor, principal investigator (PI), co-PI (if applicable), team members and collaborators identified in the proposal?
- Are staff time, facilities, equipment, materials and other expenses (if applicable) costed?
- Is a full economic cost presented?
- Is a résumé provided for each team member? Is there a description of how their experience, skills and expertise fit the project?

- Are the team members' role, responsibilities and deliverables clearly described?
- Are plans for the effective management of the team described?
- How will supervision, support and staff development be undertaken?

IMPACT

- Has the potential for impact been identified in the proposal? Has evidence of this been supported by the literature and/or other reliable sources?
- Have potential users and beneficiaries been identified in the proposal?
- How will representatives of potential users and beneficiaries be involved in the study? Is there evidence that contact has been made with them and agreement about their participation sought? What are their roles and time commitment?
- Has a dissemination and communication plan been described? What is the overall approach/strategy of the plan? Has any particular model/framework been used to underpin the approach?
- Have the activities to communicate and engage with potential users and beneficiaries been outlined?
- Are these activities appropriate, varied and coherent?
- Have the impact activities been costed in the proposal?

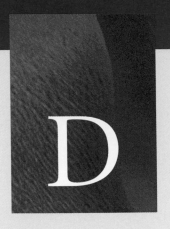

D CHECKLIST FOR MIXED METHODS STUDIES IN RESEARCH PROPOSALS

In addition to the relevant items in appendices A, B and C, the following questions should be answered in proposals for mixed methods studies:

- What is the rationale for choosing a mixed methods design? (e.g. What will the different methods, as opposed to a single method, add to the study?)
- What type of mixed methods design is selected for this study (e.g. concurrent)?
- Is there evidence that the different methods have been carefully selected (e.g. why a survey, case study or ethnography)?
- Is there a clear plan of how the different methods relate to one another and are integrated?
- Are all the different methods (and phases) sufficiently described?
- Is there evidence in the proposal that the team includes researchers experienced in quantitative and qualitative methods?
- How will the findings be analysed and integrated?

INDEX

■ ■

Page numbers followed by "*b*" indicate boxes, "*f*" indicate figures, "*t*" indicate tables.